Strike
Back
at Cancer

Stephen A. Rapaport, a successful businessman and author, has devoted a major portion of his time to the battle against cancer since losing his mother to the disease in 1970. He has helped raise over one million dollars for cancer research, travelled worldwide for two and a half years compiling the data for this book, and presently serves on the Board of the Leukemia Society in southern Fairfield County, Connecticut, where he resides with his wife and two children. Mr. Rapaport has been knighted by the Vatican for his charitable endeavors.

STRIKE
BACK
AT CANCER

What to Do and Where to Go
for the Best Medical Care

STEPHEN A. RAPAPORT

A SPECTRUM BOOK

PRENTICE-HALL INC., Englewood Cliffs, New Jersey 07632

Library of Congress Cataloging in Publication Data

RAPAPORT, STEPHEN A.
  Strike back at cancer.

  (A Spectrum Book)
  1. Cancer. 2. Cancer—Hospitals—Directories.
3. Oncologists—Directories. 4. Cancer patients
—Rehabilitation—Societies, etc.—Directories.
5. Cancer—Information services—Directories.
I. Title.
RC261.R36   616.9'94   78-13257
ISBN 0-13-852764-4

Suggestions for hand and arm care after mastectomy on pages 51–52, five tables in Appendix D (Mortality for Five Leading Cancer Sites; Mortality for Leading Causes of Death; How to Estimate Cancer Statistics Locally; Reference Chart; and Trends in Age-Adjusted Cancer Death Rates), and the Member listings and affiliations in Appendix C are courtesy of the American Cancer Society and are reprinted with permission.

Editorial/production supervision and interior design by Maria Carella
Manufacturing buyers: David Hetherington, Cathie Lenard

A SPECTRUM BOOK

Printed in the United States of America

10 9 8 7 6 5 4 3 2 1

PRENTICE-HALL INTERNATIONAL, INC., *London*
PRENTICE-HALL OF AUSTRALIA PTY., LIMITED, *Sydney*
PRENTICE-HALL OF CANADA, LTD., *Toronto*
PRENTICE-HALL OF INDIA PRIVATE, LIMITED, *New Delhi*
PRENTICE-HALL OF JAPAN, INC., *Tokyo*
PRENTICE-HALL OF SOUTHEAST ASIA PTE., LTD., *Singapore*
WHITEHALL BOOKS, LIMITED, *Wellington, New Zealand*

Dedicated to the late Ms. Pat Allen, who gave great service to the International Union Against Cancer and to the American Cancer Society in their worldwide fight against this dread disease

and

to a loving mother and grandmother whom cancer took from us, too.

INTERNATIONAL CANCER
INFORMATION BUREAU

The International Cancer Information Bureau is an organization dedicated to the collection and dissemination of the latest information on cancer research and treatment. Much of the data contained in *Strike Back At Cancer* was derived from the efforts of this organization.

International Cancer Information Bureau's chief goal is to provide timely information to those individuals who could benefit the most from it—the cancer patient and his family. Our researchers are in constant communication with leading cancer centers, research laboratories, scientists, oncologists, and rehabilitation organizations throughout the world devoted to the discovery and implementation of interdisciplinary treatment modalities—modalities which in some cases could mean the difference between life and death.

The vehicle that the Bureau intends to use to deliver this invaluable information is a periodic Newsletter which will be available on a subscription basis.

Other important purposes of the ICIB are to serve as a forum for the exchange of pertinent data between concerned groups and individuals, promote cancer education and preventive measures through seminars, conferences, and a speaker's bureau, as well as raising and distributing funds for specific cancer research projects.

To those individuals and groups who wish to be placed on our mailing list or would like to receive additional information about our informative Newsletter, please fill out and return the coupon below.

- -

Mail to: International Cancer Information Bureau
21 Charles Street
Westport, CT 06880

Name _____
(Print)

Address _____
\#   Street

City & State _____ Zip _____
City   State

Tel. No. _____   Date _____

I am a   ( ) Patient   ( ) Institution
( ) Family Member   ( ) Other
( ) Doctor

Contents

WHO IS FIGHTING CANCER?

APPENDIXES

A

International Directory of Leading Cancer Treatment Centers| 107

B

Organizations Devoted to Rehabilition of Cancer Patients and Their Families 324

C

International Directory of Qualified Oncologists and Research Specialists

D

Some Cancer Statistics 474

GENERAL INFORMATION ABOUT CANCER

Introduction

Strike Back at Cancer has been written with a single purpose: to help cancer patients and their families help themselves.

How do we intend to do this? Very simply, with information—specific information that can mean the difference between life and death for thousands of cancer patients every year.

This is a factual book. If our purpose had been simply to bring hope to cancer patients, we could have done so very easily by overlooking certain facts and misrepresenting certain others. We have done neither. There is no escaping that cancer is a major and tragic health problem, and no way to measure the degree of suffering it inflicts upon its victims and their families throughout the world. On the other hand, an objective view of all the facts that relate to cancer today does indeed give us reason for hope.

What's more, there are far more options open to the cancer patient today than most people realize. No longer does cancer have to be synonymous with death. More people are engaged in cancer research today than ever before—with more than one billion dollars a year being spent on cancer research in the United States alone.

Never before in history has any disease been the object of an investigation as intense or as universal in scope. And it's paying off. In the United States, cancer remains the second leading cause of death, after heart disease, but the percentage of cancer patients surviving the disease—and surviving in a normal, pain-free manner—is increasing at a dramatic rate. The survival rate—and survival is defined as a period of five years in which the disease does not recur—of skin cancer patients is more than 92 percent, when the disease is detected early enough and treated properly. Among localized-breast-cancer patients, the survival rate under the same conditions is now up to 85 percent. With uterine cancer patients, the figure is 81 percent; and with colon and rectum cancer patients, the figure is 70 percent.

There is every reason to believe that the survival rate for those cancers just mentioned, as well as other cancers, will continue to grow in years to come. Hardly a week goes by when a new finding does not emerge from a cancer research center somewhere in the world—the development of a new anticarcinogenic drug, a revolutionary surgical procedure, a new program of radiotherapy, a new application of immunotherapy—any one of which could represent the breakthrough needed to do for cancer what vaccination did for smallpox and what the Salk vaccine did for polio.

Exactly when this breakthrough will occur, no one can predict. There is as yet no known cure for cancer and no known preventive measure. So, until the time comes when the war against cancer is finally won, the sole aim of the cancer patient is to stay alive for as long as possible and in as pain-free a manner as possible.

All of which brings us to this book. Of all the factors that affect the survival rate of cancer patients, none is more crucial than the timing and the quality of diagnosis and treatment. If the quality of diagnostic and treatment techniques were uniform throughout the world, a cancer patient would not have reason to overly concern himself with this aspect of his condition. But this is far from the case.

Were you aware that the difference in survival rates between some institutions treating the same form of cancer can be as high as 60 percent to 70 percent? Were you aware that many institutions that routinely treat cancer patients are using methods and equipment that were outdated five years ago? Were you aware that most of the hospitals throughout the world lack the equipment and the know-how to provide their cancer patients with the best and most modern care?

Strike Back at Cancer examines this situation. Listed in detail in this book are those institutions and cancer centers located throughout the world that are presently doing the *best* work in cancer and achieving the *most favorable survival rates.* We have selected these places very carefully, basing our decisions on visits and on detailed discussion with many of the world's leading cancer specialists. Each listing will tell you everything you need to know about each individual institution, including whom to contact if you want to receive the care these places provide.

Being aware of these particular cancer treatment centers is only one element in the overall strategy that will increase the survival chances of today's—and tomorrow's—cancer patient. Cancer has a psychological dimension not present in other diseases—a dimension that one leading physician has referred to as "cancerphobia." "Unfortunately when it comes to cancer," Dr. F.J. Ingelfinger wrote in a *New England Journal of Medicine* editorial in December 1975, "American society is far from rational. We are possessed with fear. Cancerphobia has expanded into a demonism in which the evil spirit is ever present, but furtively viewed and spoken of obliquely. American cancer-phobia, in brief, is a disease as serious to society as cancer is to the individual—and morally more devastating."

Strike Back at Cancer is a frontal attack on cancer-phobia. Working under the assumption that ignorance breeds fear, we have presented in this book all the information a cancer patient needs to understand his condition and to deal with his disease in as rational—and effective—a manner as is possible. The antidote to fear is power, and, as Francis Bacon once wrote, "Knowledge and human power are synonymous."

A SUMMARY OF INFORMATION SOURCES

The information presented in *Strike Back at Cancer* was gathered from, and contributed by, many of the outstanding individuals and institutions in the fields of cancer treatment and research throughout the world. For over two years, the people most directly involved with compiling this information have visited many of the leading cancer centers, interviewing and establishing relationships with specialists in virtually every phase of cancer care. They have also met with nearly every concerned governmental agency, physician group, hospital group, rehabilitation association, and charitable organization. Some of the Comprehensive Cancer Centers, like Roswell Park Memorial Institute in Buffalo, have made the heads of each department available to us, and others, such as Memorial Sloan-Kettering Cancer Center in New York, have opened up their research facilities, libraries, and photographic files to us. The response of the medical establishment to our overtures in every instance has been overwhelmingly favorable. Indeed, no aspect of the project up to now has been more encouraging to us.

Below is just a partial listing of some of the individuals and institutions whose contributions have made this book possible:

Dr. Gerald Murphy, *Director*
Mrs. Eileen Simas, *Communications Officer*
Roswell Park Memorial Institute

Dr. Lewis Thomas, *President*
Mr. Gerald Delaney, *Information Officer*
Memorial Sloan-Kettering Cancer Center

Dr. David Carr, *Director*
Mayo Foundation

Dr. Gordon Zubrod, *Chairman*
Dr. Oleg Selawry, Asst. Dir.—Pulmonary Oncology
Mr. Lawrence Strum, *Public Relations Director*
Comprehensive Cancer Center—Florida

Dr. William W. Shingleton, *Director*
Dr. Diane McGrath, *Communications Coordinator*
Duke University Cancer Center

Dr. Timothy R. Talbot, *President*
Fox Chase Cancer Center

Dr. William B. Hutchinson, *Director*
Fred Hutchinson Cancer Research Center

Dr. Samuel G. Taylor, III, *Director*
Illinois Cancer Council

Dr. John R. Durant, *Director*
Ms. Gloria Goldstein, *Information Officer*
University of Alabama Cancer Center

Dr. Carl Mason, *Director of Development*
Ms. Peggy Bee, *Ass't to the Director*
USC–LAC Cancer Center

Dr. R. Lee Clark, *President*
Mr. Stephen Stuyck, *Information Coordinator*
University of Texas System Cancer Center

Dr. Howard P. Rusch, *Director*
Wisconsin Clinical Cancer Center

Ms. Marion E. Morra, *Communications Officer*
Yale University Cancer Center

The Communications and Scientific Writers Staff
National Cancer Institute

Dr. Delafresnaye, *Director*
The International Union Against Cancer–Geneva

Dr. Takashi Sugimura, *Director*
Dr. Hirayama, *Head of Epidemiology*
National Cancer Center, Tokyo

Directors of the major cancer treatment and research centers in Japan
Dr. H.C. Ho, *Director*
Queen Elizabeth Hospital, Kowloon, Hong Kong
(Chairman of Hong Kong Anti-Cancer Society)

The American Cancer Society

The Governors and Executive Secretaries of many of the Federation of Clinical Oncologic Societies

The Directors of the major rehabilitation associations (i.e. United Ostomy Association, The National Leukemia Society, The International Association of Laryngectomees, etc.)

The American College of Surgeons

All of these plus dozens of other specialists and organizations in the cancer field and thousands upon thousands of hours in research and compilation have provided us with a project which we feel will become the most important information source for the individual, or family of an individual afflicted with cancer, the millions of uninformed persons concerned about cancer, and the hospitals and medical community at large requiring a directory of doctors and institutions involved in cancer care, research, and rehabilitation.

1

Coming to Grips
with Reality

Few experiences in life are more terrifying than the discovery that you—or someone you love—has developed cancer. And with good reason. Cancer is an awesome disease; it presently kills people in the United States alone at the rate of 1,068 per day—roughly one death every eighty seconds. No one can measure the physical and emotional suffering that these statistics embody, and no thinking person can minimize the tragic proportions of the cancer problem.

But probably the most tragic aspect of the situation in cancer is not that so many people are suffering and dying, but that so many people are suffering and dying *needlessly*. For, while it is true that no one knows yet what it is that causes cancer, and no one has yet developed a "cure" for the disease, it is also true that there are millions of people throughout the world who have, or have once had, cancer and are living normal, pain-free lives. Contrary to popular belief, cancer is *not* necessarily a terminal disease. Detected early enough and treated properly, it has a more favorable prognosis than many other diseases. To put it another, much blunter way, with many cancer patients, it is not so much the disease that kills them as their ignorance about it.

THE NATURE OF CANCER

Cancer is hardly a new medical phenomenon. Evidence of the disease has been isolated in prehistoric fossils. Cancer can take any one of a hundred or more different forms, but in every case the basic nature of the disease is the same: the growth and spread throughout the body of cells that don't contribute in any positive way to normal body functioning, but do monopolize the body's energy sources in a way that encroaches on and eventually destroys normal cells.

We do not know yet what causes cancer cells to develop. There is a growing suspicion that cells of a cancerous nature are constantly being formed in the body, but, in most cases, are dealt with by the body's immunological system before they can inflict damage. But whatever its source, a cancer cell tends to reproduce itself at a much faster rate than a normal cell; and it is primarily for this reason that once a group of cancer cells—that is, a malignant tumor—starts to grow in any area of the body, the surrounding, healthy cells are invaded and eventually starved out.

In their early stages, most types of cancer can be treated effectively through either surgery or radiation. Surgery removes that portion of the body that is affected with the cancerous cells, and radiation destroys localized cancer cells by interfering with their ability to divide and reproduce themselves. The problem inherent in both surgery and radiation, however, is that in both instances healthy tissue, as well as the cancerous tissue, is affected by the treatment. This is why early detection becomes so crucial. The smaller the area affected by the cancer, the smaller the area of healthy tissue affected by the treatment.

In many situations, cancerous cells will so dominate a particular organ or a particular part of the body that removal of that organ becomes the only surgical procedure that holds a promise for recovery. Depending on the organ, this type of surgery can have either a profound or minimal effect on body functions after the operation.

But the greatest danger in cancer is that the disease will spread beyond the local area and attack other parts of the body. This spreading phenomenon is known as *metastasis,* and the further this process has taken place, the slimmer are the chances for survival. Neither surgery nor radiation treatment has proven particularly effective in the treatment of cancer patients whose conditions have reached the metastasized state. But even among these patients, the chances of survival are beginning to show dramatic improvement, thanks mainly to the development of new drugs that have demonstrated an ability to retard or suspend completely the growth of cancer cells. This form of cancer treatment is called *chemotherapy.* According to knowledgeable estimate, roughly 15 percent of cancer patients who, as recently as two or three years ago, would have been given only a few months to live, are being kept alive—and without pain—for a much longer period as a result of this new drug therapy. Chemotherapy is providing the hope among many researchers that even before a comprehensive cure for cancer is found, science will discover means of helping cancer patients live relatively normal lives even while affected with the disease, in much the same way that heart patients can stay alive if they make certain changes in life-styles.

THE TREATMENT DILEMMA

Despite the widespread nature of cancer, only a small percentage of general physicians throughout the world knows enough about the disease to treat it effectively; and an even smaller number, known as *oncologists,* specialize exclusively in cancer treatment. What's more, only a small majority of hospitals throughout the world has the equipment or adequately trained personnel needed to give the cancer patient the full benefit of what is presently known about the disease.

This situation will undoubtedly begin to show dramatic changes over the next several years as more and more knowledge about cancer filters down to the level of the general physician and as more and more hospitals acquire the technology and the expertise to implement new cancer treatment techniques. In the meantime, however, we are presently being victimized by our own shortsightedness. Until very recently, cancer was, and in some places still is, a subject that no one wants to talk about. The main reason is the conviction among most people that since the disease is incurable anyway, why go out of your way to find out if you have it? For years now, organizations like the American Cancer Society have been trying to dispel this notion and have attempted to alert the general public to the fact that we are not helpless in our fight against cancer.

The reasons these campaigns have not been more successful are many and complex, but most relate to the point just mentioned: the refusal or the inability of the average person to look the cancer problem squarely in the eye. Probably the most incredible dimension of the cancer story today is that in the United States alone, there are dozens of medical centers specializing in cancer that are staffed with the foremost experts in this disease and are equipped with the newest diagnostic treatment equipment—yet they remain underutilized.

Money is not the issue. No cancer patient has ever been turned away from a federally operated cancer center because he didn't have the financial resources to pay for the treatment. The *real* issue is the reluctance and lack of knowledge of too many general physicians in areas throughout the country to make adequate use of these services. In all too many cases, by the time a cancer patient is finally advised to seek help at a center specializing in cancer treatment, his condition has deteriorated past the point at which any of the initial treatment procedures could be expected to produce favorable results. Therefore, the need for major medical center consultation should be of prime importance to the individual diagnosed as having cancer.

2

Recognizing Cancer's Seven Warning Signals

No factor is more important to the survival of a cancer patient than early detection. Cancer is not an incurable disease. There are millions of people today throughout the world living normal and pain-free lives even though, at one time, they suffered from cancer. Why have they survived when others have not? In virtually every instance, it is because their condition was diagnosed at an early enough stage and was treated properly.

UNDERSTANDING CANCER'S SYMPTOMS

Except in rare instances, the presence of cancer in the body will always manifest itself one way or the other. The problem is that many of the symptoms of cancer are not much different from the symptoms of a number of other minor ailments. Consequently, many victims of cancer fail to take action until their condition has gone beyond the easily treatable state. In the United States, in particular, there is a curious reluctance on the part of many people to seek medical help unless the symptoms they are experiencing are severe. What is important to remember about cancer, however, is that its early symptoms are *not* severe. Consequently, they are frequently ignored—until it is too late.

Following is a brief description of each of the seven main warning signals of cancer. Be familiar with them. If any of them persist for more than a few days, don't be embarrassed, be intelligent. *See your doctor.*

1. Change in Bowel or Bladder Habits

Changes in bowel or bladder habits are the principal symptoms for two of the most common forms of cancer: cancer of the bowel and cancer of the prostate. Prolonged constipation, diarrhea, frequent gas pains, rectal bleeding—any of these symptoms could be caused by an obstruction in the bowel—an obstruction that might be a benign polyp but also one that could be cancerous.

Prostate cancer symptoms relate mostly to urine flow. Blood in the urine, pain or difficulty in urinating, weak or interrupted flow of urine, the need to urinate frequently—each of these symptoms is a sign that the prostate gland is enlarged. In most cases, prostate enlargement is *not* cancerous; but even so, it does require medical attention.

2. A Sore That Does Not Heal

The body has its own self-healing mechanisms, so when there is a sore of any kind that is *not* healing, it could well be a sign of cancer. Skin cancers are easily detectable and are the easiest cancers to treat—providing, again, that they are discovered early. Cancers in the mouth can best be detected through regular dental checkups, although the patient should be able to tell if a mouth sore is not healing or if an unusual lump has formed in the oral cavity. Mouth cancers, like skin cancers, have a very favorable prognosis if they are detected early.

3. Unusual Bleeding or Vaginal Discharge

Unusual bleeding or discharge is a prime symptom of uterine cancer. It is an *early* sign for cancer of the *body* of the uterus, which, if caught early enough, usually results in complete recovery.

Unfortunately, vaginal bleeding is also a *late* sign for cancer of the *neck* of the uterus—that is, cervical cancer. However, the Pap Test can detect signs of cervical cancer at its earliest and most curable states. This test is painless and inexpensive. It should be taken by every woman at least once a year.

4. Thickening or Lump in Breast
or Elsewhere

Tumorous masses appear in different parts of the body from time to time in many people. Most of the time, these lumps are not cancerous. Then, again, there is always the possibility of cancer—a possibility that should never be overlooked. Women, in particular, should get into the habit of examining their breasts once a month for signs of a tumor. Many women are reluctant to perform this self-examination—mainly out of fear of discovery. Perhaps this important statistic will help ease their fears. When breast cancer is detected early, approximately 85 out of 100 women survive and show no evidence of the disease after five years.

5. Indigestion or Difficulty in Swallowing

Two forms of cancer—cancer of the stomach and cancer of the esophagus—have symptoms that are among the most common general ailment symptoms of modern life. In the case of stomach cancer, any of the following symptoms—*if they persist*—warrant a visit to the doctor: indigestion, pain, nausea, heartburn, loss of appetite, vomiting, constant belching.

Constant difficulty in swallowing is indicative of blockage and is a symptom of cancer of the esophagus. It warrants a medical checkup.

6. An Obvious Change in a Wart or Mole

An obvious change in a wart or mole could be a sign of skin cancer. For that matter, any skin area in which there is a persistent inflammation that appears to be worsening should be examined by a doctor. Be particularly watchful for any small, dark brown or black molelike growth that either becomes larger or ulcerates and bleeds. Such a growth could conceivably be a melanoma, one of the most dangerous varieties of skin cancer. Many—but not all—melanomas develop from preexisting moles.

7. Nagging Cough or Hoarseness

A persistent cough could be an indication of lung cancer, although most lung cancers are difficult to detect in their early stages. Much depends on where the cancer originates. If it strikes the air passages of the lung—the bronchi—then the consequent irritation will most likely produce a cough.

Persistent hoarseness is one symptom of cancer of the larynx—and an early one as well. Here again, if detected early enough and treated properly, there is an excellent chance for complete recovery. The trouble is that many people who have cancer of the larynx ignore the symptoms and attribute them either to a cold or to excessive smoking. A constant lump, soreness in the throat, or difficulty in swallowing are additional signs of a possible cancer of the larynx.

WHEN TO ACT ON THE WARNING SIGNALS

Drawing the lines between intelligent concern and needless worry with regard to your health is not easy. As you can see for yourself, the vast majority of the warning signals that indicate the possibility of cancer are common, and, in some cases, are also symptoms of far less serious conditions. The key factor in these signals is their *persistence*. We all get coughs and indigestion from time to time. We all get skin irritations and mouth sores. What's more, few of us can afford the luxury or even have the time to see a doctor every time one of these symptoms occurs.

Let common sense be your guide. Once any condition continues for more than a few days, it is a sign that your body is telling you something. Don't ignore it. Check with your doctor, and don't let the possibility that your doctor may indeed discover cancer prevent you from taking the early action that can save your life.

3

Treating

Cancer

BASIC METHODS OF TREATMENT

Surgery

Surgery is the most common primary treatment used in the majority of cancer cases. The basic idea is simple enough: the cancerous mass is removed. But the overall subject is a good deal more complex.

In the first place, some cancers are located in areas of the body that are inaccessible through conventional surgical techniques. Then, too, surgical procedures frequently involve not only the removal of the cancerous mass, but also of the organs to which this mass has attached itself. In some cases, such as prostate cancer, the organ is not directly connected to survival. In other cases—colon cancer, for instance—artificial means can be used to compensate for the loss of the organ. Obviously, however, there are organs in the body whose function cannot be duplicated through artificial means. Thus, while it may get rid of the cancer, surgery involving the removal or serious disruption of these organs produces dire consequences of its own. In addition, there is the general trauma to the body that major surgery creates and the often profound psychological effects that the removal of the organ—however unessential it may be to survival—can be on a patient.

But there is yet another aspect of cancer surgery that you should know about. As we mentioned earlier, primary cancer sites tend to spread, forming secondary malignancies known as *metastases*. It is now generally accepted that surgery, in and of itself, can sometimes cause an increase in metastases by spreading the cells that were originally at the surgical site throughout the body cavity.

These reservations apart, surgical procedures have proven most successful for tumors involving the lung, colon, stomach, bowel, liver, and skin. The techniques used in these procedures have improved considerably over the years, and surgeons are now able to perform most cancer operations with more precision and with less general risk than ever before. At the same time, however, cancer specialists are now openly questioning whether much of the surgery now being done represents the best approach.

Probably the biggest controversy at present surrounds surgery involving breast cancer. Breast cancer, of course, is a major killer of women; but it isn't the breast cancer itself that does the damage. It's the spreading that forms in the lymph nodes of the breast. Most surgeons take the position that whether or not the spreading shows up under X-ray diagnosis, *micrometastases* already exist. Therefore, the accepted conservative surgical procedure is to remove the entire breast, the lymph nodes located in the armpit, and, most often, the pectoral muscles—a procedure known as *radical mastectomy*. Lately, however, some surgeons have been reporting success with much less radical procedures which remove as little actual tissue as possible, and follow the surgery with extensive radiation therapy.

Although certain studies indicate that less radical mastectomies, followed by radiation, are at least as effective as radical mastectomies in the treatment of breast cancer, most of the cancer establishment remains uncomfortable with the new approach. The problem seems to be that there is no sure way at present to tell just how far breast cancer has spread in individual cases.

A number of major studies in this area are currently going on, and hopefully answers will begin to emerge in the not too distant future. But all pros and cons notwithstanding, most cancer specialists recommend that when a cancer patient is told that he or she needs surgery, a second opinion should be sought. Indeed, second opinions are now routinely required by certain medical insurance companies before they will approve the payment. Remember, too, that there are many different types of surgeons—general surgeons, orthopedic surgeons, neurosurgeons, eye surgeons, vascular surgeons, and so forth.

It is generally agreed that if surgery is necessary, you should seek out an oncological surgeon specializing in the particular part of the body that is affected by the cancer.

Radiation Therapy

Radiation therapy refers to the use of energy—generally light rays—in very high, concentrated doses to destroy cancer cells. X rays are a form of radiation. So are cobalt rays and radium rays. These forms of energy penetrate deep into the body cavity without inflicting damage to the skin surface.

As a weapon against cancer, radiation therapy was originally used as an adjunct to surgery. It is still frequently used in concert with surgery (along with chemotherapy), but it has now emerged as a treatment unto itself. Radiation therapy is now used as the primary treatment for cancers involving the cervix, head and neck, larynx, prostate, and skin, among others. But it is also being used to shrink tumors prior to cancer surgery, to simplify the surgical procedure. It is being used, too, simply to contain cancer growth in patients whose tumors do not lend themselves to other treatment. Finally, one of the major uses of radiation therapy is as an anti-metastatic measure in areas where a cancer may not be visible but is nonetheless likely to spread.

The chief attraction of radiation as a cancer therapy is that, unlike surgery, it doesn't produce disfigurement, and, generally speaking, is a much less complicated procedure. Unfortunately, radiation doesn't just affect cancer cells; it affects "normal" cells as well by destroying their ability to reproduce. Because most cancer cells are more susceptible to radiation than are normal cells, and because cancer cells multiply at a much faster rate than normal cells, they are a better target for radiation.

Because radiation poses a threat to normal cells, the primary challenge of radiation therapy has always been to administer treatment in a way that destroys as many cancer cells while destroying as few normal cells as possible—a kind of therapeutic balancing act. Early radiation therapy didn't always strike the optimum balance. For one thing, the body's reaction to high doses of radiation produces a terribly discomforting side effect known as *radiation sickness* whose chief symptom is nausea. What's more, the imprecision of early techniques often left noncancerous organs near the cancerous area permanently damaged.

But many recent advances, some in diagnostic procedures and others in the administration of radiation therapy itself, have minimized these negative aspects of the treatment. Now that radiation therapy can be administered to a cancerous area at different angles the effects of radiation sickness have been minimized. And the use of "megavoltage" (over one million volts) and electron therapy techniques have enabled radiation therapists to be a good deal more precise in their aim so that the "fallout effect" on other tissues has been dramatically reduced. One form of cancer in particular, Hodgkin's disease, has lent itself encouragingly well to megavoltage therapy, particularly if the condition is diagnosed early. And there are heartening indications that certain forms of leukemia are better treated with radiation therapy than with chemotherapy.

Most cancer centers today are equipped with the latest in radiation therapy equipment. But just as important as the equipment used is the person administering it. Radiation therapy should always be administered by a specialist (they're known as radiation oncologists) and preferably a specialist working as part of a cancer treatment team. No two cancers are exactly alike, and no two people respond the same way to radiation therapy. Therefore, it is paramount that you receive a therapy that is tailored to your particular situation.

While the future of radiation therapy as a cancer weapon seems bright indeed, recently there have been some questions raised regarding its use as an adjunct to surgery. A study reported last year in Europe showed that women who had breast cancer surgery and no postsurgical radiation therapy fared better than women who had breast cancer surgery coupled with radiation therapy.

All in all, however, the current state of the art in radiation therapy is quite good and getting better all the time. Yes, there are side effects, but with the proper equipment and a qualified therapist, these side effects can be far less painful and inconvenient than the side effects produced by surgery and chemotherapy.

Chemotherapy

Chemotherapy is defined as the treatment of cancer with drugs designed either to arrest the growth of cancer cells or to kill them outright. Theoretically, chemotherapy represents the ideal cancer treatment—ideal because, unlike surgery or radiation, drugs can travel through the bloodstream and attack cancers throughout the body. The problem, however, is that no drug has yet been devised that can kill cancer cells selectively, without harming normal cells and without causing serious side effects.

Chemotherapy in one form or another has been in use since the late 1940s, when Dr. Sidney Farber was able to induce very short-range remissions in leukemia patients through the use of methotrexate. Since then, roughly fifty different drug substances have been used at one time or another in the treatment of different forms of cancer, no one of which has worked well enough to be classified as a cancer "cure."

The one form of cancer in which chemotherapy has enjoyed its most notable success is acute leukemia in children, although the term "success" should not be confused with "cure." A new drug regimen developed at the Roswell Park Memorial Institute involves the use of a two-drug combination of cytosine arabinoside (ara-C) and Adriamycin (ADR). In one study, reported in late summer of 1977, more than 60 percent of a group of 31 leukemia patients showed complete remission as a result of the drug therapy. Roswell Park has also reported limited successes in chemotherapy treatments for ovarian cancer and liver cancer. Again, however, it should be emphasized that all of these reports concern limited studies.

Drugs used in cancer treatment fight cancer cells in different ways. Some drugs are designed to attack cancer cells as they reproduce. Others mimic the properties of substances on which cancer cells normally depend for energy but do not yield the energy, thus "starving" the cells to death. In any event, cancer drugs are rarely used individually. They are usually used in combination, in order to take advantage of the differences between normal cells and cancer cells.

Just how effective are the current anticancer drugs in controlling cancer? It is difficult to answer this question in general terms. The feeling among most specialists at present is that drugs are most successful when they are used to kill or control very small tumors or limited metastases, but are not notably successful as the primary weapon in extensive tumor masses. Chemotherapy is used mainly today as a secondary treatment to surgery and as a postoperative strategy along with radiation. It has proven most successful on its own with acute leukemia in children, Hodgkin's disease, skin cancer, and a number of rather rare cancers such as Wilms's tumor (kidney cancer), and cancer of the testicles.

Like the challenge facing researchers in radiation therapy, the main challenge facing researchers in chemotherapy is to find cancer-killing drugs that do not destroy other cells as well and that do not produce serious side effects. Among the side effects produced by anticancer drugs are loss of hair, nausea, vomiting, and diarrhea. In addition, patients undergoing extensive chemotherapy often suffer from depression and lose much of their ability to fight off infectious disease. Some anticancer drugs affect cardiac and neural function.

Side effects vary considerably not only from drug to drug, but also from patient to patient. Therefore, the ability of a patient to withstand the side effects is a crucial factor in the use of chemotherapy. People who have a high threshold for discomfort tend to fare better on chemotherapy than people who don't.

One of the as yet unanswered questions involving chemotherapy is the long-range effect that massive doses of drugs have on the body. Since many anticancer drugs have an adverse effect on the body's immunological system, destroying the bone marrow that arms this system with its ability to fight off infection, some cancer

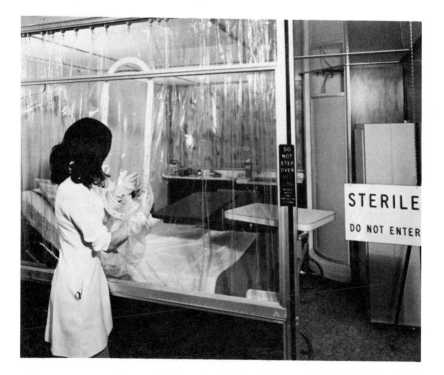

THIS IS A LAMINAR-FLOW (GERM-FREE) UNIT FOR ISOLATION OF PATIENTS UNDER INTENSIVE CANCER DRUG TREATMENT WHO MAY BE HIGHLY SUSCEPTIBLE TO INFECTION. IN THIS UNIT A PATIENT CAN BE ISOLATED FROM ALL SOURCES OF INFECTION IN A COMPLETELY STERILE AREA FOR A PRESCRIBED PERIOD OF TIME. (Courtesy of The National Cancer Institute)

patients undergoing massive chemotherapy die not of cancer but of pneumonia or some other infectious disease.

Still another unresolved question has to do with the relationship between the patient's state of mind, which can be affected by the drugs he is taking, and his general physical condition. There is some evidence to indicate that some patients taking cancer drugs "give up" because of the side effects.

In sum, chemotherapy is a cancer treatment that has produced some isolated successes in certain areas but remains, on balance, an approach that is largely in its experimental stage. The cancers that have proven most responsive to chemotherapy are leukemia, cancer of the head and neck, and Hodgkin's disease, although it would be misleading to say that there are chemical "cures" for these cancers.

Probably the most important thing to bear in mind if you or someone you know is given the choice of undergoing chemotherapy is that the treatment is highly unpredictable and that the psychological makeup and tolerance level of the patient is as much a factor in the success or failure of the therapy as the therapy itself.

Immunotherapy

The basic concept behind immunotherapy—the newest form of cancer therapy in use today—is helping the body help itself. There is solid evidence to indicate that cancer patients are notably deficient in certain cells, usually referred to as *antibodies*, whose chief function is to destroy foreign substances that find their way into the body. There is even a theory, not yet proven, that cancer strikes just about everybody; but that some people, by virtue of their immunological systems, are able to destroy the cancer cells before they can create serious damage. In any case, immunotherapy is designed to strengthen the immunological system to help it destroy cancer cells.

Immunotherapy represents the most ideal approach to cancer treatment. If it were possible to equip the body's own defense system with the weapons it needs to conquer cancer, the side effects that accompany other forms of treatment would not occur with as much frequency or severity. The problem, though, is that since scientists know only a little of how the immunological system operates, immunotherapy is still very much in the experimental stage.

At present, there are three different approaches involving immunotherapy. The most widely used, known as *nonspecific immunotherapy*, seeks to stimulate the immunological system as a whole with the introduction into the system of a special bacteriological extract.

The bacteria most widely used in this therapy is known as BCG. It is the same bacteria used in tuberculosis vaccine. Early studies involving melanoma treated with BCG have produced encouraging results, and now BCG is being used experimentally in other forms of cancer. However, it is still far too soon to assess the overall effectiveness of BCG as a primary cancer weapon. Moreover, there have been a number of side effects, including death, in some cases.

The second most widely used form of immunotherapy is known as *active immunotherapy*. This treatment uses some of the cellular material from the patient's

DRUGS USED AGAINST CANCER (AS OF SEPTEMBER 1975). (Courtesy of The National Cancer Institute)

Common name	Other names	Leukemia Acute Granulocytic	Acute Lymphocytic	Chronic Granulocytic	Chronic Lymphocytic	Adrenal cancer	Bladder Cancer	Brain tumors	Breast cancer
ALKYLATING AGENTS:									
Busulfan	Myleran			●					
Chlorambucil	Leukeran				●				●
Cyclophosphamide	Endoxan, Cytoxan		●		●				●
Dibromomannitol	DBM, Myelobromal			●					
Nitrogen mustard	HN2, Mustargen, Mechlorethamine								●
Phenylalanine mustard	L-Sarcolysin, Melphalan, Alkeran								●
Thio TEPA	TSPA						●		●
ANTIMETABOLITES:									
6-azauridine triacetate	Azaribine								
Cytosine arabinoside	Ara-C, Cytarabine, Cytosar	●	●						
5-fluorouracil	5-FU						●		●
6-mercaptopurine	6-MP, Purinethol	●	●	●					
Methotrexate	Amethopterin		●						●
Thioguanine	TTG	●	●						
MITOTIC INHIBITORS:									
Vinblastine sulfate	Velban								●
Vincristine sulfate	Oncovin		●						●
ANTIBIOTICS:									
Actinomycin D	Dactinomycin, Cosmegen, Meractinomycin								
Adriamycin		●	●				●		●
Bleomycin									
Daunomycin	Rubidomycin, Daunorubicin	●	●						
Mithramycin	Mithracin								
Mitomycin C									
RANDOM SYNTHETICS:									
BCNU	1, 3-Bis(2-chloroethyl) 1-nitrosourea							●	
CCNU								●	
Hydroxyurea	Hydrea			●					
Imidazole carboxamide	NSC-45388								
Methyl CCNU								●	
o, p' – DDD	Mitotane					●			
Procarbazine	Matulane, MIH, Ibenzmethyzin								
Streptozotocin									
HORMONAL AGENTS:	Hormonal agents are known by a variety of								
Adrenal cortical compounds:	trade names								
Cortisone			●		●				●
Hydrocortisone			●		●				●
Prednisolone			●		●				●
Prednisone			●		●				●
Dexamethasone			●						
Androgens:									
Calusterone									●
Delta-1-testololactone									●
Fluoxymesterone									●
Testosterone propionate									●
Estrogens:									
Diethylstilbestrol									●
Ethinyl estradiol									●
Other:									
ACTH			●						
Progesterone									
ENZYMES									
L-asparaginase	EC-2		●						

	Burkitt's lymphoma	Choriocarcinoma	Colon cancer	Endometrial cancer	Ewing's sarcoma	Head & neck cancer	Hodgkin's disease	Lung cancer	Melanoma	Multiple myeloma	Mycosis fungoides	Neuroblastoma	Non-Hodgkin's Lymphoma	Osteogenic sarcoma	Ovarian cancer	Pancreatic islet cell tumors	Polycythemia vera	Prostatic cancer	Retinoblastoma	Rhabdomyosarcoma	Sarcomas (general)	Stomach cancer	Testicular cancer	Wilms's tumor
Burkitt's lymphoma	•																							
Choriocarcinoma																							•	
Colon cancer				•																				
Endometrial cancer																								
Ewing's sarcoma	•																							
Head & neck cancer																								
Hodgkin's disease	•						•						•											
Lung cancer	•						•	•																
Melanoma									•															
Multiple myeloma	•									•														
Mycosis fungoides	•										•													
Neuroblastoma	•											•												
Non-Hodgkin's Lymphoma	•						•						•											
Osteogenic sarcoma														•										
Ovarian cancer	•						•						•	•	•									
Pancreatic islet cell tumors																•								
Polycythemia vera																								
Prostatic cancer	•																	•						
Retinoblastoma																			•					
Rhabdomyosarcoma																				•				
Sarcomas (general)																								
Stomach cancer																						•		
Testicular cancer	•																						•	
Wilms's tumor																								•

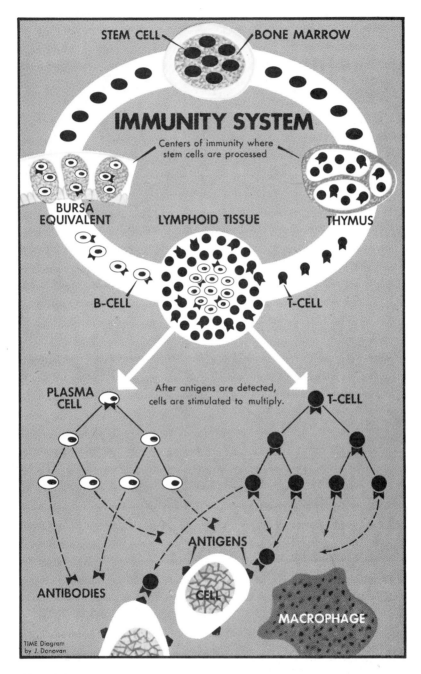

DR. ROBERT GOOD, THE PRESIDENT AND DIRECTOR OF SLOAN-KETTER-
ING INSTITUTE FOR CANCER RESEARCH, IS ONE OF THE WORLD'S LEAD-
ING AUTHORITIES ON IMMUNOLOGY. THIS DIAGRAM IS A GRAPHIC
EXPLANATION OF THE WORKING OF THE IMMUNITY SYSTEM, CREATED
FROM *TIME*'S INTERVIEW WITH DR. GOOD. (Reprinted by permission of TIME,
The Weekly Newsmagazine; Copyright Time, Inc., 1973)

own tumor in the hopes that their introduction into the system will stimulate the immune system to fight not only this material but the existing cancer cells in the body.

The third form of immunotherapy, *passive immunization,* involves the injection of immune cells from a healthy patient into a cancer patient, the theory being that these "healthy" cells will help the immunological defenses of the cancer patient.

Some success has been reported in cases involving all three of these immunotherapy approaches, but no definite pattern has yet emerged to convince researchers that these therapies should be used in lieu of other treatments that have fared much better statistically.

Nearly everyone agrees that immunotherapy carries an enormous potential as a cancer weapon. But until we understand the immunological system itself much better than we do today, it is unlikely that a breakthrough is going to occur imminently in this particular branch of cancer treatment. All the signs at present point to the growing use of immunotherapy as an adjunct to the other three main treatment regimens.

A good source of information regarding doctors, hospitals, and researchers who are active in the field of immunotherapy is Helen Nauts, Executive Director, Cancer Research Institute, 1225 Park Avenue, New York, New York 10028.

HYPERTHERMIA AND THE NEW RADIATION

The application of heat to treat disease is a very old concept. Its use in ancient Greece is described to us in the writings of Hippocrates. Throughout the ages, "heat treatment" has been prescribed for an almost endless array of ailments, and with each succeeding generation, additional knowledge has been acquired as to the curative or catalytic powers of heat.

There is evidence that heat played a strong role in the successful use of Coley's mixed toxins for cancer treatment early in this century (described in our chapter on immunology), and in the 1960s and 1970s, research and experimentation into the use of heat for the treatment of cancer has taken on new and important implications. This form of treatment is known as *hyperthermia.*

The heating of body tissue, and particularly *in situ* (within the body) tumor tissue, however, is not a simple procedure because the degree and intensity of the heat and the accuracy of the area of application are crucial to the success of the treatment. Many research groups are developing a variety of therapeutic instrumentation to create "controlled heat." Perhaps the most promising of these developments involves the use of radio frequency waves. The radio frequency "long waves," which are similar to those used in AM broadcasting, and "microwaves," similar to those used to relay television signals, produce the controlled heat of X-ray treatment, but without its undesirable side-effects. X rays produce *ionizing radiation* which affects cells in the body other than those being treated. This radiation normally causes such temporary—but usually reversible—side effects as nausea, headaches, fatigue, and general malaise, or, in some cases, the permanent destruction of a particular organ's ability to function. On the other hand, radio frequency waves such as those used in diathermy treatment for the uniform heating of injured muscles, produce *nonionizing radiation* and therefore do not induce these problems. This absence of negative side-effects offers the physician considerable latitude in the amount of treatment he can prescribe for his patient.

Presently, over fourteen major research organizations in the United States under the committee chairmanship of Richard J.R. Johnson, M.D., Chief of the Department of Radiation Medicine at Roswell Park Memorial Institute in Buffalo, New York, and other researchers and institutions throughout the world, have been studying the effects of heat on tumor tissue. The results of these studies seem to indicate that temperatures of 42°C will not harm normal tissue but will damage cancerous tissue. Although there is no proven explanation of this phenomenon, a number of leading specialists have developed a theory, discussed later in this chapter, that is gaining considerable acceptance in the medical community. Regardless of how or why it takes place, this discovery has provided cancer researchers with an important and discernible difference between normal and malignant cells that we hope will shortcut their search for methods to selectively attack and destroy these diseased cells.

Radio frequency therapy or "new radiation," as it is occasionally referred to, simultaneously heats a tumor and its surrounding normal tissue. As the tissue starts to reach the critical temperature of 42°C, the malignant cells literally begin to "burn up" at a temperature that is still within the tolerance of a normal cell. Radio frequency microwaves penetrate only short distances into the body and therefore can be used effectively on surface malignancies, such as melanomas. Radio frequency long waves are capable of complete penetration and can be utilized for deep seeded and often inoperable tumors.

One of the leading researchers in the field of radio frequency therapy is Harry H. LeVeen, M.D., Chief of Surgery at the Veterans Administration Hospital, Fort Hamilton, Brooklyn, New York. Dr. LeVeen is also Professor of Surgery at Downstate Medical School in Brooklyn. In the early 1970s, Dr. LeVeen began to search for a new method of treatment for inoperable lung cancer, one of the most difficult of all malignant diseases to treat. Its symptoms usually do not appear until the tumor has already grown beyond an operable state. Dr. LeVeen began to test the use of long radio waves to treat lung cancers as well as other inoperable tumors in the body cavity. During the next few years, a series of custom-designed radio-wave generators were developed, modified, and rebuilt, and in 1975 serious treatment of patients commenced. The results reported so far are quite encouraging. Many patients have recovered completely. Others are in a "controlled" condition—their tumors no longer growing and no evidence of metastasis. Most patients have experienced relief of pain, increase in appetite and energy levels, and a sense of well-being (the technical term for such improvement is *palliation*). Of those patients who died, the autopsy studies showed that their tumors had *necrosed,* or died, and that an immunoresponse was occurring at the time of death. This is one of the most significant aspects of radio frequency treatment reported to date.

Most widely used cancer therapies* are known to be immunosuppressive. Their action on cells suppress the activity of the immune system, the defense mechanism that the body uses to fight off all types of disease. Consequently, many cancer patients under treatment succumb to illnesses which would normally have been repelled by a responsive immune system. Radio frequency therapy hopes to eliminate this additional treatment problem.

Another important discovery about hyperthermia's effectiveness may also have come from the experimentations of Dr. LeVeen and his colleagues. In studying blood flow through tumors and healthy tissue, it was found that the movement of the blood through the tumorous tissue was very slow and torturous. Dr. LeVeen reasoned that by applying heat uniformly to an entire section of the body containing a tumorous mass, the tumor itself would heat up more rapidly than the surrounding normal tissue simply because the healthy tissue would remain cooler owing to its more rapid blood flow, the body's normal response to increasing internal heat. In contrast, the blood flow through a tumor is so slow that it is unable to effectively dissipate the excess heat. Subsequent animal studies have verified this theory and clinical studies on humans appear to confirm it. Additional research has indicated that this form of hyperthermia may be particularly effective against tumors that exist in or are adjacent to organs with a substantial blood supply, such as the lung and the liver.

A number of oncologic specialists now utilizing radio frequency therapy are:

Harry H. LeVeen, M.D.
Veterans Administration Hospital
Fort Hamilton
Brooklyn, New York

Joseph Washburn, M.D.
University of Nebraska Medical Center
Omaha, Nebraska

Herbert Johnson, M.D.
Tampa Memorial Hospital
Tampa, Florida

Ray Ridings, M.D.
Southeast Missouri Hospital
Cape Girardeau, Missouri

John Durant, M.D.
University of Alabama Medical Center
Birmingham, Alabama

John Stehlin, M.D.
The Stehlin Foundation for Cancer
    Research
St. Joseph's Hospital
Houston, Texas

M.L.M. Boone, M.D.
University of Arizona Medical Center
Tucson, Arizona

G.M. Hahn, Ph.D.
Stanford University School of Medicine
Palo Alto, California

I.H. Kim, M.D.
Department of Radiation Therapy
Memorial Sloan-Kettering Cancer Center
New York, New York 10021

J.A. Dickson, M.D.
Royal Victoria Infirmary
Newcastle-on-Tyne, Great Britain

Horst M. Mechlem, M.D.
Krankenhaus Vizentinum Ruhpolding
Munich, West Germany

J.A.G. Holt, M.D.
Radiotherapy Center
21 McCourt Street
Leaderville, Western Australia

*Not including immuno-stimulating drugs described in the chapter on immunology.

Microwaves and Melanomas

Melanomas are tumors of—or near—the surface of the skin. Although they start out as simple growths or warts, they frequently develop into difficult and intractable malignancies. The use of microwave heating (hyperthermia) for treatment of melanomas is very promising. The microwaves are applied through special applicators directly in contact with the skin. Since these waves are very short, they are absorbed directly into the tissue and into the tumor. The applicators are designed to prevent the skin from burning while the tumor itself is heated to a critical temperature of between 42.5°C and 43.0°C.

Doctors using this procedure have reported some very impressive initial results. As is usual with new techniques, most of the patients treated were advanced cases; and while there have been many reports of complete tumor eradication and wound healing, this clinical work is relatively new. It will take several more years and many hundreds of additional treatments before the total value of the treatment can be ascertained.

Some of the researchers actively working on the use of microwaves to treat melanomas are:

Richard Johnson, M.D.
Roswell Park Memorial Hospital
Buffalo, New York

J. Mendecki, Ph.D.
Bronx Montefiore Hospital
Bronx, New York

John Holt, M.D.
Institute of Radiotherapy and Oncology
Leaderville, Western Australia

W.T. Joines, Ph.D.
Duke University
Durham, North Carolina

G.M. Hahn, Ph.D.
Stanford University School of Medicine
Palo Alto, California

Arthur Guy, Ph.D.
University of Washington Medical Center
Seattle, Washington

J.E. Robinson, M.D.
Martha V. Filbert Radiation Center
University of Maryland Hospital
Baltimore, Maryland

The Stehlin Foundation for Cancer Research

A completely unique use of hyperthermia has been developed by Dr. John Stehlin at the Stehlin Foundation for Cancer Research in Houston, Texas. This institute is one of the most remarkable cancer treatment and research centers in the world today. It is a relatively small center compared with the major Comprehensive Cancer Centers listed in this book; however, its innovative research and treatment methods are impressive.

The institute utilizes a unique technique called *perfusion,* especially in the treatment of intractable melanomas of the arm or leg. The blood supply of the affected limb is isolated from the rest of the body by pumping it through a heart-lung machine. There it is oxygenated and heated so that the tumor is perfused with "hot" blood. Anticancer drugs are then added to the heated blood in order to treat the tumor directly, without causing the drugs to circulate through the rest of the body.

In this way most of the induced and unpleasant side-effects of standard chemo-therapy treatment are eliminated. Although this method has been employed primarily against melanomas, the institute has also achieved a degree of success treating other body tumors with the same technique.

Nude Mice Stand-Ins

The Stehlin Foundation has been very successful in breeding large numbers of "nude mice," so called because they grow no hair. These mice are mutants that are born without a *thymus gland,* a genetic defect which means that the nude mouse has no immune system and is therefore incapable of fighting off even the simplest infection. Consequently, the nude mouse cannot reject human tumor cells injected into its body, and it is therefore an invaluable experimental animal. No other laboratory in the world has been as successful in breeding these mice in large numbers because of the absolute controlled and sterile conditions necessary for their survival. They are used for a wide variety of cancer experiments, but in the Stehlin Treatment System the mice primarily act as "stand-ins" for patients under treatment.

Tissue from a patient's tumor is removed and transplanted or injected into up to 100 nude mice. These transplants become viable living tumors in the mice in approximately twelve days. They are then checked by chromosome studies to verify that they are the same as the parent human tumor and have not been altered by transplantation to the nude mice. Once the tumors are viable, different chemo-therapeutic and immunological drugs are tested on these mice to see which anti-cancer drug—or combination of drugs—is most effective in treating the tumor. Thus the nude mouse serves as a stand-in "guinea pig" for the patient in determining which treatment will be most effective for him. Over the last few years, the clinical results of this program appear to be equal to, or better than, those of other cancer treatment centers and are steadily improving, as the Stehlin specialists gain more experience in combining the nude mouse "stand-in" system with perfusion and hyperthermia.

Once again, it is important to note that although this procedure has been in use since 1972, most of the patients treated at the Stehlin Foundation for Cancer Research have had extensive previous therapy. It will be necessary to continue experimentation with this promising new program for a considerable length of time and with a more expanded patient base to determine exactly how effective the treatment is and whether the patients presently in remission will achieve a permanent, "cured" status.

Whole-Body Hyperthermia

In this chapter we have endeavored to cover the use of heat in the treatment of selective body areas afflicted with cancer. During the past few years, researchers from several different countries have also been experimenting with methods to monitor the effects of heat applied to the entire body of a cancer patient. One of the original researchers in this field is R.T. Pettigrew, M.D., of Western General Hospital in Edinburgh, Scotland. Dr. Pettigrew's treatment procedure involves insulating the entire body of a patient and increasing the body temperature to 42.5°C. Initial reports from Dr. Pettigrew indicate that the treatment has a palliative effect on his patients, relieving pain and discomfort, but that the maximum dosage is quite limited by the patient's physiological tolerance. However, Dr. Pettigrew does report that *whole-body hyperthermia* appears to be even more effective when used in conjunction with anticancer drugs and X-ray treatment.

The National Cancer Institute in Bethesda, Maryland has also started experimental studies into whole-body hyperthermia. Their experiments use a type of rubber space-suit to induce a uniform increase in body heat. At this time there are no published reports of their findings or information available as to whether they are using hyperthermia in conjunction with other standard treatment methods.

Another leading research institute, Roswell Park Memorial Institute in Buffalo, New York, is using rubber suits to insulate patients, not dissimilar to those used for deep sea diving; and Dr. Harry H. LeVeen, who was mentioned earlier in this chapter, utilizes a rubber sheet during treatment to create an overall low-grade fever in his patients.

There are many other researchers throughout the world who are working with heat in the treatment of cancer. We have tried to cover some of the principal ones in this section. For additional information, contact Ronald Atkinson, Ph.D., at the National Cancer Institute in Bethesda, Maryland 20014. Another source of information on hyperthermia is Helen Nauts, Executive Director, Cancer Research Institute, 1225 Park Avenue, New York, New York, 10028.

4

Laetrile: The Cancer Enigma

In the past few years, the Laetrile controversy has had more publicity than any other subject in the cancer field. Articles have appeared in major newspapers and magazines. Interviews and special reports have been broadcast on television. Debates have been conducted on radio and in the public forum. Why the fuss, what has generated so much conflict? Does it work? These are difficult questions. On one side of the controversy, doctors, researchers, government agencies, heads of major cancer-research institutions, and scientists claim there is no evidence that Laetrile is effective in treating cancer. The Food and Drug Administration says that Laetrile, an unapproved drug, cannot be sold in the United States. They have indicted many of its proponents, from profit-motivated traffickers to reputable physicians. On the other side of the controversy, a large number of cancer patients, treated with Laetrile outside of the country, claim they have been helped or cured and that their futures depend on receiving regular supplies of Laetrile. This conflict has resulted in unprecedented events in American medical and legal history.

Laetrile has been used to treat cancer for the last twenty years. Throughout its history, it has been controversial and generally illegal in the United States. Consequently, most of the doctors and clinics that treat cancer patients with

Laetrile are located outside the country. One major center for such treatment is in Tijuana, Mexico. Another well-known center is in Hanover, Germany. Additional centers are operating in the Philippines, South America, Jamaica, and other localities. The two major production centers are in Mexico and Germany.

Laetrile itself is a chemical substance called amygdalin, extracted and purified from the pits of apricots. It comes in two forms—tablets and an injectable solution. Prior to its notoriety, it was used principally as a food and candy additive. During the mid-1960s, the substance was promoted in California as a cure for cancer patients. After California health authorities took action against the Laetrile proponents, a clinic was set up over the border in Tijuana, Mexico. Terminal cancer patients who had no alternative treatment left to them tried the drug. Since then, increasing numbers of people have gone to Mexico and Europe to seek treatment with Laetrile. Those who felt they were helped and were unable to obtain continuing supplies of the substance through legal channels in the United States, wound up purchasing it in the black market. This led to a confrontation between government agencies upholding the existing law and a growing cadre of individuals, convinced that Laetrile was beneficial.

In the past few years, the government's actions have resulted in a polarization and consolidation of the pro-Laetrile forces. The best-known pro-Laetrile organization is the Committee for Freedom of Choice which claims 40 Chapters and 60,000 members. This group has developed sufficient political power to help create a remarkable legal precedent. Through its lobbying efforts, laws have been passed in sixteen states (as of this date) which allow cancer patients to use Laetrile as a treatment if they so choose. In most states, these laws were passed by an overwhelming majority of the legislators. There is every indication that similar laws will be passed in another six states within the next few months.

An examination of the positions, attitudes, and arguments on both sides of this controversy indicates that establishment doctors and experts are opposed to Laetrile. They claim that no evidence exists in animal or clinical studies to support any possibility that the substance is effective. They further claim that, although Laetrile is probably safe and there is no evidence that it is dangerous or toxic (although a few deaths have been reported from the substance), patients who use it may forsake other treatments which might control or even cure their cancer.

Proponents claim that they are patients who are in possession of well-documented records regarding their own cases and that Laetrile has proven helpful to them. They are upset with the system and their doctors. After listening to their testimony, state legislators have usually favored "freedom-of-choice" bills for these people, in spite of the fact that the state bills they have passed are in direct conflict with federal food and drug laws.

It is difficult to comment on the value of Laetrile. There are good reports and acknowledgments from many doctors that the substance seems to relieve pain for a significant number of cancer patients. Frequently, doctors who prescribe Laetrile also prescribe special diets and a complete change in nutritional habits for their patients. To what extent does this contribute to any patient benefit? No one knows for sure. One thing is clear. It is difficult for doctors to conceive that Laetrile could be effective for a person with uncontrolled malignancy rampaging through his or her body in the form of massive inoperable tumors and extensive metastases.

The National Cancer Institute has only recently indicated that it is trying to approach the problem in an unbiased fashion in order to finally determine whether or not there is any anticancer value in Laetrile and what it might be.

To date, we have found that information regarding Laetrile has frequently been presented in an emotional, biased manner, a point that should be considered by anyone who is investigating the subject.

Sources of Information

American Cancer Society
777 Third Avenue
New York, New York, 10017

Cancer Control Society
2043 North Berendo
Los Angeles, California

The Association for Alternative
Cancer Therapies
101 West 12th Street
New York, New York

5

How to Live with a Cancer Patient

The misery of cancer is not confined to its victims alone. For every person who contracts cancer, there are other people—chiefly family members—whose lives are profoundly affected as well. The effects, of course, will vary from family to family, and a great deal will depend upon the nature of the cancer and the personality of the patient. One thing, however, is certain. The better the people surrounding a cancer patient are able to understand the psychological dynamics that affect both the patient and themselves, the more effectively they will be able to cope with the situation, difficult and tragic as it may be. We hope this chapter will help increase this understanding.

HOW MUCH SHOULD THE PATIENT KNOW?

Probably the biggest decision a family affected by cancer must make is how truthful to be with the cancer patient. Years ago, before the cure rate for cancer began to rise, it was common practice to conceal the nature of the patient's condition from him.

Nowadays, however, more and more doctors are encouraging a candid approach, particularly in cases where the prognosis seems reasonably favorable. Many doctors have found that by not informing a patient that he does indeed have cancer, it is often difficult to convince that patient to undergo the necessary treatment soon enough to provide a good chance for recovery. It's been found, too, that patients who have had successful treatment but have not been told that their condition was malignant are often reluctant to take the periodic checkups a person with a history of cancer should take as a basic health precaution.

Where the real problem arises, however, is in situations where the disease has spread to such an extent that doctors hold out little or no chance of recovery. Should a person who doctors believe has, at most, a year to live be informed of this fact? Unfortunately, there are no black and white answers to this question. There are undoubtedly people who would be much better off knowing the exact nature of their condition, to better structure their life accordingly. Such people would probably sense, anyway, that they have not been told the truth and would very likely react far worse than they would have had they been properly informed in the first place. On the other hand, there are many people who are simply unable to deal with the knowledge that they are suffering from a fatal disease. Such people, when confronted with the truth, are very likely to slip immediately into such a depressed—and perhaps suicidal—state that whatever time they might have had to live is, for all intents and purposes, lost.

Many psychiatrists and psychologists who have examined this problem are now recommending what might be described as judicious candor, or, as one psychologist once put it, "truth in small doses." It is one thing to tell a person that he has cancer, and something else again to tell him that his chances of recovery are all but nil. Cancer is an extremely unpredictable disease, and there isn't a cancer specialist anywhere in the world who can't recite story after story of patients who are still living despite the fact that years ago their conditions were diagnosed as terminal, with death expected within months.

Therefore, your first obligation, as a person who is close to a cancer patient, is to do whatever you can to prevent the patient from giving up hope entirely. This does not mean misleading the patient by going through an elaborate charade to give him the impression that he's being cured. It means, instead, constantly reassuring the patient that everything possible is being done to bring about an improvement in his condition and maintaining his hope. As recently as 1919, children who were diagnosed as diabetics had little or no chance of reaching adulthood. Two years later, insulin was discovered and diabetes, though still serious, was virtually eliminated as a killer of children. Who can say for certain that a similar discovery might not occur in cancer within months, thus renewing life for thousands upon thousands of "terminal" patients whose faith and hope kept them alive those extra couple of months to make the difference!

UNDERSTANDING THE
CANCER PATIENT

Thanks to a growing number of psychological studies, we now know a lot more about the psychological changes that cancer patients undergo than we had previously. This new knowledge should help the families of cancer patients to better understand and thus deal more effectively with the changes in the patients' personality that almost always take place.

The first thing you have to realize is that, like anybody inflicted with a condition that is more serious than a mild cold, a cancer patient almost always undergoes what psychiatrist Paul H. Brauer has described as "an immediate and revolutionary reorientation of all his drives and interests." Says Dr. Brauer, "The only thing that matters to the patient is getting well. . . . Naturally, although the members of the 'normal' family want a return to health almost as much as the patient, this focus is neither so sharp nor so exclusive for them."

Apart from this shifting of priorities, it is difficult to generalize about the different types of psychological reactions cancer patients have, but there seem to be certain patterns that most cancer patients fall into in one degree or another. Some people show incredible degrees of strength and stoicism, rarely revealing their fears and their needs—fearful, above all, of becoming a burden to their families. In others, the reaction is totally different. The patient becomes more and more helpless and more and more demanding. In between these extremes are any number of reaction levels that range from shame to fear to a paranoia that sometimes manifests itself in violent outbursts—the patient convinced that he is being victimized by a conspiracy whose chief design is to end his life as soon as possible.

One extremely important factor in a cancer patient's psychological reaction to his condition is the organ—or organs—affected by the disease.

Cancer specialists are only now beginning to fully appreciate this aspect of cancer and, as a result, are tailoring treatment strategies accordingly. Radical surgery is not being performed as summarily as in the past, as more and more doctors have come to realize that for some people, the specter of disfigurement is a more fearul prospect than death. Thus, even in those cases in which a patient has been treated "successfully," the psychological reaction to the removal of a breast or a limb can be severe—as severe in its own way as the reaction to the news that the patient's condition is terminal.

In summary, a person suffering from cancer will almost always undergo a very noticeable change in personality. The nature and extent of the change and the length of time it takes for the patient to regain his "normal" personality will depend, in large part, on his psychological makeup. But a crucial aspect in this process as well is the psychological reaction and the response of his family.

UNDERSTANDING OURSELVES

Just as cancer patients show a variety of psychological reactions upon the realization of their condition, so do the friends and family of the patient respond in a variety of ways. There are, of course, the natural reactions of grief and sympathy, but these reactions are frequently mixed with emotions that some people have difficulty understanding and dealing with.

One of the most common of these reactions is guilt. It is extremely difficult to see someone we care for very deeply suffer without experiencing pangs of guilt. This is particularly true of the parents of young cancer victims, but can apply as well to other familial relationships. In situations like this, it is very natural to look back and regret the things we didn't do to make the person now suffering from cancer happier and more secure.

There isn't much you can do to prevent feelings of guilt from arising. But by recognizing, however, that the guilt feelings are doing nothing to benefit the patient, we can begin to channel these feelings into acts that will make a meaningful difference to him or her.

Curiously enough, another common reaction among the family members of cancer patients is resentment. Serious illness of any kind invariably disrupts the routine of a household. Everyone has careers, hobbies, interests, and relationships that they find themselves having to subordinate in order to care for the cancer patient. It is only normal to feel some resentment because of this sacrifice. Most people, however, are able to accept the infringement upon their own lives with understanding and compassion. Accepting the responsibility that has been thrust upon us and recognizing that whatever sacrifices we are making are minimal compared to those of the patient can often keep resentment down to a very manageable minimum. Additional help in this area can often be found through membership in one of the organizations devoted to rehabilitation of cancer patients and their families, listed in Appendix B of this book.

RELATING TO THE PATIENT

Every situation created by cancer has its own individual ramifications. Depending upon the personalities involved, a very serious condition can sometimes be less disruptive to a family than a relatively mild condition. The nature of the family relationship before cancer has struck, the financial circumstances of a family, the degree of religious conviction in the household—each of these factors can, of itself, shape the psychological climate within the household that finds itself coping with a cancer patient.

Above all, the people who surround a cancer patient must maintain emotional control—particularly in direct dealings with the patient. Remember that the patient himself is undergoing an emotional trauma. His moods will very likely be unstable and often extreme. Responding to these emotional extremes with emotional outbursts of equal intensity will only exacerbate the problem. The patient needs understanding, assurance, and an atmosphere of emotional stability. Give vent to your emotions in private or in the company of close friends, but don't subject the patient to them.

Another goal for the family caring for a cancer patient is the maintenance of as close a level of normalcy within the household as possible, according to the special needs of the patient. In their natural desire to make the patient as comfortable and as secure as possible, many families make the mistake of changing the normal household routine so drastically that the patient, instead of being grateful, feels uneasy and uncomfortable in the knowledge that his condition has become so burdensome to the family. The self-image of a cancer patient suffers enough from his condition alone. The last thing he needs is the additional loss of self-esteem that arises from the feeling of helplessness.

Even in extreme circumstances—those in which a cancer patient becomes an invalid—it is possible to keep the household going in a reasonably normal fashion. If the patient requires constant looking after, there's no reason that everyone in the household must be on constant call. Tasks should be divided equally among family members.

Wherever possible, encourage the cancer patient to pursue whatever normal activities he is physically capable of doing. Even when the prognois is very favorable, a cancer patient will frequently experience difficulty reestablishing a normal rhythm in his life—and the reasons are frequently more psychological than physical. A temporary state of psychological withdrawal is to be expected; but if it is prolonged, it is up to you and your doctor and, if necessary, a psychological counselor, to help the patient help himself.

Keep an open mind about the source of the patient's inactivity. A patient's decision to stay at home rather than attend a function he regularly attended before he was sick, may really be rooted in a basic logistical problem: he doesn't want to drive or doesn't want to bother a friend to pick him up. You can provide no greater service to a cancer patient than to furnish the seemingly unimportant bits of help that enable the patient to regain a sense of normalcy to his life.

Be understanding. There is a very delicate balance between overindulging a cancer patient and neglecting him, and it is sometimes difficult for a family to strike this balance. To be sure, a cancer patient needs sympathy and assurance. But more important, he needs to regain the self-esteem that is almost invariably lost when a person is directly affected by cancer.

Never confuse physical dependency with mental weakness. The fact that a cancer patient is temporarily confined to his bed does not mean that he cannot assume an active role in the making of family decisions. Denying a cancer patient this role increases his feeling of helplessness and further depletes his self-respect.

WHEN YOU NEED HELP

Not all families can deal equally effectively with the psychological pressures that cancer invariably produces. Sometimes the psychological—and practical—problems are so intense and complicated that even the best-adjusted families find it impossible to cope with them.

Fortunately, there are numerous agencies throughout the country that offer help to families who find themselves in this situation. This help may take the form of a volunteer nurse who will come into your home and teach you how to make the patient more comfortable. Or it may take the form of psychological counseling designed to help the various family members relate to the cancer patient in a more positive manner. Whatever the problem, there are people who will help. Your best source of information for this help is your local chapter or representative of the American Cancer Society.

SPECIFIC
TYPES
OF CANCER

6

What You Should Know About Cancer of the Breast

Breast cancer is almost exclusively a women's disease, although there are isolated cases of it occurring in middle-aged and older men. It is the most common form of cancer among women, and in the 40 to 44 age bracket, the number-one cause of death. There has been a great deal of publicity about breast cancer in recent years—primarily because of the news that surrounded Betty Ford's and Happy Rockefeller's experiences with it. But there remains a larger number of women whose fear of the disease prevents them from taking the routine measures that lead to early detection.

THE NATURE OF BREAST CANCER

Breast cancer usually appears in the form of a small, painless lump in the breast which occasionally adheres to the skin, and, in some cases, ulcerates. Breast cancer characteristically metastasizes to the lymph nodes in the armpit or to the chain of lymph nodes beneath the junction of the breastbone and ribs. As long as the condition doesn't spread *beyond* these nodes, the condition is usually operable and curable. And of course the more localized the condition is, the more favorable the prognosis will be.

DETECTING BREAST CANCER

In recent years, enormous strides have been made in detection techniques for breast cancer, and these advances have had a very significant impact on the breast-cancer survival rate. The most important development has been the establishment by the American Cancer Society, together with the National Cancer Institute, of a network of Breast Cancer Detection Screening Centers throughout the country. As of this writing there are twenty-seven such centers in different parts of the country capable of screening hundreds of thousands of women every year—and at no cost.

What differentiates these centers from standard medical centers is the sophistication and variety of their equipment and diagnostic procedures. Most breast cancers today are detected by either women themselves or their physicians during routine examinations, but the screening techniques utilized by these centers, among them mammography and xeroradiography, are able to detect tumors *before* they have grown large enough to be detected by a physical examination. With these small growths, cancer has normally not yet spread to the lymph nodes. Of the 1,850 women in whom disease was detected, 592 had these miniscule tumors.

Recent studies conducted by the American Cancer Society and the National Cancer Institute point up the meaning of this difference. In one study, it was found that the number of women whose breast cancer had been detected at a screening center and treated successfully was almost 70 percent higher than the number of conventionally diagnosed breast cancer patients whose treatment had been judged a success. Translated into survival figures, this number represents tens of thousands of lives each year. In yet another study, it was found that less than 3 percent whose cancer had been detected by mammography before the tumor had become visible died of breast cancer within the five-year follow-up period.

Recently, however, the National Cancer Institute has indicated that mammography testing will be restricted to women over fifty, except in cases of patients who had had cancer or a family history of breast cancer. Their recommendation came in response to studies which showed that repeated exposure to the radiation from mammography may, in fact, increase a woman's susceptibility to breast cancer.

A new technique, however, for the detection of breast cancer has recently been tested at the Memorial Sloan-Kettering Cancer Center which appears to be highly effective and completely safe. The technique is known as *Graphic Stress Telethermometry*. The test does not use radiation but instead measures the variations in temperatures over the entire breast area. So far, it has proved to give an 80 percent accuracy rate for the detection of malignant tumors and almost 100 percent for benign tumors. If further testing corroborates these findings, this revolutionary testing procedure will undoubtedly be available in the 27 Breast Cancer Detecting Screening Centers.

BREAST CANCER DETECTION DEMONSTRATION PROJECT (AS OF SEPTEMBER 1974).
(Courtesy of The National Cancer Institute)

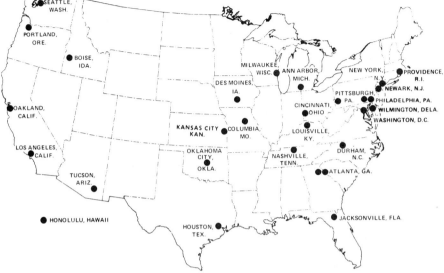

In any case, the evidence is overwhelming. Women who undergo regular annual checkups at Breast Cancer Detection Screening Centers are far less likely to die of breast cancer than women who undergo conventional examinations. Above is a map indicating the geographical locations of the Breast Cancer Detection Demonstration Projects, an Introduction to the program, and a listing of the Detection Centers and their Project Directors. If there is no center near you, contact your local American Cancer Society or representative to find out if a new center has opened in your area, or where you can get similar testing at a nearby institution.

THE BREAST CANCER DETECTION DEMONSTRATION PROJECT*

In 1973 the National Cancer Institute (NCI) and the American Cancer Society (ACS) cosponsored and initiated the Breast Cancer Detection Demonstration Project (BCDDP). The Project is designed to demonstrate to the medical profession and to the public the application of periodic screenings in the detection of early breast cancer. Funds are provided by NCI contracts and ACS grants. Twenty-seven projects supporting 29 BCDDP screening centers have been set up in selected cities throughout the United States. For demonstration purposes the centers have been

*Reproduced from the National Institutes of Health Breast Cancer Detection Demonstration Project, *Manual of Procedures and Operations.*

established in various types of medical institutions. At the completion of recruitment, the entire Project will have enrolled a total of 270,000 women 35 years of age and older.

Goal and Objectives

The overall goal of the Breast Cancer Detection Demonstration Project (BCDDP) is to increase awareness of breast cancer through the demonstration of methods and techniques for early detection. It is designed to demonstrate the use of breast-screening modalities such as thermography, mammography, and physical examination in large-scale screening programs. Education of the public and the medical profession in the value and methods of recruitment and application of screening modalities and followup is of prime concern. In each project, approximately 10,000 women are being enrolled over a 2-year period. Each project will provide for five annual screenings plus five years of followup. Screenees are recruited from the population at large, and an emphasis has been placed on efforts to recruit a cross section of races, ethnic groups, and socio-economic levels, utilizing the volunteer corps of the ACS to the maximum extent. There is no charge to screenees.

The objectives of the BCDDP are:

⊕ Recruit 10,000 asymptomatic, non-pregnant women between the ages of 35 and 74 years in each of the 27 projects over a 2-year period for a total of 270,000 women in the program. (Implementation: Screening Center with ACS Volunteers)

⊕ Screen each of these women with history, physical examination, mammography, and thermography, each independently obtained and interpreted in accordance with guidelines for specific age groups. (Implementation: Screening Center)

⊕ Refer these screenees for either surgical consultation (i.e., biopsy or aspiration), early recall, or annual rescreen on the basis of overall evaluation of the combined screening modalities. (Implementation: Screening Center)

⊕ Assist all screenees in entering the medical care system. (Implementation: Screening Center)

⊕ Inform all screenees and their physicians of the results of each examination. (Implementation: Screening Center)

⊕ Examine all screenees annually by all three modalities according to age group guidelines for a total of five annual examinations. (Implementation: Screening Center)

⊕ Follow each screenee annually for 5 years after the five annual screenings. (Implementation: Screening Center)

⊕ Provide information as to the usefulness of ACS volunteers in recruiting, recalling, and following up all the participating women. (Implementation: Screening Center)

- ⊕ Utilize the lowest practicable level of radiation exposure consistent with good image quality. (Implementation: Screening Center assisted by the Centers for Radiological Physics)
- ⊕ Prepare a complete set of data forms on each screenee. Data sets will be sent to a data management center for processing and management. (Implementation: Screening Center)
- ⊕ Develop local support for continuing certain aspects of the Project beyond the NCI-ACS funding period. (Implementation: Screening Center)

Project Directors

Philip Strax, M.D., *Director*
Breast Cancer Demonstration Project
Guttman Institute
200 Madison Avenue
New York, New York 10016
(212) 830-4127

Robert L. Egan, M.D., *Director*
Georgia Cancer Management Network
1645 Tully Circle, N.E., Suite 126
Atlanta, Georgia 30329
(404) 634-1524

A. Hamblin Letton, M.D., *Director*
Breast Cancer Screening Project
Georgia Baptist Hospital
Professional Building East
315 Boulevard, N.E., Suite 500
Atlanta, Georgia 30312
(404) 681-3733

Jerry B. Buchanan, M.D., *Director*
Breast Cancer Demonstration Project
601 S. Floyd Street
Louisville, Kentucky 40202
(502) 588-5261, 64

John R. Milbrath, M.D., *Director*
Breast Cancer Detection Center
8700 W. Wisconsin Avenue
Milwaukee, Wisconsin 53226
(414) 257-5200

Thomas Carlile, M.D., *Director*
Breast Cancer Detection Center
1323 Spring Street
Seattle, Washington 98104
(206) 322-0500

JoAnn Haberman, M.D., *Director*
Breast Cancer Center
711 Stanton Young Blvd., Suite 211
Oklahoma City, Oklahoma 73104
(405) 271-4514

Elisabeth B. Ward, M.D., *Director*
Breast Cancer Detection Center
215 Avenue B
Boise, Idaho 83702
(208) 345-3590

Benjamin F. Rush, Jr., M.D., *Director*
Breast Cancer Detection Project
Department of Surgery—Room 852
65 Bergen Street
Newark, New Jersey 07107
(201) 456-4435

Larry Baker, M.D., *Director*
Breast Cancer Detection Center
Department of Surgery
University of Kansas Medical Center
39th & Rainbow Boulevard
Kansas City, Kansas 66103
(913) 588-6101

Myron Moskowitz, M.D., *Director*
Breast Cancer Detection Center
Room 10E Logan Hall Basement
Cincinnati General Hospital
Elland & Bethesda Avenues
Cincinnati, Ohio 45267
(513) 872-5335

Marvin V. McClow, M.D., *Director*
Breast Cancer Detection Center
St. Vincent's Medical Center
Barrs Street at St. Johns Avenue
Jacksonville, Florida 32203
(904) 389-7751 Ext. 8332

Harold J. Isard, M.D., *Director*
Breast Cancer Demonstration Project
Albert Einstein Medical Center
York and Tabor Roads
Philadelphia, Pennsylvania 19141
(215) 455-8400, ext. 10

Marc S. Lapayowker, M.D., *Director*
Breast Cancer Detection Clinic
Department of Radiology
Temple University Hospital
3401 N. Broad Street
Philadelphia, Pennsylvania 19140
(215) 221-4206

Bernard Fisher, M.D., *Director*
Breast Cancer Detection Center
914 Scaife Hall
University of Pittsburgh
Pittsburgh, Pennsylvania 15261
(412) 624-2671

Leslie W. Whitney, M.D., *Director*
Breast Screening Project
1200 Jefferson Street
Wilmington, Delaware 19801
(302) 428-2113

Barbara Threatt, M.D., *Director*
Breast Cancer Detection Center
396 W. Washington Street
Ann Arbor, Michigan 48109
(313) 764-1474

Donald C. Young, M.D., *Director*
Breast Cancer Demonstration Project
Iowa Lutheran Hospital
University & Penn. Avenues
Des Moines, Iowa 50316
(515) 283-5205

Fred I. Gilbert, Jr., M.D., *Director*
Breast Cancer Detection Center
545 Alexander Young Building
Bishop and Hotel Streets
Honolulu, Hawaii 96813
(808) 524-4411

Robert J. Schweitzer, M.D., *Director*
Breast Screening Center
384 34th Street
Oakland, California 94609
(415) 451-8683

Bruce Shnider, M.D., *Director*
Medical Center Cancer Screening Project
5125 MacArthur Blvd., N.W.
Washington, D.C. 20016
(202) 625-2181

Robert McLelland, M.D., *Director*
Breast Cancer Detection Project
3040 Erwin Road
Durham, North Carolina 27705
(919) 684-4397

Arthur J. Present, M.D., *Director*
Breast Cancer Detection Project
Professor of Radiology
2231 East Speedway Blvd.
Tucson, Arizona 85719
(602) 882-7492

Lewis W. Guiss, M.D., *Director*
Breast Cancer Detection Program
John Wesley County Hospital
2826 South Hope Street, Room 123
Los Angeles, California 90007
(213) 748-3111

Ned D. Rodes, M.D., *Director*
Breast Cancer Detection Project
Cancer Research Center
Business Loop 70 & Garth Avenue
Columbia, Missouri 65201
(314) 449-2711, ext. 352

Morton J. Goodman, M.D., *Director*
Breast Cancer Screening Center
2222 N.W. Lovejoy Street, Suite 171
Portland, Oregon 97210
(503) 229-7292

Herbert P. Constantine, M.D., *Director*
Breast Cancer Detection Project
Rhode Island Hospital
593 Eddy Street
Ambulatory Patient Center, Room 141
Providence, Rhode Island 02902
(401) 277-5736

M. Dee Ingram, Jr., M.D., *Director*
Vanderbilt Breast Cancer Detection
    Center
Room 110, Baker Building
110 21st Avenue, S.
Nashville, Tennessee 37203
(615) 322-3495

Duncan L. Moore, M.D., *Director*
Breast Cancer Detection Center
2000 Crawford
Houston, Texas 77002
(713) 659-8626

TREATING BREAST CANCER

Once a self-examination or a screening procedure has led to the discovery of a lump or mass in the breast, the first step is to determine as quickly as possible if the tumor is benign or malignant. Mammographs and xeroradiographs can determine the nature of a tumor with an accuracy rate of 90 percent, but there is only one foolproof way of determining if a tumor is malignant: a biopsy. The decisions you make at this state will have a profound effect on your condition—if indeed the tumor is found to be malignant.

A biopsy is a minor and routine operation, but you should exercise a good deal of care in selecting your surgeon. For your own welfare, unpleasant as it may be, anticipate the possibility of the tumor's being malignant. If the biopsy reveals no malignancy—which is the outcome in the majority of cases—you have lost nothing. However, if the tumor is judged to be malignant, the subsequent decisions are best made by a surgeon who is familiar with breast cancer and has discussed the situation with you beforehand.

WHY THE SURGEON IS IMPORTANT

The tissue that is taken from a patient during a biopsy is usually analyzed while the patient is still on the operating table. If the tissue is judged to be benign, the surgeon closes the incision and the patient is sent to the recovery room. If, however, the tumor has proven to be malignant, then the surgeon has some crucial decisions to make. Does he perform a mastectomy? And, if so, which type?

A surgeon who has had extensive experience dealing with breast cancer is far more prepared to make these decisions than a general surgeon. A knowledgeable breast-cancer surgeon will have done extensive preoperative testing to determine whether the potential cancer is localized or has already undergone metastasis beyond the lymph nodes into other sites of the body. The distinction is crucial. For example, if metastasis has gone beyond a certain stage, mastectomy becomes pointless and chemotherapy becomes the treatment most often prescribed.

An experienced breast-cancer surgeon will usually discuss with the patient ahead of time the various options open if mastectomy is called for. It is unfortunate but true that a great many mastectomies are performed in this country by surgeons who are not familiar enough with breast cancer to make the decision which will produce optimal results for the patient. There are different types of mastectomies including

SELF-EXAMINATION PROCEDURES

Whether or not you avail yourself of the cancer-screening services offered by the new screening centers, it is always a wise policy to conduct a monthly self-examination of your breasts. The time to conduct this test is a week after each menstrual period. After menopause, you should check your breasts on the first day of each month. This is the procedure recommended by breast-cancer specialists.

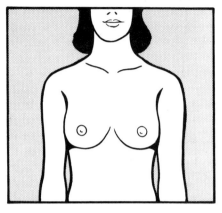

1. Stand before a mirror in a normal position with your hands at your sides. See if there is any change in the size or shape of your breasts. Look for any dimpling or scaling of the skin of your nipples. Remember, the left and right breasts of most women are *not* identical. Several months' examination will give you an idea of the normal contours of your breasts.

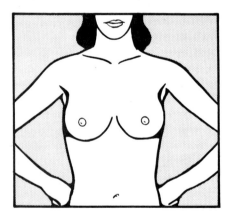

2. Raise your arms and press your hands behind your head. Look for any abnormality.

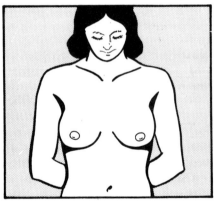

3. With your hands clasped behind your back, lean forward. Note any abnormality.

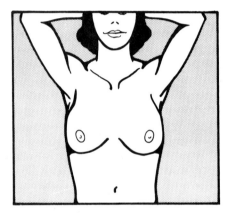

4. Place your hands on your hips, press inward, and flex your arm and chest muscles. Once again, look for any disfiguration or abnormality.

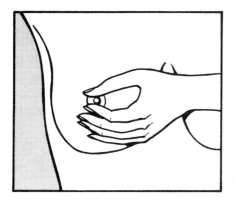

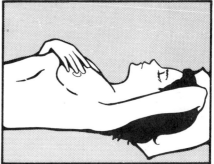

5. Using your thumb and index finger, gently squeeze the nipple of each breast. If there is any discharge, report it to your doctor immediately.

6. Lie flat on your back with a pillow under your left shoulder and your left hand tucked under your head. Using your right hand slightly cupped, feel for any lumps, thickening, hard knots, or change in the texture of your breast or skin. Start with the inner half of the left breast from top to bottom and from the nipple to the breastbone. Don't compress or pinch your breast between the thumb and fingers. This might give the false impression of a lump which does not actually exist.

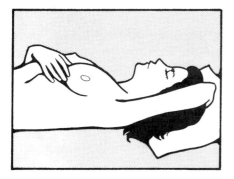

7. Examine the outer half of your breast from bottom to top and from the nipple to the left side of your chest.

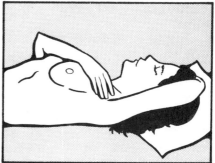

8. Take particular care to examine the armpit and the area between the breast and the armpit.

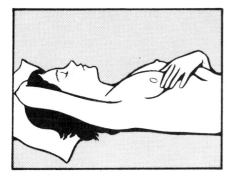

9. Place the pillow under your right shoulder, and with the right hand tucked under your head, repeat this same procedure for the right breast using your left hand to do the examination. Note: A ridge of tissue in the lower curve of each breast is normal.

Feel your breasts and armpits thoroughly, and if you find something which appears abnormal, contact your doctor as soon as possible for an examination. For the most part, most breast lumps are not serious, but all should be examined by a qualified physician for a final diagnosis and to eliminate any question of a doubt. Remember, 95 percent of breast cancers are first discovered by women themselves.

segmental, partial, and radical. A segmental (or wedge) mastectomy involves the removal of a pie-shaped section of the breast including the affiliated lymph nodes. A partial mastectomy includes removal of the entire breast, skin, and lymph nodes, but leaves the muscles intact. A radical mastectomy involves removal of the entire breast, muscles, and armpit lymph nodes. Surgeons best qualified to make these decisions are those surgeons who are accredited oncologists and who are on the staff or associated with one of the hospitals or institutions devoted to cancer treatment.

CHOOSING THE RIGHT SURGEON

The best strategy for selecting a breast surgeon is to get the recommendations of several doctors whose opinions you trust, and, if possible, talk to women who have already undergone mastectomies. Your local American Cancer Society chapter will also be a source of useful information for you, as well as the director or staff member of any of the cancer treatment institutions listed in the appendixes of this book. These sources should provide you with a list of several qualified oncologists. Try to meet personally with as many of these oncologists as you can comfortably manage. Dealing with a surgeon in whose judgment you have great confidence is an indispensable first step to breast cancer treatment.

WHAT WE'RE LEARNING ABOUT MASTECTOMIES

Numerous studies are now underway to determine which type of mastectomy represents the optimal treatment for primary breast cancer. One such study being conducted by a group called the National Surgical Adjuvant Breast Project (NSABP) has produced findings which indicate that moderate strategies, such as a segmental mastectomy, produce results that are equivalent to more radical strategies. These findings have spurred hope that breast cancer patients who previously would have been faced with total mastectomies may someday undergo a much more limited procedure with equally beneficial results. As of now, however, not enough long-range findings are available to allow for any firm conclusions.

POSTOPERATIVE THERAPIES

The determining factor in the survival rate of breast cancer patients is the presence of the disease in the axillary (armpit) nodes. In cases where the disease has *not* reached these nodes, the survival rate is presently 85 percent. These figures drop noticeably, however, in cases where the malignancy has metastasized to this area.

One recent and encouraging development in this area is a recent study, conducted by the National Cancer Institute, which showed that a drug called L-Phenylalanine mustard (L-PAM) can, when combined with a modified or radical mastectomy, significantly reduce the cancer recurrence rate among women whose cancer has metastasized to the axillary nodes. Other studies involving other anti-cancer drugs show equally encouraging results.

What is particularly significant about these studies is that they hold out new hope to breast cancer patients whose chances for survival have historically been less than 50 percent. Indications are that the L-PAM treatment, which involves the taking of the drug by mouth five consecutive days every six weeks for two years, has minimal side-effects.

ADVANCED CASES

The prospect for breast cancer patients with very advanced cases is still not bright, but better today than it has ever been. In one recent study, sponsored by the Eastern Cooperative Oncology Group, a new three-drug combination has proven to be more effective than L-PAM alone in the shrinking of cancerous tumors. Similar work is going on at the Albany Medical College of Union University and at Roswell Park Memorial Institute in Buffalo, where studies are underway to test the effectiveness of combination chemotherapy. It should be pointed out, however, that these therapies, where they have succeeded, have served to *control* the disease, not to cure it.

THE OUTLOOK

Approximately 90,000 American women will develop breast cancer this year, making it the major type of cancer among women. Fortunately, however, the survival outlook for women who do contract the disease has never been better. Advances in early detection and diagnosis have already begun to make significant inroads into the death rate, and all the evidence points to the implementation of newer and much more limited surgical techniques than have been used in the past. What's more, advances in chemotherapy hold out new hope for women whose cancer has gone beyond the primary stage.

SUGGESTIONS FOR HAND AND ARM
CARE AFTER A MASTECTOMY*

After breast surgery, which may include removal of the lymph glands in the armpit, there sometimes is a tendency towards swelling of the arm. Ordinarily, this swelling

*Prepared by the Reach to Recovery Program of the American Cancer Society.

is so slight as to be hardly noticeable, but occasionally, it is more severe. Infection can be introduced from trivial injuries, insect bites, etc. Every attempt should be made to prevent such injuries or infections, and to obtain prompt treatment.

In the event of infection of the arm, which may appear as redness, pain and swelling of any part of the arm or hand, with or without fever and feelings of illness, call for prompt consultation with your physician.

Be particularly careful when manicuring this hand, and avoid cutting the cuticles. Use a lanolin-base cream or ointment on the hand and at the base of nails to keep the cuticles soft.

It is best to suggest to the nurse or technician when a blood sample or blood pressure is taken to use the other arm. Injections and vaccinations are best avoided on that side unless specifically prescribed by a physician who is aware of the previous breast surgery.

Ordinary housework is desirable, but one should be careful to avoid burns and other such injuries.

For patients who do much sewing, it is important that thimbles be used to avoid pricking the ends of the fingers with pins or needles.

Gardening is good exercise and fun, but work gloves should be worn to protect hands from thorns and scratches.

It is wise to wear loose-fitting rubber gloves for household work, especially if hands are immersed in water for any length of time.

When carrying a heavy object, use the other arm, or better still, carry it with both hands or roll your shoulders back and balance the object on your hip. It helps your posture, too.

Sunburn, particularly if severe, can result in significant swelling and is best avoided. Keep a light scarf or kerchief with you—throw it over your arm if it is necessary for you to be exposed to the sun for any length of time. Sunbathe and enjoy, but don't burn. Any skin area which has received X-ray therapy should be protected from direct exposure to the sun.

HORMONES

Some cosmetics contain hormones. If the cosmetics that you use contain hormones, be sure to ask your physician whether you can use them. It is always important to avoid taking any medication of any kind without advice of your physician.

7

What You Should Know About Cancer of the Lung

There is no escape from the fact that lung cancer is one of the most lethal forms of disease. In the United States alone, more than 90,000 people die each year from lung cancer—more than three-quarters of them men, although the percentage of women contracting lung cancer, primarily from cigarette smoking, is increasing at near-epidemic proportions. The figure represents a tenfold increase over the statistics of fifty years ago. Moreover, the five-year survival rate for lung cancer is among the lowest of all forms of cancer. At present, the five-year survival rate is somewhere between 8 and 12 percent.

Yet, despite these bleak statistics, the overall, lung-cancer picture, is gradually beginning to brighten. As in other forms of the disease, improved diagnostic techniques have enhanced the ability of lung cancer specialists to discover lung cancer increasingly earlier. And while surgery remains the primary treatment therapy for lung cancer, there are increasing indications that a multidisciplinary approach which combines surgery with other therapies—radiotherapy, chemotherapy, immunotherapy, and new radio frequency therapy—will begin to produce a dramatic surge in the survival rate of lung cancer patients in the near future. In addition, the pattern of lung cancer is such that we know more about *preventing* it than we do about most other cancers.

THE NATURE OF THE DISEASE

The lung is an organ—actually a pair of organs—which controls breathing. Because the lung is constantly expanding and contracting, and because it has an extremely rich blood and lymph supply, cancer cells that develop in the lung have a tendency to metastasize much faster than cancer cells which develop in other organs. Whereas it may take some cancers—prostate cancer, for instance—months and even years to spread, metastasis in the lung can take place in a matter of weeks. Typically, too, lung cancers can spread to the brain, liver, bone marrow, and heart even before the symptoms of the primary tumor are discovered.

SYMPTOMS OF LUNG CANCER

The symptoms of lung cancer vary according to where in the lung the cancer develops. In many instances, there are no symptoms at all in the early stages—no symptoms, that is, until the condition has begun to spread, by which time it is generally too late for a positive prognosis. In other cases, particularly in cancers that develop in the bronchi (the air passages), the most common early symptom is a cough. But because this cough is no different from a cough from a simple cold or throat irritation, it is not until several days have passed without any cessation of the symptom that cancer might be suspected. Pain is rare in early stages of the disease, but sometimes there will be blood in the sputum. Anytime there is blood in the sputum and anytime there is a *lingering* cough, consult your doctor immediately.

DETECTING LUNG CANCER

A conventional X ray will usually indicate the presence of most lung tumors. However, even if the X rays take place every six months, the odds are against discovering the tumor before metastasis has occurred. What's more, there are some lung tumors that conventional X rays cannot isolate in the early stages. "When we're talking about conventional diagnostic methods," one cancer specialist from Roswell Park Memorial Institute says, "we're really talking about the luck of the draw. If you happen to time the examination perfectly, we have a chance of getting to the cancer before it spreads. Otherwise, even if you get a chest X ray every three months, it's still unlikely that we'll catch it early enough to do anything."

There is, however, some progress to report. New isotope-scanning techniques are proving much more effective at discovering some lung cancers in the early stages than conventional X-ray techniques. Another device being used more and more in diagnostic work is the bronchoscope—an instrument that enables a physician not only to visually examine the interior of the lung, but to take a sample of suspicious tissue as well. And one of the more promising areas at present involves a relatively

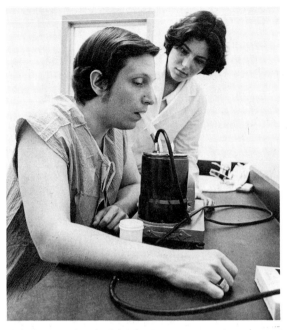

new diagnostic technique known as sputum cytology—the periodic analysis of sputum. Some researchers are now advocating a program of regular sputum analysis once every three months for men in "high-risk" categories—that is, men over fifty-five who are heavy smokers or who have a family history of lung cancer.

TREATING LUNG CANCER

The primary form of treatment for lung cancer is surgery. In cases where the tumor has remained localized, the prospects for patients who have undergone surgery are excellent, even if the surgical treatment has removed a large portion of the lung. But because the vast majority of lung cancer patients are already in various stages of metastasis by the time the surgery is performed, the emphasis in the more progressive treatment centers is on a team approach to treatment. Says Dr. Oleg Selawry, the Associate Director of Pulmonary Oncology of the Comprehensive Cancer Center for the State of Florida,

> *"What we're doing today that we weren't doing five years ago, is emphasizing individualized treatment involving not just one specialist but a whole team of specialists—the surgeon, the radiologist, the chemotherapist, the pathologist, and the immunotherapist. By doing this, we coordinate all the therapies so that we eliminate unnecessary surgery and unnecessary radiation."*

Dr. Selawry is one of a number of cancer specialists looking into chemotherapy as a possible weapon against lung cancer. His research shows promise but is still very much in the experimental stage. Much the same can be said, too, for studies currently investigating the effects of cryosurgery on lung cancer.

Dr. Paul Chretien of the NCI, Bethesda, Maryland, is presently conducting a controlled study on a new immunological drug called thymesine which is made from an extract of animal thymus glands. Although this study is quite limited, the initial results are promising. Additional information can be obtained from Dr. Chretien at the Department of Surgery of the National Cancer Institute in Bethesda, Maryland 20014.

The NCI is also conducting experiments with Vitamin A and related chemicals called artificial retinoids. However, this study is geared toward the prevention of lung cancer in high-risk groups rather than treatment of existing tumors.

Cornebacterium parvum, usually referred to as *C. parvum,* has shown significant antitumor activity when tested in animals, especially against lung cancer. It is presently being tested at a number of institutions in the United States and abroad to ascertain if its use will prevent or inhibit recurrences of lung tumors following surgery. One of the international centers investigating it is the Ludwig Institute of Cancer Research, Lausanne, Switzerland. Information can be obtained from Dr. Jan Stjernsward.

An additional new development in the treatment of lung cancer, especially in the case of inoperable tumors, is the use of radio frequency waves. The information on this new treatment regimen is covered in Chapter 4, "Hyperthermia and the New Radiation."

8

What You Should Know About Cancer of the Colon and Rectum

Cancer of the colon and rectum victimizes more people throughout the world than any other form of cancer, but because the nature of the disease and the part of the body it affects are a source of embarrassment to many people, the disease is often called "the cancer nobody talks about." This is extremely regrettable. The survival rate among patients with cancer of the colon and rectum who are treated promptly and properly is around 75 percent, making the potential for saving the lives of people affected by this particular variety of cancer among the highest of any cancer type. The *actual* survival rate, however, is around 40 percent, which means that thousands of people each year die needlessly.

Any number of conditions can interfere with the normal functioning of the colon and the rectum and thus impair the body's waste-removal machinery. Among the more common colon problems are temporary constipation (which can have a variety of causes) or hemorrhoids. Among the most dangerous is the growth of a cancerous tumor.

TUMORS IN THE COLON

The cells that make up the colon are constantly dividing and reproducing them-selves—and at a faster rate than cells in other portions of the body. Consequently, the potential for tumor growth is high in this area of the body. The majority of the tumors that form in the colon are nonmalignant polyps. They can generally be removed, without complication, by means of a relatively minor operation. Cancer-ous tumors are another story.

SYMPTOMS OF COLON CANCER

Most colon cancers appear in the last part of the colon, close to the rectum. Conse-quently, the most common symptom of colon cancer is a noticeable change in bowel habits. Diarrhea, constipation, gas pains, rectal bleeding—any or all of these symptoms, if they persist for more than several days, could indicate the possibility of cancer.

In most cancer cases, the symptoms grow progressively more severe. Gas pains in the early stages of colon cancer are noticeable sporadically at first, but as the cancer grows, the abdominal pains will become more frequent and more intense. Typically, too, colon and rectal cancers eventually ulcerate, producing blood in the stool that appears either red or black.

Rectal bleeding is also a symptom of a very common medical problem—hemor-rhoids (piles). Most of the time, rectal bleeding will indicate nothing more serious than hemorrhoids. However, ignoring rectal bleeding on the assumption that all you have is hemorrhoids is taking an unnecessary risk with your life. Any bleeding in the bowel should always prompt a visit to a physician.

DETECTING COLON AND
RECTAL CANCER

Unlike many cancers, cancer of the colon and cancer of the rectum are relatively easy to detect in most cases, even in the early stages. A simple finger probe by a physician can frequently detect the presence of a rectal tumor. Many physicians routinely use a device called the proctosigmoidoscope (commonly known as the "proctoscope"), which can probe several inches into the colon. Your phy-sician will probably make this examination during your regular checkup, but if the examination is not made, request it, particularly if you are over forty.

Another instrument, known as the *fiberoptic colonoscope,* has proven to be extremely effective in the diagnosis—and, in some cases—the removal of cancer-ous or precancerous tumors. A physician trained in the use of this instrument can examine the entire length of the colon and can detect early cancers which even X-ray studies will not reveal. The instrument can be used, in some cases, to remove suspicious growths with considerably less discomfort and inconvenience than would be caused by abdominal surgery.

If a tumor is suspected, your physician will probably recommend an X-ray examination. X-ray procedures involving the colon call for the bowel to be filled with a liquid barium compound that causes the colon and rectum to show up clearly on the X-ray film. The procedure is uncomfortable but not terribly painful.

TREATING COLON AND RECTAL CANCER

Any growth in the colon or rectal area should be treated promptly, whether it is found to be cancerous or not. Even if a benign tumor is not creating any major difficulties, there is always the possibility—and a very real one, as tests have indicated—that this benign tumor may become cancerous.

In its earliest states, colon and rectal cancer can usually be excised in the doctor's office with either a proctosigmoidoscope or a colonoscope. If, however, the tumor has progressed beyond an early stage, the most effective treatment known thus far is surgery. In a typical cancer of the colon operation, the part of the bowel containing the tumor is removed along with the contiguous segments on both sides. Generally, too, the lymph nodes that drain the area are removed as well to close off a possible route for metastasis.

AFTER TREATMENT

As long as the amount of the colon removed during a cancer operation is very small, the body can continue to function at close to normal efficiency; but if the operation involves extensive surgery, an operation known as a colostomy must be performed.

A colostomy is basically an incision made in the colon in order to create an external opening called an *ostomy* (meaning opening) or *stoma* (meaning mouth). There are several kinds of colostomies, each named for the particular segment of the colon in which it is located. A brief description can be broken down into three parts. The sigmoid or descending colostomy involves removal of a portion of the sigmoid colon so that bowel contents must be discharged through the stoma. It is usually permanent. The transverse colostomy, performed along the transverse colon, involves two kinds of surgery: the double-barrel, consisting of two separate stomas which may or may not be separated by skin, and the loop colostomy. In the latter case, a loop of intestine is brought out through a hole in the abdominal wall, and the outside of the loop is cut halfway through, creating openings to the right and left. This type of colostomy allows the lower part of the colon and/or rectum to heal and rest, and it is usually temporary.

An ileostomy involves removal of all or part of the colon. Functions formerly performed by the colon—absorption of water and electrolytes, storage and solidification of intestinal contents, and transportation of water to the outside—are carried out by bringing the end of the ileum (lowest portion of the small intestine) through the abdominal wall. In each case, the ostomate has less storage space for waste material, and the drainage must be collected in an individually fitted, properly attached appliance which is worn at all times. Under certain conditions, a sigmoid colostomy can be managed in other ways: by irrigation (enemas), dietary control, medication, wearing a pouch, or a combination of these.

Although there is little change in the digestive function, there are social and psychological questions that frequently arise. Adjustments made to living without a normal rectal or bladder opening can be compared to adjustments that one makes for eyeglasses, dental braces, or false teeth. The ostomate can settle into a normal routine, including bathroom functions which are not abnormally time consuming. Only a few additional minutes are required on those occasions when it is necessary to change and irrigate the appliance. There are no unpleasant odors. They are eliminated by means of controlled diets and specially treated appliances. Daily activities can be conducted in a normal fashion with only a few restrictions—most notably, heavy lifting, which might cause injury to the stoma. The ostomate, who will have a flatter tummy than usual, can expect to wear normal, even tight-fitting clothing and bathing suits. Baths or showers can be taken with or without the appliance. Sexual function in women is not impaired, but sexual function in men can sometimes be affected. This is a matter for consultation with a physician. Pregnancy in women with colostomies is not uncommon.

Thousands of people have had colostomy surgery without impairing their social activity. They are living productive and meaningful lives. Help with adjustments is easily obtained through ostomy chapters. These groups provide person-to-person help for new ostomates of all ages and mutual aid and moral support among their members. Most chapters meet monthly and have educational programs and group discussions. Every ostomate will find it helpful to join and be active in a local chapter. Publications that may be of help to the colostomate can be obtained from your local chapter of the American Cancer Society or purchased from the United Ostomy Association which can be contacted at 1111 Wilshire Boulevard, Los Angeles, California 90017.

THE OUTLOOK

The outlook for cancer of the colon patients continues to improve every year. Improved diagnostic techniques are helping physicians detect colon and rectal cancers in their early and most treatable stages, and improved surgical procedures have made surgery possible for patients who only a few years ago were considered too old for surgery or whose conditions were once considered too advanced. At present, nearly 80 percent of patients undergoing surgery for early cancer of the colon live at least five years after diagnosis and treatment, with most of them considered permanently cured.

In the area of nonsurgical treatment, a number of recent advances show great promise. Recent reports on drug therapy indicate that in patients whose disease cannot be treated surgically, a chemical called 5-fluorouracil—or 5-FU—sometimes reduces the size of a tumor of the colon and rectum and relieves pain for longer periods of time. Drug research in this area continues to concentrate on the development of drugs and methods of drug administration that will destory the cancer without harming the patient.

There is now evidence that radiation, administered before or after surgery, is instrumental in shrinking tumors in the colon and rectum.

None of these advances will benefit you, however, unless you take the routine measures that can lead to the early diagnosis and treatment of colon or rectal cancer.

9

What You Should Know About Cancer of the Prostate

Prostate cancer—sometimes known as prostatic cancer—attacks the small, chestnut-shaped sexual gland located just below the urinary bladder in men. It accounts for 16 percent of all cancers detected in males. It causes relatively few deaths among men under forty, but it is the third highest cause of male cancer deaths in men over fifty-five and the leading cause of cancer deaths among men over seventy-five.

Curiously, men who get cancer of the prostate carry the disease with them for many years without suffering any noticeable symptoms. Overall, 90 percent of the cases are not detected until the cancer has metastasized beyond the prostate gland. Indeed often the condition is not discovered until an autopsy is performed after death from some other cause. An estimated 15 to 20 percent of men over fifty may unknowingly be suffering from prostate cancer.

HOW THE PROSTATE FUNCTIONS

The primary function of the prostate gland is the secretion of prostatic fluid, one of several fluids that make up semen. The gland contains the first inch of the urethra, the canal which carries urine from the bladder to the penis. It also contains the muscle fibers which control ejaculation. The prostate gland is controlled, in ways not totally understood, by hormonal activity originating in both the pituitary and adrenal glands.

PROSTATE ENLARGEMENT

The prostate is quite small during adolescence, but begins to enlarge in response to hormonal activity during the twenties and thirties. The enlargement process comes to an end for many men once they reach their forties, but in many men the prostate continues to enlarge until it begins to obstruct the urethra. When this happens, the bladder's ability to empty is hampered, and action must be taken to remove the obstruction.

Although the prostate enlargement in older men is frequently tumorous in nature, the vast majority of tumors in the gland are not—repeat, *not*—cancerous and can be removed by a minor operation that has no measurable effect on sexual function. The most common noncancerous condition in the prostate is called prostatitis.

SYMPTOMS OF PROSTATE CANCER

Prostate cancer is one of the most elusive forms of cancer to diagnose because the early stages of the disease have virtually no symptoms. Most of the symptoms of the disease in its later stages relate to urinary activity. Among the specific symptoms to look out for are:

- ⊕ an unusually weak or interrupted flow of urine
- ⊕ an inability to urinate or difficulty in starting urination
- ⊕ a sharp increase in urinating frequency—especially at night
- ⊕ traces of blood in the urine
- ⊕ a difficulty in stopping urine flow
- ⊕ pain or burning during urination
- ⊕ pain in the lower back, pelvis, or upper thighs

Remember: in *most* cases the above symptoms indicate prostate enlargement and *not* prostate cancer. Nonetheless, as soon as you begin to experience these symptoms, you should see a doctor. A prostate tumor can be detected by a doctor during a routine examination, but special diagnostic tests are needed to determine if the tumor is cancerous. Methods of identifying cancerous prostate tumors have improved dramatically in recent years. Undoubtedly, when your doctor suspects cancer, he will recommend you to a cancer specialist.

TREATING PROSTATE CANCER

Except in its very advanced stages, prostate cancer has a more favorable prognosis than many other cancers. Treatment procedures have become substantially more sophisticated over the past year or so, and in the process, have minimized some of the side effects of earlier treatments.

The surgical removal of the prostate—once standard procedure in prostatic cancer—is no longer advocated by most cancer specialists as primary treatment. To begin with, most prostate tumors are inoperable by the time they are diagnosed. And those tumors which *are* operable can be treated just as effectively through *radiotherapy*—the injection of radioactive gold or phosphorus into the tumor—and without the inevitable side-effect of surgery: impotence. There is, however, a lack of radiotherapy equipment in some places, as well as a lack of physicians trained in radiotherapeutic techniques. It is reasonable to assume that some prostate cancer patients are being treated surgically only because radiotherapy is not available to them. On the other hand, there are a number of highly regarded facilities in practically every region of the country that can provide the latest radiotherapeutic treatment. Seek their advice before you submit to surgery.

Once the prostatic cancer has reached an advanced stage, neither surgery nor localized radiotherapy is enough to completely halt the disease, but there are a number of techniques that have been effective in controlling the development of the disease.

Therapies designed to control symptoms without necessarily curing the disease are known as *palliation therapy*. In the case of prostate cancer, they fall into two categories: surgical and chemical. In both instances, the goal is essentially the same: to control the supply of hormones which stimulate the growth of the cancer.

The most common surgical approach to advanced prostatic cancer has been *castration*—the removal of the testes. More radical surgical treatments include *hypophysectomy*—the removal of the pituitary gland—and *adrenalectomy*—removal of the adrenal gland. Because of their frequently severe and unpredictable side-effects, neither of these techniques is used except in those advanced cases when other more conventional treatment methods have failed. Even so, a substantial percentage of advanced prostatic cancer patients who undergo either hypophysectomy or adrenalectomy stay alive longer than they would have had they not received the treatment—and with less pain. One encouraging development in this area has been the application of *cryosurgical* (freezing) techniques to the hypophysectomy procedures. This approach achieves the same end as conventional hypophysectomies but with less danger and fewer side-effects. It should be emphasized, however, that surgical approaches like hypophysectomy and adrenalectomy are not primary therapies, and, according to most cancer specialists, should not be considered unless other treatments have failed.

Nonsurgical palliative techniques have centered around drugs which suppress the secretion of male hormones. The most common drug used in this approach is stilbestrol, the synthetic equivalent of the female hormone estrogen. Stilbestrol is used routinely in women going through menopause. It has, however, certain side effects in the treatment of prostate cancer, the most common of which is the development of feminine physical characteristics, such as enlarged breasts and fat around the hips. On the other hand, these side effects appear less severe than those experienced by patients who receive injections of cortisone to suppress the action of the adrenal glands.

It is not at all unusual for a patient with advanced prostate cancer to receive a number of palliative therapies simultaneously. It is too early to say at present which therapy is the most effective and to what degree these therapies can prolong life. What is known, however, is that younger patients tend to do better than older patients—presumably because they can deal with the side effects more effectively. In any event, in most cases, the techniques generally serve to substantially reduce pain.

THE CURRENT OUTLOOK

Although the age-adjusted death rates for prostatic cancer have changed very little over the past forty years, the prospects of prostate cancer patients have improved substantially over the past two or three years. Improved diagnostic techniques have made it easier for specialists to detect the disease at a relatively early stage. Radiotherapy has given physicians a strategy for localized cancers that does not produce impotence. And new chemotherapy research holds the promise for palliative techniques that go far beyond what is being achieved today. For example, the steroid estradiol mustard would appear to control hormone secretion more effectively than the drugs in conventional use today, and promising new findings are likely to emerge from a new chemotherapy program currently under proposal at the National Prostate Project.

At present, the crucial survival factor in prostate cancer remains early detection. For this reason, men over forty are strongly urged to have a rectal prostate examination at least once a year.

10

What You Should Know About Leukemia

Leukemia—or, as it is commonly known, cancer of the blood—is generally thought of as a children's disease. Actually, however, the disease is far more common among adults. The reason we tend to associate leukemia with children is that among children, it's the most common form of cancer. Of the nonaccidental causes of death of children between the ages of one and fifteen, cancers of all types are responsible for 20 percent. Leukemia accounts for approximately one-third of this figure.

Overall, the current outlook for leukemia is probably the brightest of all types of cancers—particularly in the specific type of leukemia that strikes children. As recently as five years ago, the condition known as acute leukemia was regarded as incurable. A recent American Cancer Society report shows that 175 persons who have had acute leukemia are alive five years later, and 100 of these have been alive for more than ten years. Leukemia researchers in general tend to be much more optimistic about the results and promise in their field than investigators in other areas of cancer. Some predict that the disease may well be under control before 1980.

THE NATURE OF LEUKEMIA

There are a number of different types of leukemia, but each type is characterized in basically the same way: the production of abnormal *leukocytes*—white blood cells. White cells are formed in the marrow—the spongy tissue that fills the center core of our bones, and in the so-called lymphoid organs: the spleen, the lymph nodes, and the thymus. Their primary function is fighting off infection and producing the antibodies that work to repel foreign substances. You might think of them as the body's prime defense system.

Leukocytes fall into various categories, the most common of which are *granulocytes*—white cells that fight infection by engulfing bacteria—and *lymphocites*—white cells that produce antibodies. Crucial as these cells are to our health, if they develop in abnormal fashion, they drastically disrupt the production of normal blood and leave the body highly susceptible to infection and hemorrhage—the two leading causes of death in leukemic patients. Particularly affected by leukemic cells are the *platelets*—the blood components that are necessary for clotting.

The two most common forms of leukemia, by far, are lymphocytic leukemia and granulocytic leukemia. Each of these diseases takes one of two forms: acute or chronic. Acute lymphocytic leukemia (ALL) is characterized by a short and severe progression of the disease. It is the most common form of leukemia in children. Acute myelogenous leukemia (AML) is similar in many ways to ALL and normally more difficult to treat. AML usually afflicts adults over twenty-five but can also affect teen-agers and younger children. Chronic leukemia, rare in children but common in adults, has a much slower progression and often takes years before its effects begin to show.

CAUSES OF LEUKEMIA

As with most cancers, the exact causes of leukemia are not known at this time, but there are a number of interesting theories. Studies involving survivors of the Hiroshima and Nagasaki atomic attacks of World War II have led some researchers to link radiation with leukemia (particularly Chronic Myelogenous Leukemia—CML) based on the fact that the incidence of leukemia among Hiroshima and Nagasaki survivors is much higher than might be expected statistically. Further studies conducted at Roswell Park Memorial Institute covering patients treated for CML between 1914 and 1975 showed that many of them had a history of radiation exposure. It's also been found that radiologists—people who work with X-ray equipment—develop leukemia at a rate that is eight times higher than doctors in other specialties. Given these statistics, many pediatricians have eliminated, as much as possible, the number of X rays given to children. However, anything that damages bone marrow, including X rays and certain toxic chemicals, can eventually lead to leukemia.

It has also been theorized that leukemia—or at least certain types of leukemia—are caused by viruses, but the results of most of the studies done in this area of research have so far been inconclusive. Certain chemicals—benzine in particular—have been mentioned as possible causative agents. Hereditary factors are also suspected of playing a role, although as yet, no one knows the precise influence.

The early symptoms of leukemia appear so gradually and are so similar to the symptoms of many common, harmless ailments, that early diagnosis of the disease is all but impossible. Fatigue, weakness, and a low-grade fever are the most common early symptoms of the disease. But even if these symptoms are linked to leukemia, there is presently no practical way to differentiate leukemia in its early stages from a typical virus or slight cold. Blood tests alone will not do the job. The most reliable way to diagnose leukemia is through an analysis of the bone marrow; however, as one cancer specialist puts it, "If we took bone marrow analysis of everyone who had early leukemia symptoms, we'd be performing ten million bone marrow operations a month."

Most leukemias are discovered after treatment for other suspected conditions fails to achieve an effect, or when the symptoms become particularly severe. Among the most common symptoms of leukemia—beyond the early stages—are severe weakness, bone or joint pain, the enlargement of the lymph nodes, liver, or spleen, and bleeding disturbances. This bleeding usually occurs in the nose and gums but can also take place internally.

DIAGNOSIS

Two diagnostic tests are used to determine the presence of leukemia. One is an analysis of the blood to determine the relative number of white cells; but a blood test alone is not enough. Along with the blood analysis, a bone marrow examination must be undertaken. Generally, tissue is removed from the marrow in the hip of a young child. It is on the basis of the white cell count in this tissue that diagnosis is made. Signs of leukemia may be evident in the gingival tissues of the mouth prior to recognition of any overt signs elsewhere in the body, according to Dr. George W. Green at the School of Dentistry of the State University of New York in Buffalo, New York.

TREATMENT

The chief weapons against leukemia at the present time are a number of anticancer drugs that interfere with the reproductive processes of leukemic cells. The drugs are effective up to a point. In more than 90 percent of the leukemia cases now being treated with chemotherapy, drugs are able to produce a very noticeable—and, in some cases, complete—reduction of symptoms. This reduction is known as *remis-*

NORMA WOLLNER, M.D. (SECOND FROM LEFT) EXAMINES PATIENT WITH
PEDIATRIC RESIDENT (FAR RIGHT), WHILE MOTHER AND PEDIATRIC
NURSE OBSERVE. (Courtesy Memorial Sloan-Kettering Cancer Center; reprinted
with permission)

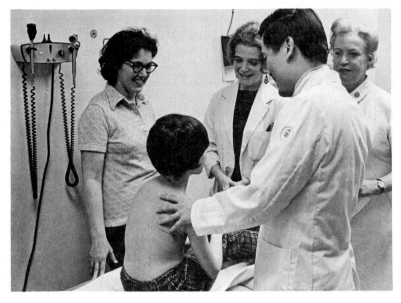

NORMA WOLLNER, M.D. (SECOND FROM LEFT) EXAMINES PATIENT WITH
PEDIATRIC RESIDENT (FAR RIGHT), WHILE MOTHER AND PEDIATRIC
NURSE OBSERVE. (Courtesy Memorial Sloan-Kettering Cancer Center; reprinted
with permission)

sion, but it is only part of the leukemic treatment strategy. The other—and more
telling—part is maintenance: keeping the patient free of leukemic cells

It is virtually impossible to predict how long remission will last. In some children, the remission lasts for months. In others, it lasts for years. And even when
relapses occur, successive remissions are most often obtained, although they are
more difficult to achieve and maintain than the initial remission. One of the reasons
the relapses occur is that some leukemic cells are able to avoid the effects of the
chemotherapeutic drugs by, in effect, "hiding out" in the central nervous system.
Recognizing this, leukemia patients are now being given a special type of chemotherapy designed to prevent these cells from spreading into the central nervous
system.

The chemotherapy used on leukemic patients does have side-effects. Some of
the drugs produce weight gain. Other drugs have a profound effect on the patient's
mood. Temporary loss of hair is another common side-effect. The side-effects of
individual drugs tend to vary from patient to patient, and a key phase of leukemia
treatment is the periodic changing of medication to limit the severity of the
side-effects.

More serious than these side-effects are the physical complications that frequently arise—chiefly infection and hemorrhage. The susceptibility to infection
arises because of the depletion in the normal white cells. Hemorrhage arises because of the reduction in the number of platelets. Here too, however, modern
treatment approaches are reducing these complications.

All in all, the prospect for leukemia patients today is far more favorable than it has ever been before. In 1960 the life expectancy of the typical leukemic child was only one year. Today, approximately 25 percent of all children with acute lymphocytic leukemia are given a life expectancy of ten years or more, and close to 50 percent of children with this disease have a life expectancy of five years. A new drug treatment program for children afflicted with acute lymphocytic leukemia, developed by Dr. Arnold J. Freeman, Chief of Roswell Park Memorial Institute's Pediatrics Department in Buffalo, New York, and currently being tested at 100 international hospitals and cancer institutions has increased the survival rate from 50 to 75 percent in clinical testing. They have achieved these results by administering high doses of *methotrexate,* thereby eliminating radiation therapy, and reducing the side effects by using an antidote called *citrovorum.*

Among adults however, the statistics are not as favorable. Chronic leukemia—the most common form of leukemia among adults—does not respond to drug treatment in a manner comparable to acute leukemia, and the life expectancy of most chronic leukemic patients is now said to be about three to four years following diagnosis.

The good news, however, is that the progress in the fight against leukemia over the past ten years has been dramatic, with institutions such as Roswell Park Memorial Institute and others achieving a "cure rate" of 70 to 85 percent on many types of leukemia. There is real hope that we are on our way to controlling leukemia in most of its forms within the next decade.

11

What You Should Know About Oral Cancer

Oral cancer is not as widespread as many other forms of the disease, but the number of oral cancer patients throughout the world is gradually on the rise. Most researchers agree that the cause is the increased rate of smoking coupled, in many instances, with alcohol consumption. Smoking itself is believed to be the singularly most important environmental cause of oral cancer. However, when combined with alcohol, the statistics of cancer seem to increase substantially. The conclusions of a ten-year study at Roswell Park Memorial Institute in Buffalo, New York, showed that women who use tobacco and alcohol may develop oral cancer as much as fifteen years earlier than their abstaining counterparts.

The overall cure rate of oral cancer is presently around 35 percent. This figure would unquestionably be higher if more dentists were alert to its early symptoms, if more people practiced self-examination, and if more patients themselves sought treatment before the cancer had spread. With the possible exception of skin cancer, no form of cancer is more visible in its early stages and more accessible to treatment than oral cancer.

One of the most encouraging aspects of the oral cancer picture is the current emphasis on and development of posttreatment reconstruction and rehabilitation techniques. "Up until a few years ago," says Dr. Norman G. Schaaf, an oral cancer specialist from Roswell Park Memorial Institute, "even patients who were cured often had such severe handicaps—an inability to speak or problems with swallowing—that a normal life was all but impossible. We've reached the stage now where our goals in this disease are not only to cure the patient of the cancer, but to do whatever is necessary to help the patient live as close to a normal existence as possible."

SYMPTOMS OF ORAL CANCER

Up until a few years ago, the chief symptom for oral cancer was thought to be mouth sores or ulcers, but oral cancer specialists today are trained to look for many different types of symptoms. Chief among these are:

- ⊕ sores that do not heal within two weeks
- ⊕ white, red, or dark patches in the mouth
- ⊕ any swelling or growths
- ⊕ pain or loss of feeling in any area of the mouth
- ⊕ repeated bleeding for no apparent cause.

Some of these symptoms are not necessarily accompanied by pain. Generally dentists are better able to discover oral cancer symptoms than general physicians, who do not normally give oral examinations. See the following photographic spread on self-examination procedures.

DIAGNOSTIC PROCEDURES

The standard procedure in situations where oral cancer is suspected is a biopsy—a removal of a portion of the tissue under suspicion and laboratory diagnosis of it. Other procedures—radiograms, for instance—are being utilized more often in diagnostic procedures, but only as an adjunct to the biopsy.

In most instances, if your dentist discovers what he considers to be a suspicious lesion in your mouth, he will refer you to a specialist who will perform the biopsy. Occasionally a dentist will conduct the biopsy himself and *then* refer you to an oral cancer specialist. Normally, it takes around five days for the final biopsy. Prompt attention to suspicious tumors is crucial because oral cancers have a tendency to mestastasize rapidly to the glands in the neck. Once this happens, the prognosis dims considerably.

TREATMENT

The standard treatment for oral cancer is surgery or radiation therapy, or a combination of both. New treatment strategies are presently in the developmental stage; among them cryosurgery, chemosurgery, and chemotherapy. If the tumor is small enough, a dental surgeon may administer treatment. Usually, though, oral cancer surgery is performed by a head and neck surgeon. Ideally, all cancerous conditions in the oral cavity should be treated by a head and neck surgeon *with specific training in cancer.*

The factor that will most determine the type of treatment in a typical oral cancer case is the type and size of the lesion. If the oral tumor is benign, its simple removal is all that is required. Very small malignant tumors can also be dealt with by means of relatively minor mouth surgery, although localized radiotherapy may also be used as well.

Large tumors that have not yet spread to the neck are generally treated with a combination of surgery and radiotherapy, with more and more cancer specialists advocating radiotherapy whenever possible, except in cases where the patient is a heavy smoker or heavy drinker, has poor dental hygiene, or suffers from poor nutrition. Tumors of the neck generally require radical surgery, with large doses of radiotherapy shortly after the operation.

The extent of the surgery will depend on the nature and extent of the cancer. If the cancer has been diagnosed early enough, the amount of tissue removed during treatment will be minimal, and the aftereffects relatively mild. In more serious cases, however, surgery may involve the removal of large portions of the mouth and perhaps the inner tongue. It was not very long ago that patients who underwent these radical treatments had little hope of reestablishing any degree of normalcy to their lives; but of late a "team" approach has been instituted in the rehabilitation of oral cancer patients. The work of specialists in speech therapy, physical therapy, occupational therapy, and reconstructive surgery, coupled with the continuing development of prosthetic devices, have made a profound positive impact on the outlook for oral cancer patients who have undergone radical treatment. Patients who have had their tongues removed have learned how to speak without them. Even though the removal of the tongue makes chewing impossible, new liquid diets have given patients a chance at life that was previously denied them. These and many other rehabilitation procedures are getting more and more handicapped oral cancer patients out of the nursing homes and hospitals and back into a meaningful existence.

POSTTREATMENT EFFECTS

Even when the treatment of an oral cancer patient is successful, the physical and psychological aftereffects can present enormous problems, although their ramifica-

SELF-EXAMINATION PROCEDURES

The following are seven basic self-examination procedures* for early detection of oral cancer. A mirror and adequate lighting are necessary for the self-exam.

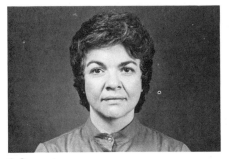

1. Symmetry
Look at your face and neck. The right and left sides are normally symmetrical; this means they have the same shape. Any differences in shape, such as a lump or swelling on one side, should be noted.

If similar lumps, bumps, or other features are found at the same place on both sides of the face, neck or inside the mouth, they are probably normal.

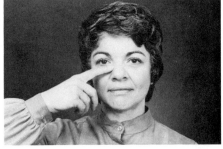

2. Face
Inspect the skin of the face, neck and lips. Look for changes in skin color, lumps, or sores. If glasses are worn, remove them and look closely at the area around the eyes and the bridge of the nose. Replace glasses.

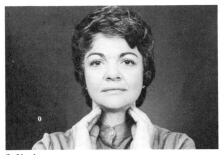

3. Neck
With your fingers press along the sides and front of the neck to detect any lumps or tenderness. (As in Step 1, use symmetry to help identify normal features.)

4. Lips
Any dentures or partials should be removed at this point. Pull the lower lip down to view any possible sores or color changes. With your fingers feel for any lump which may not be seen. Repeat procedure for upper lip.

5. Cheek
Use your fingers to expose the left inner cheek surface to observe any white, red or dark patches. Place your thumb on the inside of your cheek and your index finger on the outside. Gently squeeze your cheek between your fingers; check for any lumps or areas of tenderness. Repeat procedure for right cheek.

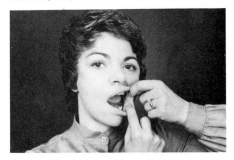

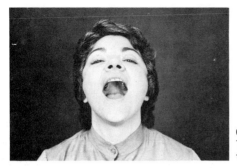

6. Roof of the Mouth
Tilt the head back and open the mouth wide to observe any color differences or lumps.

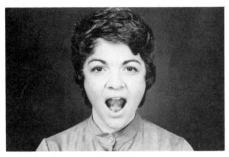

7. Floor of the Mouth and Tongue
Place the tip of the tongue to the roof of the mouth. Inspect the floor of the mouth and under-surface of the tongue for any color changes or sores. Examine the floor of the mouth by gently pressing with your finger to detect any abnormal lump or swelling.

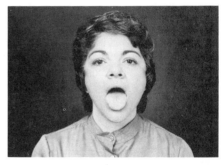

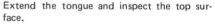

Extend the tongue and inspect the top surface.

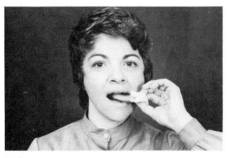

Using a gauze compress or a tissue, gently but firmly grasp the tongue and pull it forward to view the sides. Any swelling or color changes should be noted.

*Funded by the National Cancer Institute, U.S. Department of Health, Education, and Welfare, and prepared by Eastern Great Lakes Head and Neck Cancer Control Network and the Department of Oral Medicine of the State University of New York at Buffalo.

tions are easing every year. In patients with very serious oral cancer, treatment may leave a very obvious facial deformity, a speech impediment, an inability to swallow, or perhaps a breathing problem. Until the early 1960s little thought was given to these postoperative problems, and as a result, many "cured" oral patients chose to isolate themselves from the rest of the world.

The picture today has changed demonstrably. Nowadays, when oral cancer specialists talk of treatment and cure, rehabilitation is assumed to be a necessary element in the process. Many things have happened over the past fifteen years to brighten the outlook for the oral cancer patient whose treatment has left a major disability. Today more surgeons have appreciably more skill in reconstructive techniques following surgery. Dramatic advances have taken place in the field of prosthetic technology as well, for instance, the development of artificial tongues.

It should be emphasized, however, that the reconstruction process can only take place when the patient receives the services of a *team* of specialists. This team approach generally involves not only the surgeon who performs the initial operation but also a plastic surgeon, a prosthodontist, an oral surgeon, and other oral specialists whose involvement will minimize the aftereffects. Ideally, these reconstructive specialists should become involved with the case at an early stage in the treatment so that their contributions can be coordinated with the work of the surgeon whose primary concern is the removal of the cancer.

The degree to which these specialists can minimize the aftereffects of oral cancer treatment will depend, of course, on the nature of the cancer and the extent of the surgery and/or radiotherapy. "We have to think in relative terms," Dr. Schaaf says. "In very serious cases, a patient is never going to be one hundred percent of what he was before; but in most instances, we can help the patient enough so that he *can* function in society. The days of assuming that a 'cured' oral patient might have to spend the rest of his life in a nursing home is over."

WHO IS FIGHTING CANCER?

12

The National
Cancer Institute:
Its Programs,
Centers,
and Accomplishments

This chapter describes the National Cancer Institute and the nineteen hospitals or cancer care institutions that have been designated as Comprehensive Cancer Centers by the National Cancer Institute. These centers have met the highest criteria of excellence set forth by an outstanding panel of cancer specialists and are, in the opinion of many experts, the finest research, cancer care, and patient management institutions to be found in the world. In the execution of their role as Comprehensive Cancer Centers, they have also been responsible for a large percentage of the new therapy regimens which are slowly but surely bringing us closer to the eventual cure for cancer. If you, as a cancer patient, are able to apply, through your physician, to any of these institutions for in- or outpatient care, you can feel confident that you are in the best professional hands and will be afforded the maximum opportunity for proper treatment.

A complete listing of the National Cancer Institute's centers can be found in the first part of Appendix A.

There is very little doubt that cancer, in all its forms, can and will be conquered in the foreseeable future. With billions of dollars in government and private funding being distributed to hundreds of research centers and hospitals and supporting the work of tens of thousands of dedicated cancer clinicians, doctors, and researchers throughout the world, the "cancer vaccine" or "miracle drug" may be just around the corner. However, tomorrow's cure is just today's dream. For the cancer patient, the reality of today is simply to stay alive.

Because of the multiplicity of cancer and the treatment unique to each body site, obtaining the proper medical care at the right institution is of primary importance. New discoveries in cancer treatment and cure are occurring almost daily in hospitals and laboratories around the world; but unfortunately, the knowledge of these successes and the techniques utilized in performing these new methods of treatment are often disseminated only at the annual meetings of particular medical societies or in articles written for scientific journals. In some instances, this valuable, potentially lifesaving data is interchanged; but usually this interchange takes place only between the largest and most highly recognized research, diagnostic, and cancer control hospitals and universities, where, because of the availability of equipment and personnel, parallel testing and corroborating treatment can be carried out. It may be months or even years before the technology related to these new and revolutionary cancer treatments and cures is made available to secondary institutions or the medical community at large; and even then, they are often unable to implement the use of this invaluable information, owing to their lack of adequate funding, unavailability of proper equipment, and insufficiently trained personnel.

In the United States alone, where perhaps the greatest amount of cancer research is taking place, of over 7,000 hospitals, only about 10 percent are adequately equipped and staffed to treat the many different forms of cancer, and an even smaller number are considered by the American College of Surgeons as being first-rate in available equipment, trained staff, and diagnostic, treatment, and postoperative cancer care programs. It has been ascertained in recent studies that some hospitals achieve up to a 25 percent higher rate of cure for certain diseases* than do others. This makes the selection of a hospital or specialized cancer care center by a cancer patient or his doctor even more acute. The level of treatment may determine the length of his life.

CANCER CLINICAL RESEARCH CENTERS PROGRAM

In 1962 the National Cancer Institute in Bethesda, Maryland, which is a branch of the Health, Education, and Welfare Department of the United States Government, realized that because of the relative scarcity of specialized cancer treatment centers, a great many cancer patients were receiving their initial care through their private physicians or through general treatment clinics. These clinics and doctors were often immersed in the busy day-to-day activities of their extensive medical practices and seldom had the opportunity to become familiar with modern cancer diagnostic

*Not necessarily limited to cancer.

and treatment procedures. As it became evident that continued research was making long-term remissions possible and extending the lives of many cancer patients, it became essential that rapid steps be taken to apply these techniques to as many cancer sufferers as possible.

The National Cancer Institute implemented this need by establishing the Cancer Clinical Research Centers Program in 1962. During the next eight years, this program was expanded to include medical schools, specialized cancer facilities, practicing physicians, and community medical services—all participating in an integrated program of cancer research and training.

COMPREHENSIVE CANCER CENTERS

The results of this program were so dramatic that in 1971 Congress authorized the establishment of the National Cancer Program, allotting funds to the National Cancer Institute necessary to launch the most effective attack on cancer ever undertaken. Its main thrust was to create a network of Comprehensive Cancer Centers that would link together cancer screening, detection, diagnosis, treatment, rehabilitation, and continuing care in conjunction with community-oriented organizations, local hospitals, and physicians. Through this network, a nationally compatible data gathering and exchange system is being set up to disseminate to qualified doctors and institutions everywhere the most recent techniques of diagnosis and therapy necessary for the proper treatment of their cancer patients. By merging this leadership in cancer control and the diagnostic and treatment resources ordinarily available only in major medical centers and universities with community-based hospitals, professional and lay groups, and local and state health organizations, and locating the central facilities within the geographic availability of the majority of the nation's population, it is hoped that the suffering and mortality rate of those afflicted with cancer will be radically reduced and eventually eliminated.

As this program expands over the next few years and more centers are established throughout the country, there should be no reason why any American who develops cancer cannot receive the finest care available at the nearest Comprehensive or Specialized Cancer Center or from one of the cooperative member hospitals or cancer specialists linked to the national cancer information network.

In addition to the National Cancer Institute, each year The American Cancer Society and other charitable institutions and foundations provide considerable financial support through grants, to many individuals, experimental groups, schools, and hospitals involved in all facets of cancer detection, research, treatment, and rehabilitation; however, in the author's opinion, nowhere is this money being more wisely spent than in the creation and support of the aforementioned Comprehensive Cancer Centers and their network of cooperative hospitals and universities. It is to these large, extensively equipped, professionally staffed, and interconnected institutions, which have met the highest possible criteria in every area of cancer research and control, that a patient can be referred by his personal physician or medical group for the absolute finest in cancer care. There, as an inpatient or outpatient, he has the greatest possible opportunity for remission, cure, and long life. No longer need a cancer patient ask the question: "Where can I go for treatment?"

In order to qualify as a Comprehensive National Cancer and Demonstration Center, the National Cancer Advisory Board has determined that each applicant institution must have the following characteristics:

⊕ The center must have a stated purpose that includes carrying out of basic and clinical research, training, and demonstration of advanced diagnostic and treatment methods relating to cancer.

⊕ The center must have an environment of excellence in basic science which will assure the highest quality in basic research.

⊕ The center must have high-quality interdisciplinary capability in the performance of diagnosis and treatment of malignant diseases.

⊕ The center should have or should develop an organized cancer detection program.

⊕ The center must maintain a statistical base for evaluation of the results of its program activities. For this purpose, records should be developed which will standardize disease classification to enable exchange of information between institutions.

⊕ The center should provide leadership in developing community programs involving active participation by members of the medical profession practicing within the area served by the center.

⊕ The center must have a strong research base (fundamental and applied) and related training programs, with an organizational structure which will provide for the coordination of these activities with other facets of the center's program.

⊕ The center must have an administrative structure that will assure maximum efficiency of operation and sound financial practices. The administration should include responsibility for program planning, monitoring, and execution as well as preparation of the budget and control of expenditures. Administration and management would include staff appointment and space allocation, the intent being that such a center will have the authority to establish the necessary administrative and management procedures for carrying out its total responsibility as defined in the criteria.

⊕ It is a requirement that each center group have sufficient beds for cancer patients to give the program cohesion, identification, and favorable facilities for the clinical research program to be carried out. In general it is expected that existing inpatient facilities will be committed for this purpose.

Since the institution of this program, a total of 19 Comprehensive Cancer Centers have been established and are in operation. They are listed in Appendix A.

SPECIALIZED CLINICAL
CANCER CENTERS

A second and most important activity of the National Cancer Institute is the establishment of Specialized Clinical Cancer Centers. These centers usually involve clinical investigation and radiation programs (i.e., therapy, biology, and physics) or programs in cancer biology. These centers should have the following characteristics:

⊕ A defined organization plan to coordinate cancer-related activities.
⊕ A qualified Director of the Cancer Program serving on a full- or part-time basis.
⊕ Sufficient autonomy to fulfill its program responsibilities: the center should be recognized as a major function within the organizational structure of the parent institution.
⊕ Physical facilities which, so far as possible, promote collaboration among the constituent programs.
⊕ Sufficient staff (full-time as well as part-time), space, and facilities to ensure successful scientific and administrative operation of the center.
⊕ A Scientific Advisory Committee to ensure adequate review of the programs. This committee may include both internal and external members.

Many of these centers have inpatient and outpatient capabilities and are available for consultation, training, and demonstration. Those that are affiliated with the established Comprehensive Cancer Centers or are listed as one of the "Leading Cancer Treatment Centers" are listed in Appendix A.

CANCER CLINICAL COOPERATIVE
GROUPS PROGRAM

In addition to establishing and coordinating the activities of the Comprehensive Cancer Centers and the Specialized Cancer Centers, the National Cancer Institute funds and supervises an almost unbelievable variety of projects concerned with the conquest of cancer. One of the most important applications of this funding takes place under the auspices of NCI's Clinical Investigations Branch of the Division of Cancer Treatment, under the directorship of Dr. Vincent J. Devita. It is called the Cancer Clinical Cooperative Groups Program.

Through the CCCG Program, NCI provides tens of millions of dollars in grants to carefully selected universities, hospitals, cancer clinics, cancer research centers and foundations, and individual investigators for continuing therapy research and treatment of specific types of cancer. There are presently 436 such institutions with over 2,450 investigators located throughout the United States, Canada, Denmark, France, Israel, Mexico, Peru, Puerto Rico, South Africa, Sweden, and Switzerland.

Each of these institutions is funded for research studies into a particular category of cancer disease or tumor type, and are assigned to their own Clinical Cooperative Group. A distinguished cancer expert is the chairman of each group. He or she coordinates their studies, receives their findings, and prepares a periodic report on their progress for the National Cancer Institute. In many instances, a large or particularly qualified institution may be a member of more than one study group and may consequently be reporting to more than one group chairman. Some of these centers are presently providing their cancer patients with outstanding, innovative cancer management developed in their own facilities. These Cooperative Groups and their chairmen are listed in Appendix A.

ACCOMPLISHMENTS OF DIRECT BENEFIT TO PEOPLE SINCE 1971*

Since the enactment of the first National Cancer Act in 1937, tremendous strides have been made in the battle against cancer under the sponsorship of the National Cancer Program. Below are enumerated those accomplishments, reported by HEW in June 1977 that were achieved from projects, both national and international, that have come to fruition since 1971.

⊕ A new treatment strategy of giving anticancer drugs postoperatively to women with breast cancer and a high risk of recurrence has significantly lowered the recurrence rate among such patients. One breast cancer study used the drug, L-PAM, as a post-operative treatment; another used a three-drug combination called CMF. There is great and justifiable cause for optimism in these results, because experience has shown that prolonged tumor-free survival leads to increased survival rates. About 90,000 women develop breast cancer each year in this country alone. And about 33,000 will die with this disease this year. Breast cancer kills more American women than does any other disease, often at prime ages of their lives. These dramatic results can only mean that many American women, who would have died, may live virtually normal lives and have normal life expectancies.

⊕ A study of the treatment of breast cancer with less radical surgery has shown to date that it may be as effective as radical surgery. If the trend continues, the results will lead to treatment tailored to the individual patient and in many cases significantly different from the traditional radical surgery.

⊕ With the use of postoperative drug treatment with either high doses of methotrexate followed by an antidote (citrovorum factor) of Adriamycin, a new drug, the two-year survival rate for osteogenic sarcoma has been increased

*As reported by the U.S. Department of Health, Education, and Welfare.

significantly. Osteogenic sarcoma, a tumor of the bone, occurs most often in young people.

⊕ More than 50 percent of children with acute childhood leukemia treated at various centers in the nation now survive more than five years without disease. In 1972, I reported that in the best of institutions and under the best of circumstances more than 90 percent of children with this disease could be alive 5 years after diagnosis. At that time, only about 25 percent of American children had access to this kind of treatment. From a recent study of the availability of the modern treatment strategies, I am pleased to report that the majority of patients are receiving the currently accepted treatment regimens. Even this accessibility will be improved, not only for acute lymphocytic leukemia, but for other childhood cancers as well.

⊕ The addition of immunotherapy to chemotherapy (drug treatment) in patients with acute myelogenous leukemia has led to a temporary prolongation of remission duration over that observed in patients treated with drugs alone. In immunotherapy, agents are used to stimulate the immune defense system of the patient.

⊕ Preliminary observations indicate that immunotherapy combined with surgery may improve survival. If living BCG organisms (bacillus Calmette-Guerin) are put into the chest cavity of patients following surgery to remove early lung cancers, there may be a decrease in the rate of tumor recurrence and a prolongation in survival, compared with patients being treated with surgery alone. A large-scale study of the usefulness of this form of immunotherapy in lung cancer is being initiated.

⊕ With the treatments now available at certain centers, more than 90 percent of patients with early Hodgkin's disease, and about 70 percent with advanced disease, are surviving five years. Many of these are free of disease and are expected to live normal lifetimes. Recent update of these data shows that those achieving a complete remission with anticancer drugs have a 66 percent chance of remaining free of disease up to 10 years. This success is reflected in a decrease of cancer deaths in national mortality data among young adults.

⊕ Some patients with various types of advanced non-Hodgkin's lymphomas (diffuse histiocytic and nodular mixed lymphomas) can be cured (have survived up to nine years without evidence of disease) by use of drug combinations. The application of these combinations to patients with early disease in conjunction with radiotherapy is being studied.

⊕ It is firmly established that chemotherapy combined with surgery and radiotherapy is curative in 80 to 90 percent of patients with Wilms's tumor, a previously fatal childhood cancer of the kidney.

⊕ The use of drugs and X-ray therapy in treatment of Ewing's sarcoma, another type of cancer that afflicts children, has led to markedly improved survival of patients with this disease.

⊕ Progress has been reported in the treatment of some types of advanced malignant melanoma, a relatively rare form of skin cancer, by chemoimmunotherapy, a combination of an anticancer drug (DTIC) and a killed bacterial vaccine (BCG), which stimulates the immune defense system of the patient. Immunotherapy with BCG alone appears useful in preventing recurrences in patients with operable melanoma who ordinarily would have a high risk of recurrence.

⊕ The first successful combination drug treatments (i.e. ability to induce remissions) of advanced cancers of the colon-rectum and stomach have been reported. A drug combination found effective for advanced cancer of the colon-rectum was 5-FU, vincristine (a plant alkaloid), and a derivative of a class of compounds called nitrosoureas. The new drug is methyl-CCNU. Improved responses have also been obtained with 5-FU and methyl-CCNU on patients with advanced stomach cancer.

⊕ Important developments in the supportive care of cancer patients include transfusions of blood components, such as platelets to prevent hemorrhage and white blood cells to treat infections; and laminar flow rooms to provide an environment that protects patients against infections.

⊕ A test that predicts the response of patients with recurrent breast cancer to treatment with hormones has been developed and is in clinical trial. Presence of a protein (estrogen receptor protein) in the tumor predicts a positive response to removal of hormone sources (ovaries, adrenals, or pituitary gland). Between 40 and 50 percent of breast cancers have cells containing the receptors. Absence of the protein, indicating that there would be no response to hormone treatment, will spare a patient a useless operation. Such patients can instead be given therapy with anticancer drugs.

⊕ CCNU and BCNU are members of a new chemical class of anticancer drugs now being developed. CCNU has been approved as a prescription drug and is available for general medical practice. These drugs can penetrate the so-called "blood-brain barrier," and are therefore very important in the treatment of primary and metastatic brain tumors.

⊕ Adriamycin, a new anticancer drug, was approved as a prescription drug by the Food and Drug Administration in 1974 for use in cancer patients. Adriamycin has the widest spectrum of activity of any anticancer drug against human solid tumors, and is the most active single agent against advanced breast cancer. It has been incorporated into the treatment plans for breast cancer, bone cancer, other sarcomas and lymphomas. Adriamycin has also been shown to be effective against a heretofore drug-resistant tumor, bladder cancer.

⊕ DTIC, a new anticancer drug discovered and developed by the National Cancer Institute, became available as a prescription drug in 1975. It has activity against malignant melanoma.

⊕ Maytansine, a plant recently discovered by scientists in the National Cancer Institute drug development program, has high activity against leukemia in laboratory animals. Preliminary clinical trials have been started against this and other cancers.

⊕ Chlorozotocin, a new agent identified within the past two years, is a nitrosourea derivative with considerably less bone marrow toxicity than the other nitrosourea anticancer agents. It is being tested in preliminary clinical trials.

⊕ There have been clinical reports of tumor regression with the use of heat, and these have been supported by experimental data demonstrating that hyperthermia kills tumor cells in laboratory animals and cell cultures. The mechanism of this phenomenon is not well understood. But it appears that heat may induce selective lethal injury to cancer cells; and that this effect is dependent on the temperature and time of heat exposure. Clinical trials with whole body hyperthermia are in progress.

⊕ The addition of a new drug, cis-platinum (II) diamminedichloride to a drug combination already in use has improved still further the significant response rate of a very malignant tumor of young adults, testicular cancer. Last year it was reported that a high rate of response by testicular cancer patients was produced by a combination of vinblastine, an alkaloid isolated from the periwinkle plant, and bleomycin, an antibiotic first used in Japan and commercially available as an anticancer drug in the United States since 1973. When the new drug was given in addition to bleomycin, vinblastine, dactinomycin, and cyclophosphamide, responses were observed in 90 percent of the patients. It is likely that at least 50 percent of the patients with advanced testicular cancer will survive longer than two years, and that some will be cured.

⊕ Progress has been observed in early results from combined chemotherapy and radiotherapy of small cell carcinoma of the lung, which accounts for about 20 percent of lung cancer cases.

⊕ In radiation therapy, a 10-year study was reported in which total body irradiation of a small group of patients with chronic lymphocytic leukemia resulted in complete disappearance of clinical symptoms of the disease and increased survival time in some patients. This is the first time remissions have been reported of sufficient degree to alter the course of the disease in a significant number of patients.

⊕ Nineteen Comprehensive Cancer and 64 Specialized Centers located around the country are a national resource for interdisciplinary basic research, clinical research, training, demonstration, continuing education of health professionals, and cancer information. Many of these Centers carry out a broad spectrum of cancer research and treatment. Others emphasize special fields, such as pediatric cancer or interdepartmental studies in immunology and immunotherapy. The Centers also focus the nationwide effort to pass on quickly the best in modern knowledge about cancer treatment to trainees in health professions and to the practicing physicians who frequently are the first to care for the great majority of cancer patients.

⊕ Cancer Information Services have been developed through the 15 Comprehensive Cancer Centers to provide cancer information to health professionals, cancer patients, and those at risk to cancer. Toll-free telephone service and resources for cancer information are being established at the Centers.

⊕ The Clinical Cooperative Group program, which has been in existence for some years to conduct clinical trials primarily of drugs, has been expanded to emphasize combined treatment research including surgical oncology, radiation oncology, chemotherapy, and immunotherapy. Much effort has been expended to integrate the activities of the Clinical Cooperative Groups into the total clinical treatment program of the National Cancer Institute. In various clinical trials, we have influenced the treatment of 280,000 cancer patients, and about 28,000 of these were entered in clinical trial protocols. This is important because these 280,000 patients were seen and evaluated by expert oncologists and were provided the best medical advice available, even though only 1 out of 10 actually entered a clinical trial.

⊕ The cancer control program is supporting demonstration projects involving networks of cooperating community physicians and hospitals linked to major hospitals to disseminate the latest information and techniques in the diagnosis, treatment, and rehabilitation of breast cancer (12 networks); head and neck cancer (7 networks); and childhood leukemia and lymphoma (7 networks).

⊕ The cancer control program implemented two community-based cancer control programs in urban and rural communities with populations totaling 5.6 million people. The purpose of these programs is to test whether coordinated cancer control efforts are more effective than a fragmented approach. The range of cancer control techniques, from prevention through continuing care and rehabilitation, will be demonstrated. The intent of these programs is not to provide health care but to encourage organizations that do provide it to improve cancer care. The Metropolitan Detroit Cancer Control program will integrate community efforts involving cancers of the breast, uterine cervix, colon-rectum, and head and neck. The University of New Mexico Cancer Research and Treatment Center will focus on cancers of the breast, uterus, and colon-rectum. It is hoped that a model cancer control system that could be adapted by other communities will become available from these demonstration programs.

⊕ The International Cancer Research Data Bank Program (ICRDB) is actively promoting worldwide exchange of information among cancer scientists. The ICRDB Program is operating an on-line computer information retrieval system called CANCERLINE (Cancer Information on-Line). It links the computer system at the National Library of Medicine in Bethesda with terminals in more than 500 locations in the United States and in several countries throughout the world. CANCERLINE presently contains some 65,000 abstracts of worldwide published papers dealing with cancer therapy and carcinogenesis. Information on more than 16,000 ongoing cancer research projects and clinical cancer therapy protocols are being processed and added to the data base for on-line use by research investigators and clinicians worldwide. This is in direct compliance with directives from the Congress in 1971 and 1974.

⊕ A nationwide breast cancer detection demonstration program cosponsored with the American Cancer Society, encompassing 27 projects, is under way in 25 states. Some 270,000 women have been examined and of these, about 1600 have been found to have cancer.

⊕ More than 35 States are cooperating through their Health Departments in a uterine cervical cancer screening program, giving the Pap test to women at high risk who have not previously had it. By the end of fiscal year 1977, an estimated 750,000 screenings will have been performed. [From the first] 550,000 women [who] have been screened, 780 women have been found to have cancer of the uterus. Not only early stages of cancer, but abnormal changes in the cervix may be identified five to ten years before symptoms of cancer appear.

⊕ A prototype cell-sorting machine has been able to analyze cervical cytology specimens and identify more than 90 percent of the abnormal specimens. This is a significant step toward the goal of automation of the reading of Pap test specimens. The cell-sorting machines under development are designed to scan specimens rapidly and select those with abnormal cells for subsequent analysis by trained personnel.

⊕ Use of an improved fiberoptic endoscope, a flexible instrument that permits determination of the location and extent of the tumor, is assisting the detection of cancer of the colon in earlier stages. The instrument is also proving valuable in the diagnosis of cancer of the pancreas.

⊕ Six radiological physics centers were established to assist medical physics practice in cancer detection, diagnosis and treatment, such as monitoring and standardization of quantity and extent of radiation given. This important quality control mechanism has served as a model that will benefit the millions of Americans undergoing diagnostic radiologic procedures yearly, and the more than 400,000 cancer patients receiving radiation therapy yearly.

⊕ Computer-assisted X-ray tomography is a new technique that has revolutionized the diagnosis of brain tumors and other brain diseases. It is a technique for making a series of cross-section radiographs of brain tissues. It permits location of tumors in a way not previously observable by X ray. Computerized tomography is being adapted to the diagnosis of cancer in other parts of the body.

⊕ A large study featuring cell examination of sputum and chest X rays to detect lung cancer in heavy smokers without symptoms of the disease has screened approximately 20,000 individuals and found some 150 cancers. The study has already shown that early lung cancer can be detected in this way and that the fiberoptic bronchoscope can diagnose the exact location and extent of the tumor for surgical treatment. Many of the tumors were small enough that survival is expected to be better than usual in patients with lung cancer.

⊕ A cancer control project is supporting observation of at least 4,000 young women, born between 1943 and 1963, who were exposed before birth to a drug, DES [di-ethyl stilbesterol], which their mothers received to prevent [miscarriages] during pregnancy. The young women will be followed for five years or more for cancer and other abnormalities of the genital tract. The detection and diagnostic procedures developed in this study may then be applied to the larger population at risk.

⊕ The NCI supported a workshop on the late effects of irradiation to the head and neck in infancy and childhood, in cooperation with the National Institute of Arthritis, Metabolism and Digestive Diseases at NIH and the Bureau of Radiological Health of the FDA. This workshop brought together experts in various aspects of the subject to assess the present state of knowledge. Reports have been prepared for practicing physicians and the public to provide information relating to identifying populations at risk of thyroid cancer, optimum frequency for re-examination, indications for various types of treatment, and the best procedures for followup. Only a small fraction of the at-risk individuals will develop cancer, and in adults, the tumors usually grow slowly and are easy to detect and cure.

⊕ New chemicals found to be carcinogenic include vinyl chloride, chlordane, trichloroethylene, ethylene dibromide, heptachlor, DES, Kepone, chloroform, and TRIS-BP (a flame-retardant used in fabrics).

⊕ An association was reported between the use of oral contraceptives by young women and the development of liver tumors. Most of the tumors were benign and a few were cancerous. The number of women with liver tumors is a very small percentage of the estimated 35 million American women who take or have taken the pill. The NCI is cooperating with other Federal agencies in efforts to gather more data on the association. Because of the delayed action of tumor-inducing substances, there is a possibility of a higher occurrence of liver cancers in the future, as compared with the small number reported to date. A warning statement as to the possibility of liver tumors has been added to the labeling of oral contraceptives approved by Food and Drug Administration.

⊕ Public attention has been drawn to reports that women taking female sex hormones to ease the symptoms of menopause have a five-fold greater risk of cancer of the lining of the uterus (endometrium) than women who do not take these hormones. The FDA has approved new package labeling suggesting low-dose, short-term use with appropriate monitoring for this type of cancer.

⊕ To counteract the increasing consumption of tobacco, less hazardous cigarettes have been developed and evaluated in newly developed inhalation smoking machines. These cigarettes are now in wide use. With their decreased tar and nicotine content, these cigarettes should have a beneficial impact on reducing the number of new lung and other cancers.

⊕ Progress has been made in developing relatively quick, inexpensive laboratory techniques for identifying potential cancer-causing chemicals for test in the laboratory animal test systems. We are evaluating one procedure in which test chemicals are injected into pregnant hamsters; the embryos are removed and their cells grown in the laboratory. Evidence of cancerous transformation can be detected in as little as two weeks instead of the usual three or more years and at a cost of $1,000 instead of $200,000. The cancerous transformation is confirmed by the ability of the cells to produce cancer when injected into healthy hamsters. In another test, the ability of a chemical to cause genetic mutation in bacteria in cultured cells could be a warning of its possible cancer-causing activity and the need for comprehensive long-term testing in laboratory animals. It is hoped that a battery of different kinds of short-term test systems, including the use of cultural human cells, will be developed and validated in the next few years to speed up the testing of suspected carcinogens. These studies are important to enable investigators more rapidly to obtain definitive information on which regulatory or other actions can be taken to protect people from specific carcinogens in the environment.

⊕ Tests are in progress on some 290 chemicals to determine their cancer-causing ability in laboratory animals. The compounds are selected on the basis of level of human exposure, the chemical structure, and preliminary information of their biological activity. Among the chemicals being tested are pharmaceuticals, industrial chemicals, pesticides and agricultural chemicals, and in addition, natural materials, food additives, and a variety of other environmental chemicals and intermediates.

⊕ A series of monographs, *Evaluation of Carcinogenic Risk of Chemicals to Man,* has been published by the International Agency for Research on Cancer with direct support and collaboration from the National Cancer Institute. These volumes bring together the results of testing of many chemicals for their cancer-causing ability, provide a quick reference for investigators, and prevent unnecessary duplication of testing. Ten volumes have been published covering more than 270 substances for which there is a significant human exposure and some published evidence of carcinogenicity in animals and/or man. An eleventh volume, covering epoxides and miscellaneous industrial chemicals, is being prepared.

⊕ Publication of an *Atlas of Cancer Mortality for U.S. Counties: 1950-1969* has pinpointed geographic concentrations of cancer throughout the country. High cancer death rates were found in industrial counties such as those concerned with production of chemicals and certain types of heavy machinery. These findings have led to numerous inquiries from communities throughout the country anxious to identify their cancer-causing problems, and they will continue to be analyzed by institute scientists to identify high-risk counties and groups of people. We shall identify environmental factors in the causation of cancer and important host/environment interactions.

⊕ An atlas of geographic variations in cancer mortality among nonwhites, based on county-by-county death data between 1950 and 1969, was produced as a companion volume to the atlas published on cancer mortality among whites. The major United States nonwhites are Blacks, American Indians, Chinese, and Japanese. A similarity in geographic patterns of cancer for whites and nonwhites was particularly striking for cancers of the breast, colon, rectum, and esophagus. Compared with other racial groups, Blacks experienced high rates for cancer of the mouth, throat, esophagus, stomach, pancreas, larynx, lung, bladder and cervix, and multiple myeloma. American Indians experienced high rates for cancer of the gallbladder, bile ducts, and liver; Chinese, for cancer of the nasopharynx; and Japanese for cancer of the stomach.

⊕ The high death rate for melanoma, a rare type of skin cancer, in the Southern United States supported the view that excessive exposure to sunlight is a factor in that type as well as other skin cancers. High mortality for stomach cancer found for both sexes in the North Central States corresponds closely with the geographic concentrations of people with ancestors from Austria, the Soviet Union, and Scandinavia. This pattern may be related to the dietary preferences of these population groups. Stomach cancer rates in these countries of origin are also higher than the United States.

⊕ Cancers of the colon and rectum, which may be related to diet, were found at above-average rates in the Northeast and in urban areas along the Great Lakes. Low rates were found in the southern and central parts of the United States. Breast cancer showed a similar pattern, suggesting that this disease may have an environmental factor in common with cancers of the large intestine.

⊕ A surprising finding was high mortality rates for lung cancer along the Gulf Coast from Texas to the Florida Panhandle. This finding suggested that environmental factors, in addition to cigarette smoking, may contribute to lung cancer deaths in these predominantly rural and seaport areas.

⊕ A statistical association was established between the amount of beef consumed in the diet and an increased occurrence of colon cancer. This information was obtained in a study of colon cancer among Hawaiian residents of Japanese descent. The risk of colon cancer for persons who no longer ate Japanese-style meals but had adopted Western-style meals was about twice that of persons whose diet had remained relatively unchanged. The findings in this study are not considered sufficient to label beef consumption as cancer causing, but they assist in the planning of research in different population groups on the complex sequence of events leading to colon cancer.

⊕ The SEER Program (Surveillance, Epidemiology, and End Results Reporting) is monitoring the trends in cancer incidence, changes in diagnostic and treatment priorities, and associated survival rates of cancer patients. This program provides continually updated information on cancer statistics in the United States and serves as a direct check on how well (or how badly) we are doing.

⊕ A report has been published on trends in survival rates of patients with cancer. One-year survival results for patients with diagnoses made during 1970–71 suggest that improvement in the five-year survival observed during the 1960s for many forms of cancer will be sustained. Continued reporting of survival for patients treated in the 1970s is expected to demonstrate that recently introduced therapies have been increasingly effective.

⊕ A cancer control prevention project for workers in Tyler, Texas, exposed to asbestos and another one for workers in Louisville, Kentucky, exposed to vinyl chloride, both proved carcinogenic substances, provide medical surveillance and health education to the workers and their families to assure early detection of precancerous lesions and early cancer. Through programs such as these, models will be developed for monitoring high risk workers exposed to carcinogens and for identifying procedures that will provide early warning of an impending malignancy.

⊕ An occupational cancer information and alert program was initiated through an interagency agreement with the Occupational Safety and Health Administration of the Department of Labor. This is important because it will provide a means for making available to the workers of the country information and training aimed at reducing the risk of cancer.

⊕ The cancer control program is supporting the training of health professional groups to assist in continuing care and rehabilitation of cancer patients. These groups include an estimated 3,600 physical and occupational therapists, rehabilitation teams, maxillofacial prosthodontists, enterostomal therapists, and nurse oncologists.

⊕ Scientists within and outside the National Cancer Program have found again that fluoridation of drinking water does not contribute to a cancer burden for people. This information has also been confirmed and reiterated by the Royal College of Physicians of the United Kingdom. This is also important because continued fluoridation of water will help curb what many have called the most prevalent disease of people—dental caries.

13

Other Treatment Centers, Rehabilitation Organizations, and Professional Organizations

OTHER LEADING CANCER TREATMENT CENTERS

Aside from the Comprehensive Cancer Centers and Specialized Cancer Centers covered in the previous chapter, there are dozens of other hospitals and cancer treatment institutions that have extensive research programs and that provide outstanding treatment, rehabilitation, and continuing care for the cancer patient. Many of these have world-renowned medical personnel on their staff, and many specialize in particular areas of surgery and treatment. Still others are closely affiliated with a nearby Comprehensive Cancer Center and have access through the "outreach program" to all the latest research findings and technical data to enable them to provide parallel services to the center itself. There are very few geographical areas in the United States in which a cancer sufferer cannot locate a hospital or institution of outstanding caliber in which to place his faith and future.

Naturally, we would all desire to be cared for at the leading facility for our particular cancer. In "Picking the Absolutely Top Places for Medical Care in the

United States," an article which appeared in the June 1975 issue of *Mainliner* Magazine, the author, Edwin Kiester, Jr., combined the data gathered in three important national surveys conducted over the past ten years with doctors themselves, who were asked what they thought were the top places for medical care, with information he obtained through personal interviews with a number of other influential cancer specialists. He reported these findings as they pertained to cancer as follows:

In cancer treatment, the doctors' favorite is Roswell Park Cancer Institute in Buffalo, New York, one of four comprehensive cancer research and treatment centers which are the model for a projected nationwide network of cancer hospitals to spearhead the government's war on the disease. One reason Roswell Park is rated ahead of its counterparts—Memorial Sloan-Kettering Hospital in New York, Anderson Hospital in Houston and City of Hope in Duarte, California—is that it is preeminent in male cancers of the prostate, bladder, lung and colon. Memorial is noted for treatment of leukemias and the lymphomas, cancers that typically strike the young; Anderson, for cancers of the breast and female reproductive system and for many rare varieties.

Each of these institutions is identified with certain aggressive and pioneering types of surgery. Memorial has led the way in immunotherapy research, seeking to turn the body's immune system to the destruction of cancer cells. Anderson is known for chemotherapy, or drug treatment. Other hospitals have established themselves as centers for certain types of cancer. They include Tufts–New England Medical Center (melanoma, a virulent form of skin cancer); Moffitt Hospital, San Francisco (brain tumors); the University of Arizona (cancer of the bone marrow); Stanford (lymphomas). For a rare but exceeding savage cancer called eyelet-cell carcinoma of the pancreas, Ohio State University in Columbus is the choice. *

It would be impossible of course for Roswell Park Memorial Institute to accommodate everyone in the United States who had cancer of the prostate, or Moffitt Hospital, with its 22 beds allotted for cancer care, to treat all the patients diagnosed as having brain tumors. Even the University of Texas M.D. Anderson Hospital and Tumor Institute, which is one of the largest Comprehensive Cancer Centers in the country and which received 7,000 new cancer patients last year, can treat only the equivalent of less than 10 percent of its native Texans who are suffering from cancer.

However, if there are beds available, M.D. Anderson and the eighteen other Comprehensive Cancer Centers *will* accept patients who are properly referred by their private physicians or local hospitals regardless of their places of residences. Hundreds of thousands of patients from every state in the United States and from numerous countries have been treated at the nineteen Centers. Financial inability to pay is also not a deterrent. In some cases, a full third of the patients treated at

*Edwin Kiester, Jr., in *Mainliner,* vol. 19, June 1975, pp. 28-30.

a Comprehensive Cancer Center have been medically indigent and have therefore received treatment absolutely free.

With the knowledge that there are these and other outstanding institutions that are capable of giving the finest treatment for a particular form of cancer, it is incumbent on the cancer sufferer or his doctor to at least apply to these treatment centers for admission if inpatient care is required, or for consultation and outpatient care. You will find each and every one of them compassionate and willing to help in any way possible, even to recommending an alternate and equally qualfied cancer center or hospital for the patient's particular cancer disease.

Consulting with the National Cancer Institute, the American Cancer Society, the International Union Against Cancer, the American College of Surgeons, and other organizations and individuals devoted to the cancer issue, we have been able to assemble a combined and cross-referenced list of institutions that we feel offer the best possible detection, diagnostic, treatment, rehabilitation, and continuing care programs in the United States. (A similar listing for countries throughout the world is contained in the final part of these appendixes.*) Wherever possible, we have prepared a résumé of pertinent information relating to each institution, including wherever possible, but not limited to, the types of cancers treated, the available facilities and size of staff, and the name, address, and phone number of the director of each institution. There is no reason why any American suffering from cancer cannot gain admission to one of these hospitals or treatment centers and receive the finest, up-to-date therapy administered by highly trained cancer specialists.

Appendix A includes a synopsis of each of the 121 hospitals and treatment centers that our research and cross-referencing have shown to provide therapy, research, and patient management services equal to, or approaching, the quality of those available at the 19 Comprehensive Cancer Centers. Each of these institutions has highly skilled staff physicians and oncologists experienced in the latest treatment regimens for each of the anatomical sites of cancer. For the most part, they have extensive diagnostic and therapeutic equipment and the trained, technical personnel necessary to administer this equipment. After early recognition, proper treatment is the most important factor in controlling and curing cancer, and the hospitals covered in this section are among the leaders in the world in this area.

REHABILITATION ORGANIZATIONS

Today, throughout the world, there are thousands of local groups made up of cancer patients, former cancer patients, and people interested in helping cancer patients. Most of these groups are affiliated with national and international

---

*In an endeavor of such magnitude it is inevitable that several fine cancer care institutions may have been omitted.

organizations that generally are devoted to one particular area of cancer. The specific services offered by these groups vary from place to place, but the function of each group is basically the same in each case: providing information and moral support to cancer patients. In some instances, these groups provide financial aid to families in need.

Following is a brief description of each major organization and a listing of its individual chapters broken down alphabetically into countries and cities.

The Leukemia Society of America

The Leukemia Society of America
Executive Director: Meade P. Brown
National Headquarters
211 East 43rd Street
New York, New York 10017
(212) 573-8484

The Leukemia Society of America is a national organization with branch chapters in 25 states and more than 50 cities. A large percentage of its members are either individuals affected with leukemia or parents of leukemia patients. While the principal function of the organization is the raising of funds for research, at the local level, the Leukemia Society offers a variety of special services for families affected by leukemia, not the least of which is direct financial aid to families who cannot afford the continuing cost of treatment. The chartered chapters of this organization are listed in Appendix B.

The United Ostomy Association, Inc.

The United Ostomy Association, Inc.
1111 Wilshire Boulevard
Los Angeles, California 90017
(213) 481-2811

The United Ostomy Association is a national organization with branch groups and clubs located throughout the United States and Canada. The association is organized and is run by people who have had ostomies (see page 329) and acts as a clearinghouse for ostomy information and resources. On a national scale, the United Ostomy Association provides lecture material, literature, and a quarterly magazine prepared specifically for the more than 1,500,000 ostomates in North America. On a local level, clubs provide a variety of services, much of it geared toward helping new ostomy patients. The organization is a charter member of the International Ostomy Association, which comprises ostomy associations from eleven countries. The chapters of this organization are listed in Appendix B.

International Association of Laryngectomees

International Association of Laryngectomees
777 Third Avenue
New York, New York 10017
(212) 371-2900

The International Association of Laryngectomees, sponsored by the American Cancer Society, has affiliated clubs in virtually every city of the country, as well as in Europe, Asia, Africa, South America, and Australia. The clubs are made up of cancer patients for whom treatment has left a serious voice handicap. Functions and programs vary from organization to organization, but generally the groups meet once a month and offer members professional voice therapy. Clubs also offer members a directory of sources, supplies, and books designed to accelerate the rehabilitation process and to minimize the psychological impact that laryngectomees invariably face. The clubs work closely with cancer treatment centers and also with all agencies, public, private, or governmental, related to the rehabilitation of laryngectomees. The chapters of this organization are listed in Appendix B.

The American Cancer Society, Inc.

The American Cancer Society, Inc.
National Headquarters
777 Third Avenue
New York, New York 10017
(212) 371-2900

The American Cancer Society is perhaps the most important nongovernmental organization in the world dedicated entirely to the conquest of cancer. Through their 58 divisions, affiliates, and thousands of volunteers, they solicit and dispense tens of millions of dollars in research grants and patient aid services. Many rehabilitation programs are available to those who have been afflicted with cancer at no cost to the patient. Several of these programs are the "Reach to Recovery" breast rehabilitation program for women who have had mastectomies, and the "Ostomy Rehabilitation Program." For further information about these and other American Cancer Society programs and services, contact one of their divisions listed on the following pages or your local Cancer Society volunteer. The chapters of this organization are listed in Appendix B.

The Candlelighters Foundation

The Candlelighters Foundation
123 'C' Street, S.E.
Washington, D.C.
(202) 544-1696, 483-9100, 337-5543

The Candlelighters is an international organization of self-help groups formed simultaneously in Washington, D.C., Florida, and California in about 1970 to help families of pediatric cancer patients meet and deal with the emotional stress of their experiences. The membership is composed primarily of parents of children who have had, do have, or are cured of cancer. Membership is open to any family member and to any person interested in seeking to aid in the control, cure, and ultimately the conquest of cancer in children. Participating members provide personal assistance to one another in times of unusual stress and give the support that can come only from those who share a common experience. A growing number of groups have youth auxiliaries with membership open to teen-age cancer patients and teen-age siblings of cancer patients. The organization consists of separate and independent chapters and affiliates which maintain communications through a quarterly national newsletter distributed by the Candlelighters Foundation, set up as a nonprofit organization in 1976, and through bimonthly group letters. Since the foundation's organizations and leaders fluctuate constantly due to the voluntary nature of the Candlelighters, it is not possible to include a list of chartered chapters and members here. For more information on the Candlelighters or the chapter nearest you, contact Mrs. Grace Ann Monaco, President, at the above-listed address.

PHYSICIANS AND RESEARCH SPECIALISTS

No decision has more bearing on a cancer patient's prospects for recovery than his choice of physician. While there is no shortage of qualified doctors in the United States, there *is* a shortage of physicians and surgeons with the background, the training, and experience needed to provide high-level cancer care. Physicians who specialize in cancer are known as *oncologists*. With very few exceptions, a cancer patient is always better off in the hands of a qualified oncologist than with a physician who treats cancer simply as part of his or her overall practice. There is little doubt that a substantial percentage of cancer fatalities each year could be prevented if cancer patients were treated by cancer specialists.

The question of finding out whether a physician specializes in cancer is frequently a problem for the average cancer patient. For this reason, we have compiled a listing of oncologists throughout the world whose training, background, and professional affiliation give them special qualifications in particular areas of cancer treatment care. The chief source of information for these listings has been professional membership societies in the cancer field. Not every cancer specialist in the world is necessarily a member of a professional society, but the vast majority of specialists not only belong but are active in each organization. Each of the organizations from whom we've gathered information has a highly specific set of membership qualifications. The chief qualification is an active involvement in—and knowledge of—the field to which the organization addresses itself. All the physicians listed have had extensive training in their particular specialty and, in virtually every instance, are affiliated with a major cancer treatment center.

Appendix C lists these oncologists throughout the world. The United States listings have been broken down alphabetically into states and cities. The foreign listings have been broken down by countries and cities. Each of the names in the Geographical Listing in Appendix C is followed by a set of initials which indicate the physician's professional affiliation(s). Below are descriptions of each organization. There is also a geographical list of members of these organizations who are Ph.D.s specializing primarily in research.

PROFESSIONAL ORGANIZATIONS

Society of Surgical Oncology, Inc. (SSO)

Society of Surgical Oncology, Inc.
Executive Secretary:
Condict Moore, M.D., Professor of Surgery
University of Louisville School of Medicine
Preston Walnut
Louisville, Kentucky 40201
(502) 588–5555

Originally known as the James Ewing Society when it was officially organized in 1940 (the name was changed in 1975), the SSO is an international organization comprised of physicians who specialize in various areas of cancer diagnosis, treatment, and research. To qualify for membership, a physician has to be board certified and must have had papers published in at least two major medical journals within the previous ten-year period. In addition, a physician must be formally identified in his particular specialty and must specialize. There are approximately 650 members.

Society of Gynecologic Oncologists (SGO)

Society of Gynecologic Oncologists
Executive Secretary: William T. Greasman, M.D.
Director, Oncology Division
Dept. Obstetrics & Gynecology
Duke University Medical Center
Box 3079
Durham, North Carolina 27710
(919) 684–8111

The SGO is a select group of obstetricians and gynecologists who have specialized for at least three years in gynecologic-oncology (or have completed three years training in the field) and are currently in a responsible position in a gynecologic service that offers complete cancer care. To qualify for membership, a physician must be a Diplomate of the American Board of Obstetrics and Gynecology and a Fellow of the American College of Obstetricians and Gynecologists. All the members of the group are associated with treatment centers that have an organized gynecological oncology team, with regularly scheduled meetings and a tumor registry as part of their activities. The society has approximately 120 members.

The American Society of Clinical Oncology, Inc. (ASCO)

The American Society of Clinical Oncology, Inc.
Executive Secretary: Brigid G. Leventhal, M.D.
Associate Professor of Oncology and Pediatrics
Johns Hopkins Hospital
601 North Broadway
Baltimore, Maryland 21205
(301) 955-5000

The ASCO, incorporated in 1965, is the largest society within the American Federation of Clinical Oncologic Societies. Membership is open to experienced physicians of any nation who have a "predominant" interest in the diagnosis and total care of cancer patients, who are directly involved in cancer care, or, in some cases, have made significant contributions to the field. The chief function of the organization is the circulation of information and ideas relating to cancer diagnosis and treatment and the promotion of communication between oncologists working in various areas of cancer. The society holds an annual meeting and publishes papers presented at the meeting. There are more than 1,000 members.

The American Association for Cancer Education, Inc. (AACE)

The American Association for Cancer Education, Inc.
Executive Secretary: Richard F. Bakemeier, M.D.
University of Rochester School of Medicine and Dentistry
601 Elmwood Avenue
Rochester, New York 14642
(716) 275-2121

Organized in 1966 by the coordinators of the Undergraduate Cancer Teaching Grants from the National Cancer Institute in Bethesda, Maryland, the AACE brings together individuals involved with cancer teaching or training in all the varied institutions in which teaching and training programs are conducted. To qualify for membership, a person has to be actively involved in cancer education. The association has approximately 350 members.

American Radium Society, Inc. (ARS)

American Radium Society, Inc.
Executive Secretary: Alfred S. Ketcham, M.D.
Division of Oncology
University of Miami School of Medicine
P.O. Box 520875
Biscayne Annex
Miami, Florida 33152
(305) 547–6545

Founded in 1916, the American Radium Society is made up of physicians and allied scientists interested in or involved with radiation therapy as it relates to cancer. To be eligible for membership, a physician must be a graduate of a recognized medical college and a member in good standing of his or her local medical community. In addition, members must be either working in—or else have completed—an AMA-approved training program in a cancer-related field. The society's objectives deal primarily with promoting the scientific study of radium and other sources of ionizing radiation and linking these studies with therapeutic applications to cancer. There are approximately 500 members.

American Society for Head and Neck Surgery (ASHNS)

American Society for Head and Neck Surgery
Executive Secretary: Jerome C. Goldstein, M.D.
Division of Otolaryngology
Albany Medical College
Albany, New York 12208
(518) 445–3125

The American Society for Head and Neck Surgery is made up of surgeons whose practice and research are concentrated on the head and neck. To qualify for membership, a surgeon has to: (1) be certified by the American Board of Otolaryngology, Plastic Surgery, or General Surgery; (2) belong to the American College of Surgeons; (3) have two letters of reference from active members; and (4) have completed at least 35 major head and neck cases within a year of applying. The total membership is approximately 160.

American Society of Therapeutic Radiologists (ASTR)

American Society of Therapeutic Radiologists
Executive Secretary: Robert W. Edland, M.D., Associate Professor
Clinical Radiology
Gunderson Clinic Ltd.
1836 South Avenue
La Crosse, Wisconsin 54601
(608) 782-7300

Organized as a club in 1958 and established as a separate society in 1966, the ASTR is composed of physicians who specialize only in therapeutic radiology—cancer treatment that makes use of X-ray technology. The society has more than 900 members, nearly two-thirds of whom hold medical-school appointments. Its aims are to promote high standards of radiology treatment, improve the training of therapeutic radiology, and foster more research in the field.

Society of Head and Neck Surgeons (SHNS)

Society of Head and Neck Surgeons
Executive Secretary: Elliot W. Strong, M.D.
Attending Surgeon Head and Neck Service
Memorial Sloan-Kettering Cancer Center
1275 York Avenue
New York, New York 10021
(212) 794-7000

The purpose of the Society of Head and Neck Surgeons is to further the study of, and disseminate information pertaining to, the management of tumors of the head and neck (excluding lesions of the brain) with emphasis on cancer surgery. The membership, all of whom are actively engaged in the treatment of head and neck tumors, is divided into five categories: Active, Senior, Consulting, Foreign Corresponding, and Honorary. Active members must either be a diplomate of the American Board of Surgery, the American Board of Otolaryngology, a Fellow of the Royal College of Surgeons in Canada, or possess similar qualifications. Surgical members should be Fellows of the American College of Surgeons. The other categories consist of either senior-aged members or other qualified oncologists involved in head and neck tumor management. There are approximately 600 members of the Society.

APPENDIXES

A

International
Directory
of Leading
Cancer
Treatment Centers

THE NATIONAL CANCER INSTITUTE:
ITS COMPREHENSIVE CENTERS,
SPECIALIZED CLINICAL CENTERS,
AND COOPERATIVE GROUPS

Author's note: Although in our research we have attempted to be as accurate as possible in the presentation of information as of the date of publication of this book, because of the extensive, two and one-half year, worldwide compilation of names, facts and figures required to complete *Strike Back At Cancer* and due to the rapidly changing modalities of treatment, increase in available funding for equipment and research, constant changes in patient statistics, certification of new doctors, and the occasional relocation of the oncologists and allied personnel covered in this book, the author regrets any information that may be outdated or inadvertently omitted.

For the periodic updating of *Strike Back At Cancer,* if your name or the name of your institution has been omitted, please forward this and any other new information, statistics, changes of address or phone numbers, or other pertinent data to Mr. Stephen A. Rapaport, c/o *Strike Back At Cancer,* 21 Charles Street, Westport, Connecticut 06880.

Throughout this section, the abbreviation *"ft"* will be used in denoting full-time cancer personnel at the various hospitals, and *"pt"* for part-time personnel.

Under "Cancer Patient Statistics" for each institution covered in Appendix A, the number that appears below:

- ⊕ *Beds*—indicates how many beds have been set aside in that institution exclusively for the care of cancer patients.
- ⊕ *Number of In-patients*—reflects the total number of patients treated on an in-patient (hospital stay) basis during the previous year.
- ⊕ *Average Stay*—shows how many days the average patient remained in the hospital on an in-patient basis during the prior 12 months.
- ⊕ *Number of Out-patients*—indicates how many visits were made to the institution by cancer patients during the previous year for out-patient diagnosis and treatment.
- ⊕ *New Patients*—reflects the number of new cancer patients, both on an in- or out-patient basis, diagnosed or treated during the previous year.

The National Cancer Institute

National Cancer Institute (NCI)
9000 Rockville Pike
Bldg. 31, Room 10A18
Bethesda, Maryland 20014
(301) 496–6641

Director: Arthur C. Upton, M.D.

Affiliations: U.S. Dept. of Health, Education and Welfare; U.S. Public Health Service; U.S. National Institutes of Health.

Emphasis: NCI has the responsibility to establish a structure for a coherent and systematic attack on cancer throughout the United States by establishing a network of shared information, funding for research, and standards for research facilities and treatment centers. It provides financial support and coordination of all cancer-related activities throughout the country.

All areas of basic research are supported with emphasis on epidemiology, collection and analysis of results, viral carcinogenesis, tobacco and chemical carcinogenesis, screening for anticancer agents, pre-clinical pharmacology and toxicology, nucleic acid biochemistry, and tumor immunology. Clinical research in all areas is funded with studies in leukemia and other fast growing tumors and in lymphomas, tumors of the brain, cervix, ovary, breast, bladder, prostate, testis, pancreas, and colon, and head and neck cancers. Research stresses combined modalities and chemotherapy agent testing.

At NCI's Clinical Center, approximately 125 beds are set aside for cancer research and therapy. Practically all the new treatment regimens developed at the 19 Comprehensive Cancer Centers, in the NCI laboratories, and through the thousands of grant programs funded by NCI, are tested at this hospital.

Cancer control programs include chemotherapy, genital tract cancer, radiation physics centers, breast cancer and head and neck cancer treatment and rehabilitation networks, as well as rehabilitation networks, psychosocial and vocational services, and ongoing studies in high-risk factors and individuals.

Equipment:

DIAGNOSTIC	THERAPEUTIC
Nuclear medicine	12meV linear accelerator
Mammography	6meV linear accelerator
CAT body scanners (2)	Dosimetry
CT head scanners (2)	Superficial
Angiography	Simulator
Ultrasound	
Real-time ultrasound	
Gamma cameras (4)	
Fluoroscope	
Endoscope	
Bronchoscope	
Electron microscope	

Cancer Library: National Medical Library of National Institutes of Health, largest medical library in the world; Clinic Center Library.

Tumor Registry.

Professional Education: Clinical associate and research associate programs for training in all areas of basic and clinical research. Intramural research programs for visiting scientists, formal residency training in clinical and anatomic pathology. Lectures, seminars, and conferences.

The Nineteen Comprehensive Cancer Centers

ALABAMA

Birmingham: University of Alabama at Birmingham Comprehensive Cancer Center

CALIFORNIA

Los Angeles: University of Southern California Comprehensive Cancer Center (LAC–USC)
Los Angeles: The UCLA Jonsson Comprehensive Cancer Center

COLORADO

Denver: Colorado Regional Cancer Center

CONNECTICUT

New Haven: Comprehensive Cancer Center for Connecticut at Yale University

DISTRICT OF COLUMBIA

Georgetown University—Howard University Comprehensive Cancer Center

FLORIDA

Miami: Comprehensive Cancer Center for the State of Florida

ILLINOIS

Chicago: Illinois Cancer Council

MARYLAND

Baltimore: Johns Hopkins University Oncology Center

MASSACHUSETTS

Boston: Sidney Farber Cancer Center

MINNESOTA

Rochester: Mayo Comprehensive Cancer Center

NEW YORK

Buffalo: Roswell Park Memorial Institute
New York: Memorial Sloan-Kettering Cancer Center

NORTH CAROLINA

Durham: Duke Comprehensive Cancer Center

OHIO

Columbus: Ohio State University Comprehensive Cancer Center

PENNSYLVANIA

Philadelphia: Fox Chase Cancer Center

TEXAS

Houston: The University of Texas
   M.D. Anderson Hospital and Tumor Institute

WASHINGTON

Seattle: Fred Hutchinson Cancer Research Center

WISCONSIN

Madison: Wisconsin Clinical Cancer Center

Alabama: *Birmingham*

University of Alabama at Birmingham Comprehensive Cancer Center
University Station
Birmingham, Alabama 35294
(205) 934-5077

Director: John R. Durant, M.D.

Admissions: Decentralized.

Affiliations: University of Alabama Hospital system including Spain Rehabilitation Center, Children's Hospital, Veterans' Administration Hospital—all located in the Medical Center.

Emphasis: Center specializes in cancer research with treatment available for most types of cancer in all stages. It provides core services for administration, epidemiology and statistics, tissue culture, NMR, X-ray crystallography, electron microscopy, and histology. Main areas of study include viral tumor immunology, cell differentiation studies in cancer immunobiology, and new drugs and their effects for use in chemotherapy. Among community treatment projects are colposcopy clinics, a Prototype Chemotherapy Network for the state, a Prototype Network Project in Breast Cancer to facilitate early detection and treatment, rehabilitation programs, training programs for nurse practitioners, and programs in radiation dosimetry. In-Center programs include gynecologic oncology, medical oncology, surgery, radiation oncology, pediatric oncology, and pathology and rehabilitation. A statewide Medical Information Service telephone line (MIST) provides an immediate consultation facility with all specialists at the Center, and a Cancer Communications Office is part of a nationwide network providing information on existing cancer programs, agencies and services, facilities for referrals, and data on research, prevention, treatment, and detection. The new Lurleen B. Wallace Memorial Hospital, scheduled for completion this year, will further expand treatment and research facilities.

Equipment:

DIAGNOSTIC	THERAPEUTIC
Nuclear medicine	Linear accelerators (18meV and 4meV)
Mammography	Radiofrequency hyperthermia unit
Ultrasound	Cobalt
Angiography	Radium
CT head scanner	Dosimetry
Gamma camera	Supervoltage X-ray
Fluoroscope	Superficial X-ray
Endoscope	Simulator
Bronchoscope	
Colposcope	

Note: Complete range of sophisticated diagnostic and therapeutic equipment is available through the auspices of the University of Alabama, Department of Medicine.

Cancer Personnel:

M.D. AND M.D./Ph.D.: 42
Ph.D.: 32
  TOTAL: 111 full-time, 15 part-time

TECHNICAL PERSONNEL: 25 ft, 15 pt
NURSES: 12

Cancer Patient Statistics:

BEDS: 45
NO. IN-PATIENTS: 924
AVERAGE STAY: 17

NO. OUT-PATIENTS: 25,284 (visits)
NEW PATIENTS: 2000

Cancer Library: 127,995 volumes and 2100 periodicals.

Tumor Registry.

Professional Education: Center collaborates with the University of Alabama for ongoing support programs and improvement of existing oncology education. Tumor conferences bring new research and treatment plans from the Center to physicians throughout the state.

California: *Los Angeles*

Los Angeles County–University of Southern California Comprehensive Cancer Center (LAC–USC)
2025 Zonal Ave.
Los Angeles, California 90033
(213) 226–2374
(800) 252–9066

Director: G. Denman Hammond, M.D.

Affiliations: University of Southern California; Los Angeles County Department of Health Services.

Emphasis: Ongoing research programs operate in etiology, epidemiology, tumor biochemistry, pharmacology, pharmacokinetics, tumor cell biology, tumor immunology, viral oncology, molecular biology, radiation biology, and carcinogenesis. Over 70 investigators in the Schools of Medicine, Dentistry, and Pharmacy are recipients of approximately $7 million/year in contracts and grants for cancer research and training. Clinical investigations in all departments include national studies of breast, G.U., G.I., skeletal, hematologic, pediatric and gynecologic cancer, and radiation therapy, as well as studies of incidence and natural history of genital tract anomalies and cancer in offspring exposed in utero to synthetic estrogen. Existing clinical demonstration projects include an outreach program for the treatment of acute lymphocytic leukemia, a cooperative regional radiotherapy and telecopier network, and NCI-ACS demonstration project for the early detection of breast cancer. A community-based cancer control program is in operation and patient facilities are available at the Earl Carroll Cancer Clinic and Cancer Detection Clinic. Prime source in U.S. for endocurie therapy utilizing computer-designed templates for interstitial implantations at all major tumor sites for lesions beyond conventional cancer patient management and for lesions that persist or recur after a full course of radiation therapy. Once implanted, hyperthermia can be generated via RF current. Leader in electron radiography, a diagnostic technique that uses electrons for high contrast and detailed radiographs.

Equipment:

DIAGNOSTIC

Thermography
Mammography
Nuclear medicine
CAT body scanner
CT head scanner
Angiography
Ultrasound
Gamma camera
Fluoroscope
Endoscope
Bronchoscope
Electron microscope
Electron radiography
Atomic Absorption spectro-
  photometer

THERAPEUTIC

4meV linear accelerators (2)
Automated radiotherapy simulator
25meV Betatron
Cesium
Dosimetry
Orthovoltage X-ray
Superficial X-ray
High-intensity remote afterloading
  intercavity cobalt 60 unit

Cancer Personnel:

M.D. AND M.D./Ph.D.: 29 ft, 23 pt
Ph.D.: 28 ft, 33 pt
    TOTAL: 142 full-time, 64 part-time

TECHNICAL PERSONNEL: 63 ft, 7 pt
NURSES: 22 ft, 1 pt

Cancer Patient Statistics:

BEDS: 243
NO. IN-PATIENTS: 7156
AVERAGE STAY: 10

NO. OUT-PATIENTS: 49,789 (visits)
NEW PATIENTS: 1628

Cancer Library: Norris Medical Library, University of Southern California.

Tumor Registry.

Professional Education: Approximately 1500 graduate health science students are enrolled and approximately 30 postdoctoral M.D.s and Ph.D.s are undergoing full-time training in oncologic specialties in the Schools of Medicine, Pharmacy, and Dentistry in USC-affiliated hospitals. Postdoctoral programs provide training in clinical and research aspects of cancer. Two to three regional or national cancer symposia for health professionals are held annually.

California: *Los Angeles*

The UCLA Jonsson Comprehensive Cancer Center
924 Westwood Blvd.
Suite 650
Los Angeles, California 90024
(213) 825–5268

Director: Richard J. Steckel, M.D.

Affiliations: Harbor General Hospital; Wadsworth and Sepulveda V.A. Hospital;
Cedar-Sinai Medical Center; 20 additional hospitals in the Southern California
area.

Emphasis: The Center conducts basic and clinical investigations, diagnosis, and
management of adult and pediatric neoplasia and on-going professional education. The Parvum Cancer Research Laboratory, located in the Molecular Biology Institute, involves more than sixty academic investigators, researching the
broad spectrum of cellular studies, with emphasis and opportunity to bridge
basic and clinical science. The areas of expertise include viral oncology, tumor
immunology, radiation biology, and chemical carcinogenesis. The UCLA Health
Sciences faculty participates in more than fifteen cooperative clinical trials on
protocol studies with hundreds of patients at any one time. The second largest
national bone marrow transplantation program, based at UCLA, is pioneering
in autologous marrow removal. This occurs during a patient's remission, where
the marrow is banked for future transplantation when required. Multi-disciplinary
management is the norm for both solid tumors and hematologic-lymphatic cancers. Head and neck cancers, as an example, benefit from this approach, which
incorporates psychosocial counseling, speech therapy, and the services of
UCLA's maxillofacial prosthetics clinics, a regional resource for the area. Comparable services are available for all other cancer sites. The gynecology-oncology
team treats patients in six southern California hospitals and the UCLA faculty
and Cancer Center members function in sixteen affiliated hospitals. The Center
provides biostatistical consultation and study design, utilizing computerization
and data analysis techniques available to Center members. UCLA epidemiolo-
gists are involved in local, national, and international studies of cancer incidence
and causes. Graduate epidemiology students participate in field studies conducted by both this Center and the Bay Area Cancer Epidemiology Resource.

Additional cancer services include a cancer reference library, scanning and
transmission electron microscopy, consultations, tissue culture and media prepa-
rations, as well as cancer information services to the public and the professions.
The *UCLA Cancer Center Bulletin,* established in 1973, circulates bi-monthly to
eleven thousand oncology-concerned health professionals throughout the country. In mid-1978 a psychosocial telephone counseling service, with backup by
specialists, was introduced as a national prototype.

There are four National Cancer Institute therapy programs currently underway: tumor immunology, cancer epidemiology, chemical carcinogenesis, and
tumor cell surfaces. More than seventy pre- and postdoctoral students are involved, and the total number of PhD.'s and M.D.'s working in these areas
exceeds 200.

Equipment:

DIAGNOSTIC

Mammography
Nuclear medicine
CAT body scanner
CT head scanner
Angiography
Ultrasound
Gamma camera
Fluoroscope
Endoscope
Bronchoscope
Electron microscope

THERAPEUTIC

Cyclotron
Linear accelerator
Cobalt
Betatron
Dosimetry
Orthovoltage X-ray
Supervoltage X-ray
Superficial X-ray
Simulator
Hyperthermia

Cancer Personnel: There are 225 active Center members and over 1500 allied health professionals and lab technicians.

Cancer Patient Statistics (UCLA Hospital and clinics only):

BEDS: 760 (unrestricted), 42 (adult cancer), 10 (bone marrow trans-plants)   NEW PATIENTS: 1200+

Cancer Library: UCLA Bio-medical Library, 288,000 volumes, 6400 journal subscriptions.

Tumor Registry: Computerized. Contributes to California Tumor Registry, largest in the United States.

Professional Education: Postgraduate oncology refresher courses for physicians, nurses, and allied health professionals. Masters degree in nursing oncology. Mandatory education for fourth year students in UCLA School of Dentistry. Elective courses in oncology for third and fourth year students in UCLA School of Medicine. Weekly tumor conferences; 20 weekly conferences on a variety of oncologic subspecialties.

Colorado: *Denver*

Colorado Regional Cancer Center
165 Cook St., 2nd Floor
Denver, Colorado 80206
(303) 320–5921

Director: Steven G. Silverberg, M.D.

Affiliation: University of Colorado Medical Center (only academic health center in five-state area).

Emphasis: A consortium cancer center, one of three experimental models in the country, serving Colorado, Wyoming, southern and eastern Montana, western and southern Dakota, western Nebraska, and western Kansas. The area represents 1.5% of the nation's population. Thirty-seven institutions (27 community hospitals), states' departments of health and states universities are involved. The consortium coordinates and manages cancer research at bench and clinical levels, professional education, public education and information, and rehabilitation for the entire five-state area. The primary thrust is improvement of the quality of care at the community level on an outreach basis as opposed to serving as a referral point for cancer patients. Major clinical research efforts are conducted on environmental carcinogenesis owing to the region's growing importance as an energy supply center for the United States (i.e., uranium, oil, shale, coal, and natural gas). Current pollution levels in Denver are greater than those in Los Angeles County. The Colorado Clinical Oncology Group has been developed for regionalized clinical trials with volunteer services of physicians who have been privately funded in Colorado.

Equipment: *

DIAGNOSTIC	THERAPEUTIC
500 billion volt electron accelerator (Los Alamos)	Linear accelerators
	Cobalt
Mammography	Betatron
Thermography	Radium
Nuclear medicine	Dosimetry
CAT body scanner	Orthovoltage X-ray
CT head scanner	Supervoltage X-ray
Angiography	Superficial X-ray
Ultrasound	Simulator
Real-time ultrasound	Hyperthermia
Gamma camera	
Fluoroscope	
Endoscope	
Bronchoscope	
Colposcope	
Electron microscope	

Cancer Patient Statistics:

BEDS: 8100 (unrestricted in 27 Colorado hospitals)

Note: Serves 90% of all cancer patients seen. Independent oncology wards are being developed at affiliated institutions.

Cancer Library: University of Colorado Medical Library; libraries at most consortium institutions.

Tumor Registry: Central Colorado State (computerized).

*Consortium has wide range of diagnostic and therapeutic equipment at its affiliated hospitals including those in the Denver area.

Connecticut: *New Haven*

Comprehensive Cancer Center for Connecticut at Yale University
Yale-New Haven Medical Center
333 Cedar St.
New Haven, Connecticut 06510
(203) 436-1736
(800) 922-0824

Director: Jack Cole, M.D.

Affiliation: Yale University.

Emphasis: Design, synthesize, evaluate, and test new drugs in addition to researching toxic side effects of current drugs. Investigate refinements of surgical techniques and effective combinations of radiotherapy, chemotherapy, and/or
surgery. Department of Radiation Therapy sees approximately 40% of all patients treated in the state. Interdisciplinary groups join surgical teams to plan
specific treatments and rehabilitation programs and to evaluate the progress of
each patient. Expansive research is conducted in immunotherapy and the role of
host defense systems particularly in the early treatment of acute leukemia, head
and neck cancer, breast cancer, and colon-rectal cancer. Major studies are conducted in the area of cell biology, the molecular basis of genetic recombination,
and other phenomena related to ways in which viruses change cell behavior. Outreach programs disseminate information to health professionals and the lay public on cancer detection, diagnosis, treatment, and education.

Equipment:

DIAGNOSTIC
Nuclear medicine
Ultrasound
Tomography
Mammography
CAT body scanner
CT head scanner
Angiography
Gamma camera
Fluoroscope
Endoscope
Bronchoscope

THERAPEUTIC
Laminar flow rooms
Cell centrifuge
32meV linear accelerator
Cesium
Dosimetry
Orthovoltage X-ray
Supervoltage X-ray
Hyperthermia
Superficial X-ray
Simulator

Cancer Personnel:

M.D. AND M.D./Ph.D.: 100
Ph.D.: 45
   TOTAL: 370 full-time, 35 part-time

TECHNICAL PERSONNEL: 200
NURSES: 25 ft, 35 pt

Cancer Patient Statistics:

BEDS: 10 (restricted to cancer care)   NEW PATIENTS: 1263

Library: Yale University School of Medicine.

Tumor Registry: computerized statewide.

Professional Education: Medical Oncology Section is responsible for education of medical students, house staff, community physicians, and other medical personnel in the scientific basis and rationale of medical oncology and cancer chemotherapy. A yearly symposium is conducted for community physicians and a statewide Hematology/Oncology Society facilitates the development of research protocol with common and uncommon tumors.

District of Columbia

Georgetown University–Howard University Comprehensive Cancer Center
Howard University Cancer Center
Department of Oncology
Howard University Hospital
2041 Georgia Ave., N.W.
Washington D.C. 20060
(202) 745-1406

Director: Jack E. White, M.D.

Vincent T. Lombardi Cancer Research Center
Georgetown University Medical Center
3800 Reservoir Rd., N.W.
Washington, D.C. 20007
(202) 625-7118

Director: John F. Potter, M.D.

Emphasis: Basic science investigations are carried out in molecular biology, biochemistry, immunology, and virology. Scientists function as members of clinical research teams participating in projects on biochemistry of Q-B replicase, biosynthesis of actinomycin, t-RNA in neoplastic cells, purification of t-RNA, basic pharmacology of antitumor agents, DNA polymerases in human milk, *C. parvum* induction of immunity in experimental tumor systems, regulation of RNA synthesis. Treatment of all forms of cancer with specialties in surgery, irradiation, chemotherapy, and immunotherapy. Multidisciplinary treatment is emphasized. The facility functions as a tertiary treatment center. A complete program of rehabilitation is operative. All the requisite specialists in rehabilitation function on cancer teams. Clinical studies include the detection of pre-clinical breast cancer by mammography and xerography, detection of viral particles in human milk, immunologic surveillance of the cancer patient, use of high-energy neutron particles in human cancer, combination chemotherapy for nonresectable cancer of the pancreas, stomach, colon, and rectum. Use of an ACTA scanner for localizing and staging cancer and for staging and treatment of Hodgkin disease. Treatments of HSV II viral infections of the cervix, pre-irradiation laparotomy in advanced cervical cancer, and brain tumors in children.

Equipment:

DIAGNOSTIC

Mammography
Nuclear medicine
CAT body scanner
CT head scanner
Angiography
Ultrasound
Gamma camera
Fluoroscope
Endoscope
Bronchoscope
Thermography
Electron microscope
Atomic absorption spectro-
    photometer

THERAPEUTIC

Cyclotron (Naval Research Lab., Wash.)
18meV linear accelerator (2)
10meV linear accelerator
4meV linear accelerator
Cobalt units (3)
Cesium
Radium
Dosimetry
Orthovoltage X-ray (2)
Supervoltage X-ray
Superficial X-ray
Simulators (2)
High-intensity remote afterloading
    intercavity cobalt 60 units
Contact X-ray

Cancer Personnel:

M.D. AND M.D./Ph.D.: 25 ft, 50 pt, 4 volunteer
Ph.D.: 13 ft, 17 pt, 1 volunteer

TECHNICAL PERSONNEL: 66 ft, 58 pt

Cancer Patient Statistics:

BEDS: 1260 (Vincent Lombardi: unrestricted), 24 (Howard University: restricted)
NO. OUT-PATIENTS: 17,450 (visits)

AVERAGE STAY: 22
NEW PATIENTS: 530 (Lombardi), 408 (Howard)

Cancer Library.

Tumor Registry.

Professional Education: Conferences, clinics, and lectures held for all health professionals. A series of programs, in conjunction with the local health department, is conducted for the laity. A breast cancer detection clinic is in operation and other detection clinics are being expanded.

Florida: *Miami*

Comprehensive Cancer Center for the State of Florida
University of Miami School of Medicine
1400 N.W. 10th Ave.
Center House, Miami, Florida 33136
(P.O. Box 520875, Miami, Florida 33152)
(305) 547-6096
(800) 432-5953

Director: C. Gordon Zubrod, M.D.

Dept. Director: Oleg Selawry, M.D.

Affiliations: University of Miami School of Medicine; Jackson Memorial Medical Center; University of Miami, Hospitals and Clinics; Veterans' Administration Hospital.

Emphasis: Research in genetics, immunologic approaches to treatment, chemotherapy, enzyme studies, cell kinetics, organ site cancers, membrane, glycoprotein, biological markers, molecular defects in cancer cells induced by viruses, chemical radiation and repair and studies on the molecular basis of combination chemotherapy. Dr. Selawry is developing sputum cytology for early detection of lung cancer. Animal research on tumor antigens in mouse mammary cancer systems, induced bladder cancer, drug screening for anticancer agents, and immunosuppressive activity of effective therapeutic drugs. Clinical research on solid tumors, identification of markers for early detection, combined modality treatment approaches, and improved patient management and rehabilitation services.

Equipment:

DIAGNOSTIC	THERAPEUTIC
Electron microscope	13meV linear accelerator
Mammography	4meV linear accelerators (2)
Nuclear medicine	Radium
CAT body and CT head scanners	Dosimetry
Angiography	Orthovoltage X-ray
Ultrasound	Superficial X-ray
Gamma camera	Simulator
Thermography	Hyperthermia
Transverse axial tomography	

Cancer Personnel:

M.D. AND M.D./Ph.D.: 32+	TECHNICAL PERSONNEL: 30
Ph.D.: 20	NURSES: 7 (physician assts. and practitioners)
TOTAL: 89+	

Cancer Patient Statistics:

BEDS: 40 designated (110 available)	AVERAGE COST: $235.00
AVERAGE STAY: 4.5	NEW PATIENTS: 1200

Library: University Medical School Library, 100,000 volumes, 1940 periodicals.

Tumor Registry: Statewide.

Professional Education: Graduate instruction in oncology. Statewide seminars and lectures for physicians. Undergraduate course in mechanisms of disease. One- and two-year Clinical Fellowship programs.

Illinois: *Chicago*

Illinois Cancer Council
Room 700
36 So. Wabash Ave.
Chicago, Illinois 60603
(312) 346–9813, (800) 972–0586

Director: Jan W. Steiner, M.D.

Admissions: Member institutions.

Emphasis: The council is a consortium of four specialized cancer centers: Rush-Presbyterian-St. Luke's Medical Center, Northwestern University, University of Chicago, and University of Illinois, 72 other medical and health-related institutions and agencies, and 350 community-based hospitals throughout the state. This includes the Argonne National Laboratory and the Fermi National Accelerator Laboratory.

    Rush-Presbyterian-St. Luke's Medical Center has clinical programs in surgical and nuclear oncology, breast cancer, oncogenic virus, and head and neck cancer. There is a primate center for cancer research.

    University of Chicago Cancer Research Center conducts programs in virology, tumor immunology, cell biology, carcinogenesis, clinical research, radiotherapy, and radiation physics.

    Fermi Accelerator Laboratory is a high energy physics research facility with a cancer treatment center utilizing the 500 billion electron volt accelerator and proton accelerator for neutron therapy trials on radio-resistant cancers.

Equipment:

DIAGNOSTIC	THERAPEUTIC
Nuclear medicine	Linear accelerators
Mammography	Cobalt
Thermography	Isotopes
Ultravoltage X-ray	Simulators
CAT body and head scanners	Dosimetry
	Orthovoltage X-ray
	Supervoltage X-ray
	Superficial X-ray

Cancer Library: At member institutions.

Tumor Registry: Statewide.

Professional Education: Training and instruction at all levels by member institutions. Continuing education conducted by Illinois Cancer Council.

Maryland: *Baltimore*

Johns Hopkins University Oncology Center
Johns Hopkins Hospital
601 N. Broadway
Baltimore, Maryland 21205
(301) 955-3300
(800) 492-1444

Director: Albert H. Owens, Jr., M.D.

Affiliations: Johns Hopkins University and Hospital.

Emphasis: Basic areas of investigation are:
   transplantation biology—bone marrow allografts in the treatment of malignant
   tumors and diseases of marrow failure;
   cell proliferation—effects that patients' sera may have on cellular DNA synthesis;
   immunochemistry—identification of immunoglobulin abnormalities, structure
   studies, enumeration of tumor cells, amyloidosis, and human sera cytotoxic to
   human leukemia cells;
   cell biology—effects of agents on the proliferation and differentiation of hemato-
   poietic and lymphoid cells;
   pharmacology—chemistry, metabolism, and biologic interactions of antitumor
   agents (alkylating agents and the vinca alkaloids);
   biochemical virology—selectively inhibiting virus replication without interfering
   with the metabolism of the host cell;
   cell metabolism—endocrinology and biochemistry of prostatic growth and
   studies on mammalian nuclei;
   epidemiology—in process of development with viral etiology as focus.
   Disease-oriented clinical research programs include acute leukemia, lymphomas, Hodgkin disease, multiple myeloma, breast cancer, childhood neoplasia,
and aplastic anemia. A participant in the Eastern Cooperative Oncology Group,
whereby a continuity of study design has been maintained from the early controlled comparisons of single agents through the current evaluation of multiple-
drug therapy and a prolonged time of treatment. Clinical research is directed to
care for patients with disorders responsive to radiation therapy, advanced surgical techniques, chemotherapy, or combined modalities. Members of the Johns
Hopkins Psychiatric Liaison Service participate with the Center in selected clinical research, education, and patient care activities. A self-report symptom inven-
tory is currently under trial for early detection of psychiatric symptomatology
and the identification of patients in need of psychiatric treatment. A comprehensive rehabilitation service is being developed including a counseling service for em-
ployers. The Center is in the process of establishing a regional network for
cancer care and education to identify and develop practical solutions for problems related to cancer care in the community and to enhance dissemination of
recent advances in medical science. Emphasis is placed on comprehensive patient
consultation and evaluation, the provision of major therapeutic services for
treatable neoplasia, and a positive program for the total rehabilitation of
affected individuals.

Equipment:

DIAGNOSTIC

Mammography
Nuclear medicine
CAT body scanner
CT head scanner
Angiography
Gamma camera
Fluoroscope
Endoscope
Bronchoscope
Electron microscope
Ultrasound
Real-time ultrasound

THERAPEUTIC

18meV linear accelerator
4meV linear accelerator
Cobalt
Radium
Dosimetry
Orthovoltage X-ray
Superficial X-ray
Supervoltage X-ray
Simulator
Radiosensitizers
Radium
Gold
Phosphorous 32
Iodine 131

Cancer Personnel:

M.D. AND M.D./Ph.D.: 30 ft
Ph.D.: 8 ft
   TOTAL: 93 full-time, 2 part-time

TECHNICAL PERSONNEL: 46 ft, 2 pt
NURSES: 9 ft

Cancer Patient Statistics:

BEDS: 20
NO. IN-PATIENTS: 850
AVERAGE STAY: 15

NO. OUT-PATIENTS: 9350 (visits)
NEW PATIENTS: 209

Tumor Registry.

Cancer Library.

Professional Education: Instruction in oncology to medical students at all levels with prime focus on interdisciplinary programs concerned with the biology of human neoplasia and the rational basis for the optimal clinical management of patients. Interns and residents assigned on a rotational basis to the Center. Collaboration with practicing physicians through continuing education programs, conferences, and clinical review courses are offered. Clinical and laboratory fellowships are provided. In-service educational programs for nurses, technicians, and allied-health practitioners.

Massachusetts: *Boston*

Sidney Farber Cancer Center
44 Binney Street
Boston, Massachusetts 02115
(617) 732–3000
(800) 952–7420

Director: Emil Frei, III, M.D.

Affiliations: Harvard Medical School; Peter Bent Brigham Hospital; Children's Hospital Medical Center; Beth Israel Hospital; New England Deaconess Hospital.

Emphasis: Mammalian cell biology including molecular biology, cell membranes, metabolism, cytokinetics, and cytogenetics, in addition to basic and clinical tumor immunology, basic and clinical microbiology, supportive patient care, drug development, pre-clinical and clinical pharmacology, and experimental therapeutics, electron microscopy of macromolecular systems and viral carcinogenesis. Experimental studies are conducted in therapeutics, virology, microbiology, immunology, cell biology, cytochemistry, cytogenetics, cytokinetics, biological ultrastructure, pathology, bioorganic chemistry, and biochemistry. An extensive outreach program in cancer control has been developed with community hospitals in the region, in addition to interrelationships with other Harvard-affiliated institutions in the area with respect to clinical investigation, teaching, and interdisciplinary patient care. Also, major emphasis is put on Phase I, II, and III studies in various tumor types including leukemias, lymphomas, breast, G.I. tract, lung, and cervical. Program assists community hospitals to organize model cancer care systems, providing cancer patients access to local resources. Each system is used to develop programs in prevention, diagnosis, treatment, rehabilitation, and continuing care and will develop specific subprojects, i.e., cervical screening, rehabilitation. Several demonstration and pilot programs focused on interaction between community hospitals and the Center are in operation. Center representatives work with the Massachusetts Department of Public Health to develop criteria and standards to upgrade cancer management in community hospitals which are intended to become regulations under the Department's licensing authority. The Center maintains a referral relationship with New England physicians in which the referring community physician has responsibility for the follow-up care of his or her patient.

Equipment:

DIAGNOSTIC

Mammography
Thermography
Nuclear medicine
CAT body scanner (Brigham)
CT head scanner
Angiography
Ultrasound
Gamma camera
Fluoroscope
Endoscope
Bronchoscope
Electron microscope
Atomic absorption spectro-
   photometer (Brigham)

THERAPEUTIC

18meV linear accelerator (Brigham)
Cobalt   ,,
Betatron   ,,
Cesium (Boston Hospital for Women,
   Lying-in Division)
Dosimetry
Orthovoltage X-ray
Superficial X-ray
Simulator
Hyperthermia

Cancer Personnel:

M.D. AND M.D./Ph.D.:   48
Ph.D.:   28
  TOTAL: 213

TECHNICAL PERSONNEL: 117
NURSES: 20

Cancer Patient Statistics:

BEDS: 18
NO. IN-PATIENTS: 1180
AVERAGE STAY: 7

NO. OUT-PATIENTS: 18,152
NEW PATIENTS: 689

Tumor Registry.

Library: Access to the Harvard Medical School Countway Library.

Professional Education: Two-year Postdoctoral Fellowship programs in medical and pediatric oncology and pre- and postdoctoral training in basic sciences supported by education and training grants or individual Fellowship awards. Present enrollment: 27 in clinical and 14 in basic sciences.

Minnesota: *Rochester*

Mayo Comprehensive Cancer Center
200 First Street, S.W.
Rochester, Minnesota 55901
(507) 282-2511
(800) 582-5262

Director: Charles G. Mortel, M.D.

Affiliations: Mayo Foundation/Mayo Clinic, Mayo Medical School, Mayo Graduate School.

Emphasis: Ongoing programs in cellular biology, immunology, chemical carcinogenesis, oncologic virology, experimental cryosurgery, cancer cell culture of cytokinetics. Diagnosis of bronchogenic carcinoma by comparison of radiographic findings and/or sputum cytologic studies and utilization of advanced fiberoptic bronchoscopic techniques. Large-scale chemotherapy programs for breast cancer, lung cancer, gastrointestinal cancer, plasma cell neoplasms, and some soft tissue sarcomas. National Statistical Center for NCI study of women whose mothers had received diethylstilbestrol during early months of pregnancy and who may be at high risk for vaginal carcinoma. All modalities of treatment are available including medicine, surgery, chemotherapy, and radiation therapy. Subspecialties in medicine and surgery where neoplasia is part of the specialty interest. Studies involving surgery, radiation therapy, drug therapy, and immunotherapy are carried out in the management of cancer of the breast, stomach, colon, lung, and prostate and of leukemia, lymphomas, and other lesions. Large outreach program for the upper midwestern states and operations center for Central Cancer Treatment Group.

Equipment:

DIAGNOSTIC	THERAPEUTIC
Mammography	4meV linear accelerators (2)
Nuclear medicine	8meV linear accelerator
CAT body scanner	Cobalt
CT head scanner	Cesium
CT breast scanner	Radium
Angiography	Dosimetry
Ultrasound	Orthovoltage X-ray
Gamma camera	Supervoltage X-ray
	Superficial X-ray
	Simulator

Cancer Personnel:

M.D. AND M.D./Ph.D.: 50 ft, 95 pt   TECHNICAL PERSONNEL: 75 ft,
Ph.D.: 50 ft, 95 pt   140 pt
                                                          NURSES: 90 ft, 160 pt
    TOTAL: 265 full-time, 490 part-time

Cancer Patient Statistics:

BEDS: 400   AVERAGE STAY: 11
NO. IN-PATIENTS: 12,100   NEW PATIENTS: 18,500

Cancer Library: 180,000 volumes, 3100 periodicals. Mayo Medical Museum has special cancer exhibits and movies.

Professional Education: Mayo Medical School has 40 students; Mayo Graduate School has 600 residents and fellows. Postgraduate programs in oncology, surgery, medicine, and subspecialties. Outreach activities in cancer education and newspaper column, "Cancer Answers" sponsored by the Museum.

New York: *Buffalo*

Roswell Park Memorial Institute
Buffalo, New York 14203
(716) 845–2300, (800) 462–1877

Director: Gerald P. Murphy, M.D., D.Sc.

Admissions: Pat Lauck

Affiliations: SUNY at Buffalo; Niagara University; satellite facilities in suburban areas—Orchard Park, Springville, West Seneca.

Emphasis: A state-funded institution, the oldest and one of the largest cancer study centers in the world. Three major activity areas are basic research, clinical research and treatment, professional and public education. Major experimental capabilities exist in biology, physics, epidemiology, enzymology, pathology, surgery, therapeutics, immunology and immunochemistry, oncology, and animal study. A computing research section develops methods to facilitate research. Six hundred projects in operation include studies of interatomic arrangement in biologic substances at the Center for Crystallographic Research; anticancer drug development and testing at the Grace Cancer Drug Center; tobacco and chemical carcinogenesis and animal research at the Orchard Park Laboratory, interaction of cancer cells with host organism at the Cancer Cell Center; the virology of cancer at the Cell and Virus Center; and large animal research and radiation at the Springville Laboratory. Rehabilitation services use a multifaceted approach directed toward physical therapy, occupational therapy, dental and maxillo-facial prosthetics, enterostomal therapy, speech therapy, social services, surgical speech rehabilitation, and respiratory therapy. Twenty clinical research and treatment departments offer all approved methods of cancer care through inter-departmental efforts and combined modalities. Procedures include medicine, chemotherapy, surgery, radiation therapy, pathology, and immunology. In the General Clinical Research Center, clinical and pharmacologic research is applied to clinical studies within the same unit, a combined medical-surgical effort that also accepts noncancer patients. Four clinical germ-free units protect weakened patients from infection by providing a sterile environment for treatment. Dialysis and experimental techniques in kidney transplantation are available for cases of chronic renal failure. RPMI is headquarters for the National Prostatic Cancer Project and offers consulting services to 50,000 office-based physicians and dentists on all cancer problems via toll-free WATS lines. The Institute participates in Eastern Cooperative Oncology Groups, Acute Leukemia B Group, Central Oncology Group, Radiation Therapy Oncology Group and special national task forces in research on gynecologic, lung, testicular, bladder, prostatic, gastrointestinal, pancreatic, and large-bowel cancers. Numerous outreach programs are conducted through an office of cancer control activities which undertakes efforts in early detection and public education. RPMI is noted for significant contributions in the area of immunologic reactions with malignancy, the relationship between smoking and lung cancer, the first chemotherapy program, and the determination of the molecular structure of RNA resulting in the production of synthetic enzymes.

Equipment: One of the most complete diagnostically and therapeutically equipped facilities in the world including:

DIAGNOSTIC	THERAPEUTIC
Nuclear medicine	4meV linear accelerator
Mammography	6meV linear accelerator
Angiography	35meV linear accelerator
Ultrasound	Dosimetry
Thermography	Cobalt
CAT body and head scanners	Radium
Gamma camera	Superficial X-ray
X-ray spectrography	Orthovoltage X-ray

Cancer Personnel:

M.D. AND M.D./Ph.D.: 110
Ph.D.: 92
TOTAL: 605

TECHNICAL PERSONNEL: 58
NURSES: 345

Cancer Patient Statistics:

BEDS: 325
NO. IN-PATIENTS: 6989
AVERAGE STAY: 14.7

NO. OUT-PATIENTS: 70,000
NEW PATIENTS: 2955

Cancer Library: 28,000 volumes, 600 periodicals.

Tumor Registry.

Professional Education: Oncologic teaching teams are sent to New York State hospitals and conduct continuing education programs for the staff. Graduate division of the State University of New York at Buffalo offers 250 students multidisciplinary programs in the life sciences granting degrees in 10 academic areas. Research participation program for high school and college students in science careers. Speakers' bureau for community civic and social groups on cancer information. Tape library for state residents via toll-free telephone number providing information and answers to cancer questions.

New York: *New York*

Memorial Sloan-Kettering Cancer Center
1275 York Avenue
New York, New York 10021
(212) 794–7000

President: Lewis Thomas, M.D.
Robert Good, M.D., President and Director of Sloan-Kettering Institute for Cancer Research
Edward Beattie, M.D., General Director of Memorial Hospital for Cancer and Allied Diseases

Affiliations: Cornell University; Cornell University Medical College.

Emphasis: Eighty-five research laboratories are located in three laboratory buildings in New York City and one in Rye, New York. Studies are conducted in biophysics, biochemistry, cell surfaces, cellular differentiation and kinetics, cellular metabolism, drug resistance, endocrinology, experimental chemotherapy and pathology, genetics, immunology, lipids, molecular biology, oncogenesis, pharmacology, synthetic organic chemistry, and virology. Basic modalities of treatment are surgery, radiation, and chemotherapy. Concept of treatment is multidisciplinary in which teams of specialists plan patient care with one physician responsible for the patient. As an extension of this concept, task forces are established to mobilize talent for a concentrated attack on specific types of cancer. Team approach has proved effective in direct treatment of cancer and in providing supportive care for cancer patients who fall victim to other diseases while their cancer is being treated. The Rehabilitation Service in the Department of Surgery, combined with a Pain Clinic and a Nutrition Program provide for psychosocial support, restoration, support palliation, follow-up care, and education of patients. Methods-studies for diagnosis and treatment of all types of cancer, especially new agents for chemotherapy, immunotherapy, and their integration into multidisciplinary therapy with surgery and radiation; intensive study of the mechanisms of immunologic defense of the patient against cancer and of the techniques of bone marrow and organ replacement. Directs projects which include rehabilitation, nurse education, outreach service, treatment and educational programs with community hospitals, and screening for detection of early lung cancer.

Equipment:

DIAGNOSTIC	THERAPEUTIC
Mammography	12meV linear accelerator
Graphic stress telethermometry	20meV linear accelerator
Nuclear medicine	Varian linear accelerator
CAT body/head scanners	Cobalt 60 (2)
Angiograph	Cesium
Ultrasound	Radium
Gamma camera	Dosimetry
Electron microscope	Superficial X-ray
Fluoroscope	Simulators (2)
Endoscope	Hyperthermia
Bronchoscope	
Tomography	

Cancer Personnel:

M.D. AND M.D./Ph.D.:   138 ft, 23 pt, 89 volunteer
Ph.D.:   196 ft, 6 pt, 2 volunteer
TOTAL: 1472 full-time, 71 part-time, 91 volunteer

TECHNICAL PERSONNEL: 572 ft, 40 pt
NURSES: 566 ft, 2 pt

Cancer Patient Statistics:

BEDS: 610
NO. IN-PATIENTS: 9600
AVERAGE STAY: 16

NO. OUT-PATIENTS: 102,645 (visits)
NEW PATIENTS: 5157

Cancer Library: 14,090 volumes, 806 periodicals.

Tumor Registry.

Professional Education: Program for Ph.D. in biomedical sciences and M.S. in radiation physics. Student curriculum of seminars, special topics lectures, basic science courses. Hospital offers undergraduate, graduate, and postgraduate oncology training for staff who wish to gain expertise in field of cancer or to select oncology as definitive career.

North Carolina: *Durham*

Duke Comprehensive Cancer Center
P.O. Box 3814
Duke Univ. Medical Center
Durham, North Carolina 27710
(919) 684–2282, (800) 672–0943

Director: William W. Shingleton, M.D.

Affiliation: Duke University.

Emphasis: Basic research in virology, immunology, cell biology, microbiology, biochemistry, pathology, chemotherapy, and ophthalmology. Animal and laboratory isolation facilities. Clinical research in five tumor areas; gynecologic oncology studies, brain tumor research, leukemia and lymphoma, breast cancer and malignant melanoma, and prostate. Member of four clinical cooperative groups: Central Oncology Group, Southeastern Cancer Study Group, Gynecological Oncology Group and Diagnostic Breast Cancer Group. Programs in hematology, gynecology, and epidemiology; computer-based teaching program and a core radiotherapy program. Breast cancer screening, Trophoblastic Center, and community radiotherapy centers. One of world's leading centers for real-time ultrasound imagery.

Equipment:

DIAGNOSTIC	THERAPEUTIC
Thermography	4meV linear accelerators (2)
Mammography	20meV linear accelerator
Tomography	Cobalt
Nuclear medicine	Radium
CAT body scanner	Dosimetry
CT head scanner	Orthovoltage X-ray
Angiography	Supervoltage X-ray
Ultrasound (static and real-time)	Superficial X-ray
Gamma camera	Hyperthermia
Electron microscope	
Atomic absorption spectrophotometer	
Fluoroscope	
Endoscope	
Bronchoscope	
X-ray spectrography	

Cancer Personnel:

M.D. AND M.D./Ph.D.: 62	TECHNICAL PERSONNEL: 123
Ph.D.: 37	NURSES: 27
TOTAL: 249	

Cancer Patient Statistics:

BEDS*: 1000 (unrestricted), 28 (cancer protocol only)

NO. IN-PATIENT DAYS: 2929

AVERAGE STAY: 4.4

NO. OUT-PATIENTS: 153/day

NEW PATIENTS: 3100

Cancer Library.

Tumor Registry.

Professional Education: Seminars in the basic aspects of the neoplastic process. Clinical cancer education for fellows, residents, and students. Seminars and team pairing with staff experts. Research training in chemotherapy and hematology for internal specialists to conduct independent cancer research. Postgraduate training in basic immunotherapy and tumor immunotherapy. Viral oncology training for pre- and postdoctoral programs to promote careers in viral research. Cellular and molecular biology research for Ph.D. candidates.

Ohio: *Columbus*

Ohio State University Comprehensive Cancer Center
Room 357 McCampbell Hall
1580 Cannon Dr.
Columbus, Ohio 43210
(614) 422–5022

Director: David S. Yohn, M.D.

Affiliation: Ohio State University Children's Hospital, Columbus.

Emphasis: Initiated (OMEN) Ohio Medical Education Network in conjunction with 74 hospitals in Ohio, Pennsylvania, Indiana, Michigan, West Virginia, and Kentucky. Ohio State University runs seven one-week programs per year transmitting to member hospitals on 2-way audiocurrents (augmented by pre-distributed slides). The programs include lectures on most recent advances in oncology and question-and-answer sessions with the participants. The Center also maintains a pilot microwave education link tied in with two hospitals in Appalachia where attending physicians can broadcast pictures of patients' radiographs or other pertinent data and get immediate return advice on an appropriate treatment regimen. An original chemotherapy grant from NCI incorporating oncologists and nurses from five regional hospitals permit one-week, on-the-job training programs in chemotherapy applications. Major research is divided into eight interdisciplinary groups involving professional investigations by the faculty of the Colleges of Pharmacy, Biological Sciences, Medicine, Dentistry, Veterinary Pathology, and Mathematical and Physical Science (Chemistry). These groups are carcinogenesis, tumor immunology, development of chemotherapeutics, viral oncology, leukemia/lymphomas, breast cancer, neural tumors, and lung cancer.

*157 average daily cancer patient occupancy.

Equipment:

DIAGNOSTIC

Mammography
Nuclear medicine
Ultrasound
Angiography
Gamma camera
Fluoroscope
Endoscope
Bronchoscope
Electron microscope

THERAPEUTIC

Cobalt
Betatron
Cesium
Orthovoltage X-ray
Superficial X-ray
Simulator
Dosimetry
Hyperthermia

Cancer Personnel:

M.D. AND M.D./Ph.D.:   10 ft, 121 pt   NURSES: 99 ft, 3 pt
TECHNICAL PERSONNEL: 10 ft,
   280 pt
      TOTAL: 119 full-time, 404 part-time

Cancer Patient Statistics:

BEDS: 136 (cancer only),   NO. OUT-PATIENTS: 16,900
   16 (research)   NEW PATIENTS: 2008
NO. IN-PATIENTS: 4789
AVERAGE STAY: 6.5

Cancer Library: 17,000 volumes, 35 journals.

Tumor Registry.

Professional Education: Nineteen postdoctoral candidates in oncology, microbiology, and developmental chemotherapeutics. Regular workshops and seminars held for physicians, nurses, and accredited medical professionals in all subspecialties.

Pennsylvania: *Philadelphia*

Fox Chase Cancer Center
7701 Burholme Ave.
Philadelphia, Pennsylvania 19111
(215) 342–1000
(800) 952–7420

Director: Timothy Talbot, Jr., M.D.
   Paul Engstrom, M.D., Chief of Department of Medicine

Affiliation: University of Pennsylvania.

Emphasis: Originated concept of interdisciplinary research approach to the problems of malignant growth. Work involves studies of both normal and neoplastic

growth in areas of biology and biochemistry, in viruses, cells, and multicellular organisms, including man. Research emphasis on molecular structure, mechanisms of enzyme action, RNA and protein synthesis, genes, chromosomes and differentiation, structure and genetics of bacteria and viruses, the role of nutrition, the immune response, carcinogenesis, chemotherapy, and radiotherapy. The American Oncologic Hospital, the Center's treatment facility, offers surgery, radiation therapy, chemotherapy, and immunotherapy. Most forms of cancer are treated with special competence in breast cancer, tumors of the head and neck and colon and rectum, and pigmented lesions of the skin. The facility has three operating suites and access to Jeanes Hospital. It maintains a Department of Rehabilitation Medicine, with psychiatric and social services. Clinical research concentrates on the detection of transmissible agents that may contribute to the etiology of certain cancers. Work centers on the study of Australia antigen (Au), discovered in the Center's research division, and its apparent involvement as an oncogenic agent. Studies have been made to determine the relationship of Au to hepatoma and whether infection with the agent associated with Au is a factor in the development of reticulum cell sarcoma. Because there appears to be parental effects of Au, studies have been conducted to determine effects on fertility and sex ratio of offspring. Other clinical research studies on parents of children with acute leukemia. The Center, in cooperation with the Preventive Medicine Institute of New York, developed the Canscreen program for early detection, using allied-health professionals to conduct examinations based on risk factor analysis. Canscreen is now in extensive field testing. The Center serves as the focus of a network of seven community hospitals and supplies multidisciplinary training and support services for the diagnosis and management of breast cancer.

Equipment:

DIAGNOSTIC

Electron microscopes (3)
Scanning electron microscope
X-ray diffractometer
NMR spectrometers
Conventional range of diagnostic
   equipment
Mammography
Nuclear medicine
Angiography
Ultrasound
Gamma camera

THERAPEUTIC

Cobalt irradiator
Orthovoltage X-ray (2)
meV VI linear accelerator
Simulator
Conventional X-ray equipment
Cesium
Dosimetry
Radium
Superficial X-ray

Cancer Personnel:

M.D. AND M.D./Ph.D.: 25 ft, 5 pt
Ph.D.: 108
   TOTAL: 298 full-time, 44 part-time

TECHNICAL PERSONNEL: 117
NURSES: 48 ft, 39 pt

Cancer Patient Statistics:

BEDS: 94
NO. IN-PATIENTS: 2417
AVERAGE STAY: 11

NO. OUT-PATIENTS: 15,439
NEW PATIENTS: 4438

Cancer Library: 4214 volumes, 492 periodicals.

Tumor Registry.

Professional Education: Demonstration clinics for health professionals in detection and management. Annual symposia in aspects of cancer therapy and training programs in oncologic nursing.

Texas: *Houston*

The University of Texas, M.D. Anderson Hospital and Tumor Institute
Texas Medical Center
Houston, Texas 77025
(713) 792–2121
(800) 392–2040

President: Charles A. LeMaistre, M.D.

President Emeritus: Randolph Lee Clark, M.D., M.Sc.

Affiliation: The University of Texas System.

Emphasis: One of the largest research and treatment facilities contributing significantly to internationally accepted standards and equipment for cancer care. Care activities are paralleled by numerous research programs and projects carried on in more than 15 departments. Salient areas of investigation and activities include:
Department of Biochemistry—protein synthesis, immunochemistry, immunology, action and structure of pituitary hormones, and studies on carcinogenesis;
Department of Biology—effects on cells of radiation and metabolic events and studies on linkage; and the relationship between genes and neoplastic disease;
Department of Developmental Therapeutics—effect of isolated environment on cancer chemotherapy, analysis of immunology components in disease resistance and immune response to chemotherapy;
Department of Diagnostic Radiology—early diagnosis through mammography, thermography, lymphangiography;
Department of Epidemiology—search and categorization of clusters of specific types of cancer;
Department of Medicine—studies of drug regimens evaluations and regional effects;
Department of Anatomical Pathology—organ bank, cell diagnosis as related to neoplastic disease;
Department of Pediatrics—immunologic studies and usefulness of chemotherapy in disseminated and solid tumors;
Department of Physics—response of biological system to various types of irradiation in microorganisms and clinical applications of nuclides such as Californium;
Department of Radiotherapy—program in radiobiology, effect of pressure oxidation and fractionation of dosage, metabolic state of the cell evaluated in terms of type and amount of radiation;

Department of Surgery —cellular kinetic studies, program for perfusing the body with antitumor agents and clinical studies on management of types of neoplasms to be used in immunotherapy.

Studies of the head and neck are conducted with the dental school with which the Maxillofacial Center is jointly operated. The Rehabilitation Center, containing 110 beds, offers physical, psychologic, social, and vocational services to recovering patients. The Anderson-Mayfair, a patient-care apartment hotel, is operated for preliminary evaluation and consultation. UT Environmental Science Park studies the effects of biohazards on health and houses laboratories and a conference center. A "Dial Access System" gives local physicians in a multistate area current information on cancer treatment. Collaborative programs are conducted with The National Large Bowel Cancer Project, Common Computer Service Facility, Southwest Oncology Group, Regional Maxillofacial Restorative Center, The National Prostatic Cancer Project, The National Pancreatic Cancer Project, Fast Neutron Radiotherapy Program, and the Radiologic Center.

Equipment:

DIAGNOSTIC	THERAPEUTIC
Atomic absorption spectrophotometer	Cyclotron
X-ray spectrography	32meV linear accelerator
Electron microprobe	Californium 252
Thermography	Cobalt
Mammography	Betatron
Nuclear medicine	Cesium
CT scanners, head/body	Dosimetry
Angiography	Orthovoltage X-ray
Ultrasound	Supervoltage X-ray
Gamma camera	Superficial X-ray
Fluoroscope	Simulator
Endoscope	
Bronchoscope	

Cancer Personnel:

M.D. AND M.D./Ph.D.: 167 ft, 21 pt, 32 volunteer

Ph.D.: 121 ft, 2 pt, 5 volunteer

TECHNICAL PERSONNEL: 415* ft, 412* pt

NURSES: 329* ft, 12* pt, 21 volunteer

TOTAL: 1032 full-time, 447 part-time, 58 volunteer

Cancer Patient Statistics:

BEDS: 400

NO. IN-PATIENTS: 7329*

AVERAGE STAY: 13

NO. OUT-PATIENT VISITS: 334,297

NEW PATIENTS: 8089

*In 1974.

Library: 67,000 volumes, 1163 journal subscriptions.

Tumor Registry: Computerized research.

Professional Education: Primary teaching facility for The University of Texas Graduate School of Biomedical Sciences. 220 residents and pre- and post-doctoral fellows in training with allied-health professional health training. Conduct Medical Community Television System connecting 22 institutions. Annual education programs include Symposium on Fundamental Cancer Research and the clinical conference.

Washington: *Seattle*

Fred Hutchinson Cancer Research Center
1124 Columbia
Seattle, Washington 98104
(206) 292–2912

Director: William Hutchinson, M.D.

Affiliations: University of Washington; Children's Orthopedic Hospital and Medical Center; five community hospitals

Emphasis: Areas of study are epidemiology, biostatistics, biochemical oncology, chemical carcinogenesis, tumor immunology and microbiology, tumor immunology and pathology, as well as oncologic pharmacology, pathology, and cell biology, basic immunology, genetics, experimental pathology, and cancer pain research. Special programs continue in survey of cancer rehabilitation in all age groups, bone marrow transplantation, cancer immunology in melanoma, clinical pharmacology of high-dose methyltrexate with cirtrovorum rescue, generalized lymphosarcoma treatment, Phase I and Phase II chemotherapy program on new agents for cancer patients, and gynecology. Clinical Units have been established in seven area hospitals. These serve as a clinical arm of the Center, are identifiable, and are on Center protocols and data retrieval systems. Pediatric studies in cancer research are conducted at the Children's Orthopedic Hospital. Coordination of outreach programs is conducted by cancer committee chairmen in over 20 area hospitals. Collaborative programs include "SAQC" which serves as the Statistical Analysis and Quality Control Center for the retrieval of cancer patient data collected at all Centers within the United States. Also connected with the center are a Lung Cancer Study Group, concerned with immunotherapy studies of lung cancer, a Wilm's Tumor Study Group, and joint studies with Russia for gynecologic cancers.

Equipment:

DIAGNOSTIC	THERAPEUTIC
Mammography	Cobalt
Nuclear medicine	Betatron

DIAGNOSTIC	THERAPEUTIC
CAT body scanner (at associated inst.)	Cesium
Angiography	Dosimetry
Ultrasound	Orthovoltage
Gamma camera	Supervoltage
Fluoroscope	Superficial X-ray
Bronchoscope	Simulator
Cell sorter	
Cell counter	

Cancer Personnel:

M.D. AND M.D./Ph.D.: 78   TECHNICAL PERSONNEL: 189
Ph.D.: 61   NURSES: 167
  TOTAL: 495

Cancer Patient Statistics:

BEDS: 170   NO. OUT-PATIENTS: 18,578
NO. IN-PATIENTS: 2630   NEW PATIENTS: 2280
AVERAGE STAY: 20

Cancer Library: 600 volumes, 185 periodicals.

Tumor Registry: Computerized.

Professional Education: Regional Cancer Council. Programs in research training, medical oncology and pediatric oncology, tumor immunology, and biochemical oncology.

Wisconsin: *Madison*

Wisconsin Clinical Cancer Center
701C University Hospitals
1300 University Ave.
Madison, Wisconsin 53706
(608) 263–2553
(800) 362–8038

Director: Harold Rusch, M.D.

Affiliation: University of Wisconsin.

Emphasis: Research conducted on the role of enzymes in carcinogenesis, the role of steroid hormones in growth and differentiation, the role of tryptophan and nitrosamine metabolism in cancer formation. Ongoing studies in chemotherapy and radiation biology at molecular, cellular, tissue, and whole animal levels. Investigations conducted on chemical and viral carcinogenesis. Other specialties include clinical chemotherapy and radiotherapy trials, determination of steroid hormones associated with breast cancer, level of arylhydroxylases in patients with cancer, estrogen binding and breast cancer, research on childhood leukemias, cytogenics of familial cancer, and clinical pharmacology. Associated with three protocol cooperative chemotherapy programs and serves as central office for the Central Oncology Group. Cooperative clinical programs are conducted with the Medical College of Wisconsin in Milwaukee and with various hospitals and clinics throughout the state, cooperating with the State Division of Health and with the American Cancer Society for Cervical Uterine Cancer. Emphasis on locating girls whose mothers received diethylstilbestrol during pregnancy. Administration headquarters for statewide head and neck cancer program.

Equipment:

DIAGNOSTIC	THERAPEUTIC
Fluoroscope	Blood cell separator
Endoscope	4meV linear accelerators (2)
Bronchoscope	18meV linear accelerator
CAT body scanner	Cobalt
CT head/neck scanner	Cesium
Ultrasound	Simulator
Mammography	Dosimetry
Xeroradiography	250 kVP orthovoltage X-ray
Angiography	Hyperthermia

Cancer Personnel:

M.D. AND M.D./Ph.D.: 20 ft, 2 pt   TECHNICAL PERSONNEL: 96 ft, 12 pt
Ph.D.: 29 ft, 3 pt   NURSES: 32 ft
    TOTAL: 177 full-time, 17 part-time

Cancer Patient Statistics:

BEDS: 110   NO. OUT-PATIENTS: 35,097 (visits)
NO. IN-PATIENTS: 2990   NEW PATIENTS: 3120
AVERAGE STAY: 14.5

Cancer Library: 160,000 volumes, 3365 periodicals.

Tumor Registry.

Professional Education: Sponsors conferences and lectures in cooperation with the Division of Continuing Medical Education of the University. Trains residents and fellows in clinical and basic oncology. Awarded a Clinical Cancer Education Program grant by the National Cancer Institute.

Specialized Cancer Centers

RADIATION ONCOLOGY

CALIFORNIA: Stanford—Stanford University
MARYLAND: College Park—University of Maryland

MICHIGAN: Detroit–Wayne State University
NEW MEXICO: Albuquerque–University of New Mexico
PENNSYLVANIA: Philadelphia–Hahnemann Medical College and Hospital
PENNSYLVANIA: Philadelphia–Jefferson Medical College
PENNSYLVANIA: Pittsburgh–Allegheny General Hospital
VIRGINIA: Richmond–Medical College of Virginia

MEDICAL ONCOLOGY

IDAHO: Boise–Mountain States Tumor Institute
MICHIGAN: Detroit–Michigan Cancer Foundation
NEW YORK: New York–Mt. Sinai School of Medicine
NORTH CAROLINA: Winston-Salem–Bowman Gray School of Medicine
RHODE ISLAND: Providence–Roger Williams General Hospital
TEXAS: Galveston–University of Texas Medical Branch

SURGICAL ONCOLOG'

LOUISIANA: New Orleans–Tulane University

PEDIATRIC ONCOLOGY

PENNSYLVANIA: Philadelphia–Children's Hospital of Philadelphia
TENNESSEE: Memphis–St. Jude Research Hospital

MULTIDISCIPLINARY

CALIFORNIA: San Francisco–University of California, San Francisco
HAWAII: Honolulu–University of Hawaii
KANSAS: Kansas City–University of Kansas
MASSACHUSETTS: Boston–Boston University
MASSACHUSETTS: Boston–Harvard University
MASSACHUSETTS: Boston–Massachusetts General Hospital
MASSACHUSETTS: Boston–Tufts University
MINNESOTA: Minneapolis–University of Minnesota
MISSOURI: Columbia–Cancer Research Center
MISSOURI: St. Louis–Washington University, St. Louis
NEW YORK: New York–Albert Einstein College of Medicine
NEW YORK: New York–Columbia University
NEW YORK: New York–New York University
NEW YORK: Rochester–University of Rochester
TEXAS: Houston–Baylor College of Medicine
PENNSYLVANIA: Philadelphia–Temple University

Cooperative Groups

The individual Cooperative Groups and their respective chairmen are listed below. Seventeen of these Cancer Clinical Cooperative Groups are listed on the chart below with designations as to the particular disease or tumor type clinical study each one is conducting through support grants from the National Cancer Institute.

Acute Leukemia Cooperative Group B
James F. Holland, M.D.
Two Overhill Road, Suite 208
Scarsdale, New York 10583
(914) 472-0710

Brain Tumor Chemotherapy Study
  Group
Michael D. Walker, M.D.
Baltimore Cancer Research Center
3100 Wyman Park Drive
Baltimore, Maryland 21211
(301) 528-7516

Central Oncology Group
Robert O. Johnson, M.D.
Headquarters Office
University of Wisconsin Medical School
1300 University Avenue
Madison, Wisconsin 53706
(608) 262-1626

Children's Cancer Study Group
Denman Hammond, M.D.
Operations Office
University of Southern California
1721 North Griffin Avenue
Los Angeles, California 90031
(213) 226-2008

Cooperative Breast Cancer Group
Albert Segaloff, M.D.
Alton Ochsner Medical Foundation
1514 Jefferson Highway
New Orleans, Louisiana 70121
(504) 837-3000; 834-7070

Eastern Cooperative Oncology Group
Paul P. Carbone, M.D.
Operations Office
850 Sligo Avenue, Suite 601
Silver Springs, Maryland 20910
(301) 585-4602

Gynecologic Oncology Group
George Lewis, M.D.
Thomas Jefferson Medical College
Room 300
1025 Walnut Street
Philadelphia, Pennsylvania 19107
(215) 829-6507

Malignant Melanoma Clinical Cooperative
  Group
Thomas B. Fitzpatric, M.D., Ph.D.
Massachusetts General Hospital
Fruit Street
Boston, Massachusetts 02114
(617) 726-3990

National Wilms' Tumor Study Group
Giulio J. D'Angio, M.D.
Memorial Sloan-Kettering Cancer Center
1275 York Avenue
New York, New York 10021
(212) 879-3192

Polycythemia Vera Study Group
Louis R. Wasserman, M.D.
Mount Sinai Hospital
100th Street and Fifth Avenue
New York, New York 10029
(212) 650-6191

Primary Breast Cancer Therapy Group
Bernard Fisher, M.D.
University of Pittsburgh
School of Medicine
3550 Terrace Street
Pittsburgh, Pennsylvania 15261
(412) 624-2666

Radiation Therapy Oncology Group
Simon Kramer, M.D.
Thomas Jefferson University Hospital
Department of Radiation Therapy and
  Nuclear Medicine
1025 Walnut Street
Philadelphia, Pennsylvania 19107
(215) 829-6702

Radiotherapy Hodgkin's Disease Group
James J. Nickson, M.D.
University of Tennessee
Radiation Oncology Division
Chandler Building, B106
Memphis, Tennessee 38103
(901) 523-2471

Southeastern Cancer Study Group
John Durant, M.D.
University of Alabama Hospitals and
  Clinics
619 S. 19th Street
Birmingham, Alabama 35233
(205) 934-5077

Southwest Oncology Group
Barth Hoogstraten, M.D.
Operations Office
Suite 201
3500 Rainbow Boulevard
Kansas City, Kansas 66103
(913) 831-5996

Veterans Administration Cooperative
Urology Radiotherapy Research
Group
David F. Paulson, M.D.
P.O. Box 2977
Duke University Medical Center
Durham, North Carolina 27710
(919) 684-5057

Veterans Administration Cooperative
Urological Research Group
George T. Mellinger, M.D.
Veterans Administration Hospital
5500 E. Kellogg Avenue
Wichita, Kansas 67218
(316) 658-2282

Veterans Administration Lung Cancer
Study Group
Julius Wolf, M.D.
Veterans Administration Hospital
130 West Knightsbridge Road
Bronx, New York 10468
(212) 584-9604

Veterans Administration Surgical
Adjuvant Cancer Chemotherapy
Study Group
George A. Higgins, M.D.
Veterans Administration Hospital
50 Irving Street, N.W.
Washington, D.C. 20422
(202) 483-6666

Western Cancer Study Group
Joseph R. Bateman, M.D.
University of Southern California
John Wesley Hospital
2825 South Hope Street
Los Angeles, California 90007
(313) 748-3111, ext. 331

OTHER LEADING CANCER TREATMENT CENTERS IN THE UNITED STATES

ARIZONA

Phoenix: Maricopa County General Hospital

CALIFORNIA

Loma Linda: Loma Linda University Medical Center
Los Angeles: Cedars-Sinai Medical Center
    Kaiser Foundation Hospitals of Southern California
    White Memorial Medical Center
Orange: University of California, Irvine Medical Center
Sacramento: Sacramento Medical Center
San Diego: Naval Regional Medical Center
San Francisco: Mount Zion Hospital and Medical Center
    St. Mary's Hospital and Medical Center
Stanford: Stanford University Medical Center and Hospital
Torrence: Los Angeles County Harbor General Hospital

COLORADO

Denver: Fitzsimons Army Medical Center

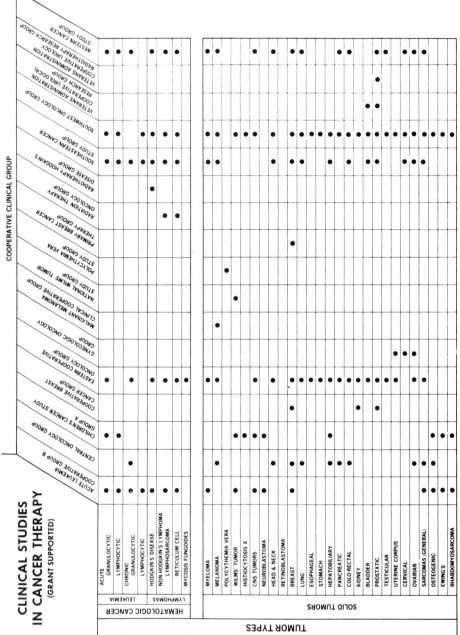

CLINICAL STUDIES IN CANCER THERAPY
(GRANT SUPPORTED)

CONNECTICUT

Bridgeport: Bridgeport Hospital
St. Vincent's Medical Center
Hartford: Hartford Hospital

DELAWARE

Wilmington: Wilmington Medical Center

DISTRICT OF COLUMBIA

George Washington University Hospital
Howard University
Walter Reed Army Medical Center

FLORIDA

Gainesville: University of Florida, Shands Teaching Hospital and Clinics
Jacksonville: University Hospital of Jacksonville
Miami Beach: Mount Sinai Medical Center
Tampa: Tampa General Hospital

GEORGIA

Atlanta: Grady Memorial Hospital
Savannah: Memorial Medical Center

IDAHO

Boise: Mountain States Tumor Institute

ILLINOIS

Chicago: Illinois Masonic Medical Center
Mercy Hospital and Medical Center
Mount Sinai Hospital Medical Center of Chicago
University of Illinois Medical Center
Evanston: Evanston Hospital
Saint Francis Hospital of Evanston
Rockford: Rockford Memorial Hospital

INDIANA

Indianapolis: Indiana University Hospitals
Methodist Hospital of Indiana, Inc.

IOWA

Iowa City: University of Iowa Hospitals and Clinics

KANSAS

Kansas City: University of Kansas Medical Center, Mid-America Cancer Center
    Program

LOUISIANA

New Orleans: Charity Hospital of Louisiana at New Orleans

MARYLAND

Baltimore: University of Maryland Hospital
Bethesda: National Naval Medical Center

MASSACHUSETTS

Boston: Beth Israel Hospital
    Children's Hospital Medical Center
    New England Deaconess Hospital
    Peter Bent Brigham Hospital
    Tufts-New England Medical Center Cancer Center
    University Hospital, Boston University Cancer Research Center
Walpole: Pondville Hospital

MICHIGAN

Ann Arbor: St. Joseph Mercy Hospital
Dearborn: Oakwood Hospital
Detroit: Henry Ford Hospital
Flint: Hurley Medical Center
Grand Rapids: Grand Rapids Clinical Oncology Program
Pontiac: St. Joseph Mercy Hospital

MINNESOTA

Minneapolis: Masonic Memorial Cancer Center, University of Minnesota, Health
    Sciences Center

MISSISSIPPI

Jackson: The University Hospital at the University of Mississippi Medical Center

MISSOURI

Columbia: Ellis Fischel State Cancer Hospital
Kansas City: St. Luke's Hospital of Kansas City
St. Louis: Barnes Hospital
    St. Mary's Health Center

NEBRASKA

Omaha: Clinical Cancer Center, University of Nebraska Hospital and Clinics

NEW HAMPSHIRE

Hanover: Mary Hitchcock Memorial Hospital

NEW JERSEY

Livingston: St. Barnabas Medical Center
Long Branch: Monmouth Medical Center

NEW MEXICO

Albuquerque: University of New Mexico Cancer Research and Treatment Center

NEW YORK

Bronx: Misericordia Hospital Medical Center
    Montefiore Hospital and Medical Center
Brooklyn: Long Island College Hospital
    Methodist Hospital of Brooklyn
    SUNY Downstate Medical Center, Kings County Hospital Center
East Meadow: Nassau County Medical Center
Mineola: Nassau Hospital
Manhasset: North Shore University Hospital
New Hyde Park: Long Island Jewish-Hillside Medical Center
New York: Cancer Center, Columbia University
    Mount Sinai Medical Center
    The New York Hospital
    New York University Medical Center
    St. Vincent's Hospital and Medical Center
Queens: Queens Hospital Center
Syracuse: Crouse-Irving Memorial Hospital
    University Hospital of Upstate Medical Center

OHIO

Akron: Akron City Hospital
Cincinnati: University of Cincinnati Medical Center
Cleveland: Cleveland Metropolitan General Hospital
Dayton: Miami Valley Hospital

OREGON

Portland: Emanuel Hospital
    University of Oregon Health Sciences Center

PENNSYLVANIA

Danville: Geisinger Medical Center
Philadelphia: Albert Einstein Medical Center, Northern Division
    Hahnemann Medical College and Hospital
    Mercy Catholic Medical Center
    Temple University Hospital
    Thomas Jefferson University Hospital
    University of Pennsylvania Cancer Center
Pittsburgh: Mercy Hospital of Pittsburgh
    St. Francis General Hospital
    Western Pennsylvania Hospital

RHODE ISLAND

Providence: Rhode Island Hospital

SOUTH CAROLINA

Charleston: Medical University, Hospital of South Carolina

TENNESSEE

Memphis: Methodist Hospital
Nashville: Vanderbilt University Medical Center

TEXAS

Dallas: Charles A. Sammons Cancer Center
    Methodist Central Hospital
    St. Paul's Hospital
Fort Sam Houston: Brooke Army Medical Center
Galveston: University of Texas, Medical Branch Hospitals
Houston: Ben Taub General Hospital
    St. Joseph Hospital
    St. Luke's Episcopal Hospital
Lackland: Wilford Hall USAF Medical Center
Temple: Scott and White Memorial Hospital

UTAH

Salt Lake City: L D S Hospital
    University of Utah Hospital

VERMONT

Burlington: Cancer Center Hospital of Vermont

VIRGINIA

Charlottesville: University of Virginia Hospitals
Richmond: Medical College of Virginia Hospitals of the Virginia Commonwealth
 University

WASHINGTON

Seattle: Swedish Hospital Medical Center
 Virginia Mason Hospital
Spokane: Sacred Heart Medical Center

WISCONSIN

Milwaukee: Milwaukee County Medical Complex

Arizona: *Phoenix*

Maricopa County General Hospital
2601 E. Roosevelt
Phoenix, Arizona 85008
(602) 267-5011

Director: William A. Markey

Admissions: Maxine MacMillan

Emphasis: Hospital has 495 acute short-term licensed beds. Owned and operated
 for the indigent residents of Maricopa County, treating all types of cancer. Diagnostic X-ray and nuclear medicine techniques and instruments.

Cancer Patient Statistics:

BEDS:	495	NO. OUT-PATIENTS:	225,000
NO. IN-PATIENTS:	10	NEW PATIENTS:	3/wk.
AVERAGE STAY:	8 days	AVERAGE COST:	$91.00

Library: 2700 volumes, 215 journals.

Tumor Registry.

California: *Loma Linda*

Loma Linda University Medical Center
11234 Anderson St.
Loma Linda, California 92350
(714) 796-7311

Administrative Assistant: John Ruffcorn

Admissions: Judy O'Connor
Thomas Godfrey, Head Oncologist

Affiliations: Jerry L. Pettis Memorial Veterans Hospital; Riverside General Hospital; Kaiser Foundation Hospital, Fontana; San Bernardino County Medical Center; Rancho Los Amigos Hospital; Children's Hospital of Los Angeles.

Emphasis: Maxillofacial prosthetics and computerized radiation therapy planning. Surgery, radiotherapy and chemotherapy, and radioactive implants. Rehabilitation center and basic immunology research.

Equipment:

DIAGNOSTIC	THERAPEUTIC
CAT head and body scanners	25 meV Betatron
Ultrasound	Cobalt 60
Nuclear medicine	Isotopes
Angiography	Radium
Mammography	

Cancer Personnel:

M.D. AND M.D./Ph.D.: 12	TECHNICAL PERSONNEL: 8
Ph.D.: 1	NURSES: 25
TOTAL: 46	

Cancer Patient Statistics:

BEDS: 90	NO. OUT-PATIENTS: 25,000
NO. IN-PATIENTS: 1825	NEW PATIENTS: 1084
AVERAGE STAY: 10	AVERAGE COST: $156.00

Cancer Library: 197,841 volumes.

Tumor Registry.

Professional Education: Postgraduate training in radiotherapy, medical oncology, and chemotherapy. Continuing medical education seminars.

California: *Los Angeles*

Cedars-Sinai Medical Center
8700 Beverly Blvd.
Los Angeles, California 90048
(213) 855-5000

Admissions: Stuart J. Marylander, James Davis

Affiliation: University of California, Los Angeles.

Emphasis: Surgery, chemotherapy and radiotherapy, and pediatric oncology.

Equipment:

DIAGNOSTIC
Thermography
Ultrasound
Whole body scanner
Chrome injection
Electron microscope
Mammography

THERAPEUTIC
Betatron
Linear accelerator
Isotopes
Simulator

Cancer Personnel:

M.D. AND M.D./Ph.D.:   22
TOTAL: 120

OTHER PERSONNEL: 98

Cancer Patient Statistics:

BEDS: 796 (unrestricted)
NO. IN-PATIENTS: 10,000

AVERAGE STAY: 7
NO. OUT-PATIENTS: 5000

Library: 276 books, 24 journals.

Tumor Registry.

Professional Education: Postgraduate training in oncology, radiology, and radiation therapy.

California: *Los Angeles*

Kaiser Foundation Hospitals of Southern California
4867 Sunset Blvd.
Los Angeles, California 90027
(213) 667–4011

Regional Medical Director: T. Hart Baker, M.D.

Affiliation: Central Association of Teaching Hospitals in Los Angeles.

Emphasis: Treatment program for all anatomic sites with specializations in gynecology, surgical and pediatric oncology, and radiation therapy. Complete prepaid
medical membership plan under Health Maintenance Organization. Foundation
is a regional cancer center consisting of eight hospital units, with specialization
in each unit, and serves one and one-half million people in Southern California.
Group cooperative studies in Eastern Oncology Group and Children's Cancer
Study Group.

Equipment:

DIAGNOSTIC
Angiography
EMI head scanner
Polytome
Conventional X-ray equipment
Fluoroscopic units
Ultrasound
Xeromammography
Nuclear medicine
Gamma camera

THERAPEUTIC
Linear accelerator
Orthovoltage X-ray
Superficial X-ray
Cesium 137
Simulator
Dosimetry
Transvaginal supervoltage X-ray

Cancer Personnel:

M.D. AND M.D./Ph.D.: 78
Ph.D.: 10
    TOTAL: 158

TECHNICAL PERSONNEL: 50
NURSES: 20

Cancer Library: In each unit.

Tumor Registries.

Professional Education: Multidisciplinary weekly conferences for 1200 doctors in group. Weekly tumor conference on all subspecialities.

California: *Los Angeles*

White Memorial Medical Center
1720 Brooklyn Ave.
Los Angeles, California 90033
(213) 269-9131

Director: Richard A. Pierce

Affiliations: Loma Linda University; Los Angeles County College, USC.

Emphasis: Treatment and rehabilitation in ear, nose and throat, and gynecologic cancers. Clinical research on breast and pancreatic cancers.

Equipment:

DIAGNOSTIC
CT scanner
Thermography
CEA
Lab Hycel-17
Electromyography

THERAPEUTIC
Betatron
Orthovoltage X-ray
Cobalt 60
Radium
Phosphorous 32
Iodine 131

Cancer Personnel:

M.D. AND M.D./Ph.D.: 5
Ph.D.: 1
TOTAL: 32

TECHNICAL PERSONNEL: 5
NURSES: 21

Cancer Patient Statistics:

BEDS: 30
NO. IN-PATIENTS: 966
AVERAGE STAY: 7

NEW PATIENTS: 430
AVERAGE COST: $140.00

Library: 43,000 volumes.

Tumor Registry.

Professional Education: Postgraduate training in radiology, oncology, surgery, gynecology and obstetrics, and cardiology.

California: *Orange*

University of California, Irvine Medical Center
101 City Drive South
Orange, California 92668
(714) 634-5678

Director: Robert W. White

Admissions: Marv Wendt

Emphasis: Comprehensive cancer treatment with chemotherapy and immuno-therapy services and research.

Equipment:

DIAGNOSTIC
Nuclear medicine
CAT whole body scanner
Gamma camera
Scintillation camera
Angiography
Isotopes
Thermography
Ultrasound

THERAPEUTIC
Linear accelerator
Orthovoltage X-ray
Supervoltage X-ray
Simulator
Dosimetry
Laminar flow room

Cancer Library.

Tumor Registry.

Professional Education: Postgraduate education and Carcinogenic Training Grant, National Cancer Institute.

California: *Sacramento*

Sacramento Medical Center
2315 Stockton Blvd.
Sacramento, California 95817
(916) 453-2011

Director: Robert B. Smith

Admissions: Jerry Lewis, M.D.

Affiliation: University of California, Davis.

Emphasis: Research and treatment in leukemia and lymphomas, chemotherapy, radiotherapy, hematology, and pediatric oncology.

Equipment:

DIAGNOSTIC	THERAPEUTIC
CT head scanner	Conventional X-ray equipment
Nuclear medicine	Cyclotron (U of C, Davis)
Gamma camera	
Scintillation camera	
Ultrasound	
Thermography	
Mammography	
Polytome	

Cancer Personnel (Hematology and Oncology Section):

M.D. AND M.D./Ph.D.:   5   TECHNICAL PERSONNEL: 5
Ph.D.:   1

Cancer Library.

Tumor Registry.

Professional Education: Postgraduate training in medical oncology and radio-diagnosis.

California: *San Diego*

Naval Regional Medical Center
Park Blvd.
San Diego, California 92134
(714) 233-2205

Director of Clinical Services: William M. McDermott, Capt.

Director of Clinical Investigations: Arthur D. Hagan, Capt.
D. Earl Brown, Jr., RADM, Commanding Officer

Affiliations: University Hospital and University of California, San Diego.

Emphasis: Associated with University of Pittsburgh on National Surgical Adjunct Breast Protocol and additional research on Rectal and Colon Cancer Protocol. Areas of specialization include pediatric hematology and oncology and surgical, gynecologic, and radiation oncology.

Equipment:

DIAGNOSTIC	THERAPEUTIC
Nuclear medicine	Cobalt
CAT body scanner	Megavoltage X-ray
Bone scanner	Orthovoltage X-ray
Brain scanner	Radium
Liver scanner	Strontium 90
Spleen scanner	Superficial X-ray
Gallium scanner	White cell transfusion
Ultrasound	Regional arterial infusion capabilities
Computerized tomography	

Cancer Patient Statistics:

BEDS: 874+ (unrestricted)

Cancer Library.

Tumor Registry.

Professional Education: Residency program in all subspecialties.

California: *San Francisco*

Mount Zion Hospital and Medical Center
1600 Divisadero St.
San Francisco, California 94115
(415) 567-6600

Executive Director: William H. Gurtner

Admissions: Nadine Brown

Affiliation: University of California, San Francisco.

Emphasis: Radiation therapy, chemotherapy, and immunotherapy treatment facilities available. Specializes in treatment of melanoma.

Equipment:

DIAGNOSTIC
CAT body scanner
Mammography
Nuclear medicine
Angiography
Ultrasound
Gamma camera

THERAPEUTIC
25 meV linear accelerator
Cobalt
Betatron
Dosimetry
Cesium 137
Orthovoltage X-ray
Superficial X-ray
Radium
Iridium

Cancer Personnel:

M.D. AND M.D./Ph.D.:   14
TECHNICAL PERSONNEL: 8
   TOTAL: 47

NURSES: 25

Cancer Patient Statistics:

BEDS: 100
NO. IN-PATIENTS: 1500
AVERAGE STAY: 5

NO. OUT-PATIENTS: 22,000
NEW PATIENTS: 850

Cancer Library: 2000 volumes.

Tumor Registry.

Professional Education: Fellowship program in medical oncology. Ten continuing education conferences and joint training program for radiation oncologists with University of California and Ralph K. Davies Medical Center.

California: *San Francisco*

St. Mary's Hospital and Medical Center
450 Stanyan St.
San Francisco, California 94117
(415) 668-1000

President and Administrator: Sister Anthony Marie

Admissions: Sister May Louise

Affiliation: The Sisters of Mercy (five hospitals in California and Arizona).

Emphasis: Primary treatment modalities in radiation oncology.

Equipment:

DIAGNOSTIC

Nuclear medicine
Gamma camera
Scintillation camera
Mammography
Ultrasound

THERAPEUTIC

Linear accelerator
Cesium 137
Radium
Iridium
Iodine 125
Superficial X-ray

Cancer Library.

Tumor Registry.

Professional Education: Resident training in radiotherapy and medical oncology.

California: *Stanford*

Stanford University Medical Center and Hospital
Stanford, California 94305
(415) 497-2300

Chief of Staff: Lawrence G. Crowley, M.D., Deputy Dean of the Medical Center

Affiliations: V.A. Hospital, Palo Alto; Valley Medical Center, Santa Clara; Children's Hospital at Stanford.

Emphasis: Center is comprised of Stanford University Hospital and School of Medicine. Stanford radiologists and physicists developed first accelerator for medical use in the Western Hemisphere. Outstanding research programs in Hodgkin disease and lymphomas with therapy combination of radiotherapy and chemotherapy. One of the leaders in the field of prostatic cancer and in cancer of the eye, throat, lung, kidney, bladder, uterus, and brain.

Equipment:

DIAGNOSTIC

Nuclear medicine
CAT body scanner
CT head scanner
Angiography
Ultrasound
Gamma camera
Electron microscope
Fluoroscope
Endoscope
Bronchoscope
Tomography

THERAPEUTIC

4meV linear accelerator
6meV linear accelerator
10meV linear accelerator
250 kVP orthovoltage X-ray
Cesium
Radium
Dosimetry
Superficial X-ray
Simulator
Hyperthermia (research)

Cancer Personnel: *

M.D. AND M.D./Ph.D.:   81   TECHNICAL PERSONNEL: 63
Ph.D.:   6

Cancer Patient Statistics: *

NO. IN-PATIENTS: 66,336   NO. OUT-PATIENTS: 41,328

Cancer Library.

Tumor Registry.

Professional Education: Residency training in all subspecialties. Annual post-graduate multidisciplinary course in clinical therapy for all physicians and surgeons in neoplastic diseases.

California: *Torrence*

Los Angeles County Harbor General Hospital
1000 W. Carson St.
Torrence, California 90509
(213) 533–2101

Director: Jerome Block, M.D.

Affiliation: University of California, Los Angeles.

Emphasis: Comprehensive cancer treatment with research in genetics, tumor markers, and endocrinologic tumors. Clinical pharmacology (specialized center).

Equipment:

DIAGNOSTIC	THERAPEUTIC
Nuclear medicine	Cobalt 60
Gamma camera	Linear accelerator
CAT scanner	Superficial X-ray
Thermography	Orthovoltage X-ray
Ultrasound	Radium
Scintillation camera	Simulator
	Dosimetry

Cancer Personnel:

M.D. AND M.D./Ph.D.:   10 ft   TECHNICAL PERSONNEL: 10 ft
Ph.D.:   5 pt   NURSES: 7 ft
     TOTAL: 27 full-time, 5 part-time

*Mostly cancer oriented.

Cancer Patient Statistics:

BEDS: 500 (unrestricted)   NO. OUT-PATIENTS: 100/wk
NO. IN-PATIENTS: 50   NEW PATIENTS: 500

Cancer Library.

Tumor Registry.

Professional Education: With UCLA and USC. Seminars and conferences in oncology.

Colorado: *Denver*

Fitzsimons Army Medical Center
Peoria and E. Colfax Sts.
Denver, Colorado 80240
(303) 341–8241

Director: Philip A. Deffer, M.D., Brig. Gen.

Admissions: Maj. Winslow F. Borzotra, M.S.C.

Affiliation: University of Colorado Medical Center.

Emphasis: Medical oncology and radiotherapy and chemotherapy treatment facilities. Care limited to active duty military personnel, retired military personnel, and dependents of active duty or retired military personnel.

Equipment:

DIAGNOSTIC   THERAPEUTIC
CAT scanner   Cobalt
Nuclear medicine   Conventional X-ray equipment
Arteriography

Cancer Personnel:

M.D. AND M.D./Ph.D.:   5

Cancer Patient Statistics:

BEDS: unrestricted (hosp. cap. 538)   AVERAGE STAY: 18
NO. IN-PATIENTS: 1117   NO. OUT-PATIENTS: 8400

Library: 30,000 volumes.

Tumor Registry.

Professional Education: Resident training in medical oncology and hematology.

Connecticut: *Bridgeport*

Bridgeport Hospital
267 Grant St.
Bridgeport, Connecticut 06602
(203) 384–3000

Admissions: Henry Tracy
 Clarence W. Bushnell, Exec. V.P.

Affiliations: Yale University; Memorial Sloan-Kettering Cancer Center.

Emphasis: Radiotherapy, chemotherapy. Specialized rehabilitation programs in breast cancer and ostomy.

Equipment:

DIAGNOSTIC	THERAPEUTIC
Mammography	Cobalt 60
CAT scanner	Conventional X-ray equipment
Proctosigmoidoscope	

Tumor Registry.

Connecticut: *Bridgeport*

St. Vincent's Medical Center
2800 Main St.
Bridgeport, Connecticut 06606
(203) 576–6000

President: William J. Riordan

Admissions: Lucia Mannello

Affiliation: Yale University School of Medicine.

Emphasis: Multidisciplinary facility with major radiation oncology and chemotherapy departments. Cooperative Computer Treatment Planning with Memorial Sloan-Kettering Cancer Center for determination of portal size and depth dose of radiation therapy. Cancer unit for total treatment including psychosocial, clerical, diagnostic, and therapeutic.

Equipment:

DIAGNOSTIC	THERAPEUTIC
Mammography	4meV linear accelerator
Nuclear medicine	300,000kV auxilliary therapy unit
CAT body scanner	Cesium
Ultrasound	Dosimetry
Angiography	Orthovoltage X-ray

DIAGNOSTIC	THERAPEUTIC
Xeroradiography	Cobalt
Gamma cameras (2)	

Cancer Personnel:

M.D. AND M.D./Ph.D.: 50 NURSES: 40
TECHNICAL PERSONNEL: 36

Cancer Patient Statistics:

BEDS: 30 (in new unit) AVERAGE COST: $116.00
NO. IN-PATIENTS: 700 NEW PATIENTS: 500
NO. OUT-PATIENTS: 1700

Cancer Library: 5500 volumes.

Tumor Registry.

Professional Education: Accredited continuing education program with Yale University including residency program in various subspecialties. Weekly lectures on all subspecialties with speakers from surrounding medical education centers.

Connecticut: *Hartford*

Hartford Hospital
80 Seymour St.
Hartford, Connecticut 06115
(203) 524–3011

President and Executive Director: John K. Springer

Admissions: Selina Daley

Affiliations: University of Connecticut; University of Hartford; Hartford College for Women.

Emphasis: Comprehensive cancer treatment with extensive diagnostic and therapeutic equipment. One thousand unrestricted beds.

Equipment:

DIAGNOSTIC	THERAPEUTIC
Conventional x-ray equipment	18meV linear accelerator
	4meV linear accelerator
	Orthovoltage X-ray
	Superficial X-ray
	Radium

Cancer Library.

Tumor Registry.

Delaware: *Wilmington*

Wilmington Medical Center
Box 1668
Wilmington, Delaware 19899
(302) 428–1212

President: James Harding

Director of Admissions: M. Weymouth

Affiliation: Jefferson Medical College, Philadelphia; University of Delaware, Nursing School.

Emphasis: Surgery, radiotherapy, chemotherapy, and breast cancer screening facility. Planned rectal cancer program.

Equipment:

DIAGNOSTIC	THERAPEUTIC
Conventional X-ray equipment	Linear accelerator
CAT scanner	Cobalt 60
Nuclear medicine	Supervoltage X-ray
Mammography	Superficial X-ray
Thermography	Isotopes

Cancer Personnel:

M.D. AND M.D./Ph.D.:   13

Tumor Registry.

District of Columbia

George Washington University Hospital
901 23rd St., N.W.
Washington, D.C. 20037
(202) 676–6000

Acting Medical Director: Dr. Dennis O'Leary, Dean for Clinical Affairs

Admissions: Madeline T. Robey

Affiliations: Children's Hospital National Medical Center, Washington; Washington Veterans' Hospital; Washington Hospital Center; Fairfax Hospital, Fairfax, Virginia.

Emphasis: Medical and surgical oncology and radiation therapy. Special research project in diagnostic tests for immunotherapy. $5,000,000 in research grants for basic and clinical research. Two thousand affiliated physicians in Washington, D.C. area.

Equipment:

DIAGNOSTIC
CAT scanners
Complete diagnostic facility

THERAPEUTIC
Full range of radiotherapeutic
equipment

Cancer Personnel:

M.D. AND M.D./Ph.D.: 16
Ph.D.: 4

TECHNICAL PERSONNEL: 26

Cancer Patient Statistics:

NO. IN-PATIENTS: 145/day
NO. OUT-PATIENTS: 50,000

NEW PATIENTS: 7200

Cancer Library.

Tumor Registry.

Professional Education: Continuing education programs for physicians, nurses, and residents.

District of Columbia

Howard University Hospital
2041 Georgia Ave., N.W.
Washington, D.C. 20060
(202) 745–6100

Director: Charles S. Ireland, M.D.

Admissions: Truman A. Clemons

Affiliation: Howard University College of Medicine.

Emphasis: Major radiation therapy program in Washington, D.C. area. Comprehensive cancer treatment. Conventional diagnostic and therapeutic equipment.

Professional Education: Physician training program with District of Columbia General Hospital, Norfolk Community Hospital, V.A. Hospital, Washington, D.C., Providence Hospital, Washington, D.C., and Greater S.E. Community Hospital, Washington, D.C. Only approved hospital with residence program for radiation therapy in D.C.

District of Columbia

Walter Reed Army Medical Center
Washington, D.C. 20012
(202) 576–3407

Director: Major General Robert Bernstein

Admissions: Colonel Max Hoyt

Affiliations: Georgetown University; George Washington University; Maryland University.

Emphasis: All surgical specialties, medical hematology/oncology, and radiation therapy. Participates in cooperative studies with NCI, Acute Leukemia Cooperative Group B, and Gynecologic Oncology Group.* Has full Social Service, Department of Psychiatry OT. Postmastectomy, ostomy, orthopedics, and psychosocial rehabilitation services.

Equipment:

DIAGNOSTIC	THERAPEUTIC
Various scopes	Clinac 4, Clinac 18
Scanners	Orthovoltage EMI 4
Radiographic equipment	Chronometric infusor
Phillips polytome body section	Laminar flow units
radiography	Cell separator
GE 1200 MA	
Ultrasound	
Sonography	

Cancer Personnel:

M.D. AND M.D./Ph.D.:   20 ft, 181 pt   NURSES: 3 ft, 225 pt
TECHNICAL PERSONNEL: 10 ft, 380 pt
   TOTAL: 32 full-time, 786 part-time

Cancer Patient Statistics:

BEDS: 80+   NO. OUT-PATIENTS: 12,350
NO. IN-PATIENTS: 2309   NEW PATIENTS: 735
AVERAGE STAY: 14

Tumor Registry.

Professional Education: Postgraduate training in hematologic, gynecologic, and head and neck oncology.

Florida: *Gainesville*

University of Florida, Shands Teaching Hospital and Clinics
Gainesville, Florida 32610
(904) 392–3261

Director: John Ives

*The latter two groups are members of study groups of the National Cancer Institute.

Affiliation: University of Florida.

Emphasis: Regional center for experimental immunology. Conducting research into reducing chemotherapeutic drug side effects by freezing bone marrow cells. Pediatric Cancer Program and radiation and drug therapy.

Equipment:

DIAGNOSTIC
Standard diagnostic equipment
CAT scanner

THERAPEUTIC
Complete therapeutic department
Linear accelerator

Cancer Library.

Florida: *Jacksonville*

University Hospital of Jacksonville
655 West Eighth St.
Jacksonville, Florida 32209
(904) 358-3272

Director: Michael J. Wood

Admissions: Leroy Smith

Affiliation: University of Florida College of Medicine.

Emphasis: Surgical oncology, chemotherapy in solid tumors. Breast study group, NASBP. Clinical research on immunology.

Equipment:

DIAGNOSTIC
Nuclear medicine
Ultrasound
Bronchoscopy
Electron microscope
CT scanner

THERAPEUTIC
Cobalt 60
Conventional X-ray equipment

Cancer Personnel:

M.D. AND M.D./Ph.D.: 14

NURSES: 2

Cancer Patient Statistics:

BEDS: 350 (unrestricted)
NO. OUT-PATIENTS: 9092

NEW PATIENTS: 500

Library: All cancer journals.

Tumor Registry.

Florida: *Miami Beach*

Mount Sinai Medical Center
4300 Alton Rd.
Miami Beach, Florida 33140
(305) 674-2121

Executive Director: Alvin M. Goldberg

Admissions: Gena Ford, Acting Director

Affiliation: University of Miami.

Emphasis: Major radiation therapy treatment facilities. Cooperative program conducted with Comprehensive Cancer Center for the State of Florida at the University of Miami.

Equipment:

DIAGNOSTIC	THERAPEUTIC
Mammography	13meV linear accelerator
Nuclear medicine	4meV linear accelerator
CAT body and head scanners	Cobalt
Angiography	Radium
Ultrasound	Dosimetry
Gamma camera	Superficial X-ray
Thermography	Simulator

Cancer Personnel:

M.D. AND M.D./Ph.D.:   20

NURSES AND TECHNICAL
PERSONNEL: 23

Cancer Patient Statistics:

BEDS: 700 (unrestricted)

NEW PATIENTS: 1500 (radiotherapy only)

Cancer Library.

Tumor Registry.

Professional Education: Seminars on all subspecialties and residency programs with University of Miami.

Florida: *Tampa*

Tampa General Hospital
Davis Island
Tampa, Florida 33606
(813) 251-7271

Administrator: William E. Mathews

Admissions: Ruth Lombardo

Affiliations: University of South Florida College of Medicine.

Emphasis: Treatment including radiotherapy, chemotherapy, and surgery with diagnostic equipment—brain scanner, nuclear medicine, and mammography.

Tumor Registry.

Georgia: *Atlanta*

Grady Memorial Hospital
80 Butler St., S.E.
Atlanta, Georgia 30303
(404) 659-1212

Director: J.W. Pinkston, Jr.

Admissions: Margaret Gaines

Affiliation: Emory University School of Medicine.

Emphasis: Medical and gynecologic radiotherapy. Specialty—enterostomal therapy. Rehabilitation center. Research in clinical trials of antineoplastic agents and combined modality trials.

Equipment:

DIAGNOSTIC	THERAPEUTIC
CT body scanner	Linear accelerator
Ultrasound	Cobalt
Conventional X-ray equipment	Orthovoltage X-ray
	Simulator
	Cesium needles

Cancer Personnel:

M.D. AND M.D./Ph.D.: 3		NURSES: 20
RESEARCH NURSES: 5		

Cancer Patient Statistics:

BEDS: 17	NO. OUT-PATIENTS: 50/wk
NO. IN-PATIENTS: 14	NEW PATIENTS: 4/wk
AVERAGE STAY: 12	AVERAGE COST: $75.00

Tumor Registry.

Georgia: *Savannah*

Memorial Medical Center
4700 Waters Ave.
Savannah, Georgia 31405
(912) 355-3200

Director: James Wood

Affiliations: Medical College of Georgia; Georgia Cancer Management Network; Southeastern Chemotherapy Group.

Emphasis: Surgery, chemotherapy, radiotherapy, and immunotherapy. Clinical research on protocols. State Cancer Tumor Clinic.

Equipment:

DIAGNOSTIC	THERAPEUTIC
Conventional X-ray	Cobalt 60 (2)
Ultrasound	Isotopes
Nuclear medicine	
CT whole body scanner	
Mammography	

Cancer Personnel:

M.D. AND M.D./Ph.D.: 4	TECHNICAL PERSONNEL: 9
Ph.D.: 1	NURSES: 4
TOTAL: 18	

Cancer Patient Statistics:

BEDS: 475	NO. OUT-PATIENTS: 16,245
NO. IN-PATIENTS: 1297	NEW PATIENTS: 8771
AVERAGE STAY: 7	

Library: 100 volumes, 10 periodicals.

Tumor Registry.

Professional Education: Postgraduate training in oncology and radiotherapy.

Idaho: *Boise*

Mountain States Tumor Institute
151 East Bannock St.
Boise, Idaho 83702
(208) 386-2222

Director: Charles E. Smith, M.D.

Affiliations: Southwest Oncology Group; University of Washington; University of Utah; Boise State University.

Emphasis: Basic clinical and cancer research. Radiation therapy, chemotherapy, and psychosocial services. Satellite chemotherapy clinics and establishment of three new tumor boards. Indigent care program available.

Equipment:

DIAGNOSTIC	THERAPEUTIC
Ultrasound	Theratron 80
X-ray simulator	18meV linear accelerator
	250kVP orthovoltage X-ray
	100kVP superficial X-ray
	Cesium
	Iridium
	Beta Eye Applicator

Cancer Personnel:

M.D. AND M.D./Ph.D.: 4 ft, 2 pt	TECHNICAL PERSONNEL: 7 ft, 2 pt
Ph.D.: 1 pt	NURSES: 4 ft, 4 pt

   TOTAL: 17 full-time, 9 part-time

Cancer Patient Statistics:

NO. IN-PATIENTS: 9	NEW PATIENTS: 639
AVERAGE STAY: 5.5 days	AVERAGE COST: $89.50
NO. OUT-PATIENTS: 19,000+	

Cancer Library: 75 journals, 311 texts.

Tumor Registry.

Illinois: *Chicago*

Illinois Masonic Medical Center
836 West Wellington Ave.
Chicago, Illinois 60657
(312) 525–2300

Executive Director: Gerald W. Mungerson

Chairman, Cancer Program: C.T. Drake, M.D.

Admissions: Dolores Spence

Affiliation: University of Illinois, Abraham Lincoln School of Medicine.

Emphasis: 560-bed short-term acute care with extensive cancer program. Referral system for amputations, laryngectomy, lobectomy/pneumonectomy, mastectomy, maxillofacial and reconstructive, neck (dissection), and ostomy surgery.

Equipment:

DIAGNOSTIC
CAT scanner
Angiography
Lymphangiography
Multiphasic screening

THERAPEUTIC
Radiation therapy
Cobalt

Cancer Patient Statistics:

NO. IN-PATIENTS: 17,176/yr
AVERAGE STAY: 8.6 days

NO. NEW PATIENTS: 450/yr
AVERAGE COST: $175.00

Cancer Library: 8200 volumes.

Tumor Registry.

Illinois: *Chicago*

Mercy Hospital and Medical Center
Stevenson Expressway at King Drive
Chicago, Illinois 60616
(312) 567-2000

President: Sister Sheila Lyne, R.S.M.

Admissions: Robert L. Rolston

Affiliations: Northwestern University Medical School—ENT Service; University of Illinois College of Medicine.

Emphasis: Treatment of pelvic, breast, and colon cancer and of lymphomas. Megavoltage radiation, chemotherapy techniques. Hematology/Oncology Unit and Tumor Clinic.

Equipment:

DIAGNOSTIC
Angiography and lymphography
Isotope scanning
Ultrasonography
Mammography
Radioimmunoassay of different
    tumor markers
Assay of estrogen receptors in breast
    cancer

THERAPEUTIC
35meV betatron
Megavoltage radiation

Cancer Personnel:

M.D. AND M.D./Ph.D.:   3 ft, 4 pt,
   7 volunteer
Ph.D.:   3 ft
   TOTAL: 22 full-time, 4 part-time,
     7 volunteer

TECHNICAL PERSONNEL: 6 ft
NURSES: 10 ft

Cancer Patient Statistics:

BEDS: unrestricted
NO. IN-PATIENTS: 967
AVERAGE STAY: 18.86

NEW PATIENTS: 552
AVERAGE COST: $150.00

Library: 178 volumes, 12 journals, 106 tapes.

Tumor Registry.

Illinois: *Chicago*

Mount Sinai Hospital Medical Center of Chicago
California at 15th St.
Chicago, Illinois 60608
(312) 542–2000

Director: M.P. Westerman, M.D.

Admissions: R. Antolak

Affiliation: Rush Medical College of Rush University.

Equipment:

DIAGNOSTIC
Conventional X-ray equipment
Isotopes
CAT scanner

THERAPEUTIC
Linear accelerator
Laminar flow facility
Conventional X-ray equipment

Cancer Personnel:

M.D. AND M.D./Ph.D.:   6 ft, 3 pt
Ph.D.:   1 volunteer
   TOTAL: 15 full-time, 3 part-time,
     1 volunteer

TECHNICAL PERSONNEL: 7
NURSES: 2

Cancer Patient Statistics:

BEDS: 28
NO. IN-PATIENTS: 400
AVERAGE STAY: 15.8 days

NO. OUT-PATIENTS: 1500/yr
NEW PATIENTS: 280/yr
AVERAGE COST: $150.00

Library: 15,000 volumes.

Illinois: *Chicago*

University of Illinois Medical Center
Division of Surgical Oncology, DMP-372
840 South Wood St.
Chicago, Illinois 60612
(312) 996-6666

Director: Tapas K. Das Gupta

Admissions: Steven Sledge

Affiliations: Cook County Hospital; West Side V.A. Hospital.

Emphasis: Treatments in malignant melanoma, breast cancer, head and neck tumors, soft tissue sarcoma, advanced pelvic tumors, G.I. tract tumors, neurofibromatosis, and retroperitoneal tumors. Division of a teaching hospital.

Equipment: Conventional diagnostic and therapeutic radiologic equipment.

Cancer Personnel:

M.D. AND M.D./Ph.D.:   21
Ph.D.:   8
   TOTAL: 45+

TECHNICAL PERSONNEL: 11
NURSES: 5+

Cancer Patient Statistics:

BEDS: 656
NO. IN-PATIENTS: 1055
AVERAGE STAY: 16.1

NO. OUT-PATIENTS: 11,169
NEW PATIENTS: 650
AVERAGE COST: $164.00

Library: 333,961 volumes.

Tumor Registry.

Illinois: *Evanston*

Evanston Hospital
2650 Ridge Ave.
Evanston, Illinois 60201
(312) 492-2000

Chairman, Dept. Surgery: Edward F. Scanlon, M.D.

Affiliation: Northwestern University Medical School.

Emphasis: Development of the T-antigen in the diagnosis and treatment of carcinoma and comprehensive cancer care and rehabilitation.

Equipment:

DIAGNOSTIC
CAT scanner
Electron microscope

THERAPEUTIC
Linear accelerator
Conventional X-ray equipment

Cancer Personnel:

M.D. AND M.D./Ph.D.: 6 ft, 15 pt,
  35 volunteer
Ph.D.: 5 ft
  TOTAL: 24 full-time, 39 part-time,
  37 volunteer

TECHNICAL PERSONNEL: 5 ft, 4 pt,
  2 volunteer
NURSES: 8 ft, 20 pt

Cancer Patient Statistics:

BEDS: 650
AVERAGE STAY: 8.5
NO. OUT-PATIENTS: 200,000

NEW PATIENTS: 750
AVERAGE COST: $150.00

Library: 20,000 volumes.

Tumor Registry.

Illinois: *Evanston*

Saint Francis Hospital of Evanston
355 Ridge Ave.
Evanston, Illinois 60202
(312) 492–4000

Director: Sister M. Alfreda, O.S.F.

Admissions: Sister M. Priscilla, O.S.F.

Affiliations: Loyola University of Chicago, Stritch School of Medicine; North-western University; The Chicago Medical School.

Emphasis: Hematologic malignancies; clinical care of breast and gynecologic malignancies and clinical care of head and neck malignancies. Most active blood component therapy facility in Chicago/suburban area.

Equipment:

DIAGNOSTIC
Ultrasound
CAT scanner head and total body

THERAPEUTIC
Cobalt 60
Iodine 125 seeds

DIAGNOSTIC	THERAPEUTIC
Cell separator providing platelets, granulocytes and therapeutic procedures	18meV linear accelerator
Nuclear medicine	
Xeroradiography	
Colposcope	
X-ray—lymphangiography, venography, arteriography	

Cancer Personnel:

M.D. AND M.D./Ph.D.: 5 ft, 6 pt   TECHNICAL PERSONNEL: 10 ft
Ph.D.: 2 ft, 1 pt   NURSES: 31 ft
    TOTAL: 48 full-time, 7 part-time

Cancer Patient Statistics:

BEDS: 331   NO. OUT-PATIENTS: 1820
NO. IN-PATIENTS: 1790   NEW PATIENTS: 555
AVERAGE STAY: 15.4   AVERAGE COST: $115.00

Library: 7800 volumes.

Tumor Registry.

Illinois: *Rockford*

Rockford Memorial Hospital
2400 N. Rockton Ave.
Rockford, Illinois 61103
(815) 968–6861

Director: Hal Maysent

Admissions: Jane Holt, R.N.

Affiliations: Rockford School of Medicine, University of Illinois.

Emphasis: Comprehensive cancer treatment including immunotherapy, chemotherapy, and radiation therapy. Equipment for mammography, thermography, and total head and body scan.

Equipment:

DIAGNOSTIC	THERAPEUTIC
Nuclear medicine	Line accelerator
CAT body/head scanner	Cobalt 60
Gamma camera	Simulator
Tomography	Dosimetry

DIAGNOSTIC	THERAPEUTIC
Mammography	Radium
Ultrasound	Cesium
Scintillation camera	Iodine
	Implants

Cancer Personnel:

M.D. AND M.D./Ph.D.: 13	TECHNICAL PERSONNEL: 55
Ph.D.: 3	NURSES: 5
TOTAL: 78	

Library: 150 volumes.

Tumor Registry.

Professional Education: Weekly conferences and seminars. Resident training in family practice.

Indiana: *Indianapolis*

Indiana University Hospitals:
  James Whitcomb Riley Children's Hospital
  Robert W. Long Hospital
  University Hospital
1100 West Michigan St.
Indianapolis, Indiana 46202
(317) 635-8431

Director: Robert Hunt

Admissions: Barbara McElroy

Affiliation: Indiana University.

Emphasis: All treatment modalities with extensive radiotherapy department.

Equipment:

DIAGNOSTIC	THERAPEUTIC
Conventional range of diagnostic equipment	40meV linear accelerator
	Cobalt

Cancer Library.

Tumor Registry.

Indiana: *Indianapolis*

Methodist Hospital of Indiana, Inc.
1604 N. Capitol
Indianapolis, Indiana 46202
(317) 924-6411

President: Jack A.L. Hahn

Admissions: Bettie Sims

Affiliation: Indiana University School of Medicine.

Emphasis: Cardiovascular, renal, neurosurgical, and oncology services.

Equipment:

DIAGNOSTIC	THERAPEUTIC
Conventional X-ray equipment	10meV linear accelerator
CAT body and head scanner	Cobalt 60
Ultrasound	250 kV unit
Tomography	
Angiography	
Nuclear medicine	
Radioimmunoassay	

Cancer Personnel:

M.D. AND M.D./Ph.D.:   7 ft, 5 pt
Ph.D.:   6 ft, 2 volunteer

TECHNICAL PERSONNEL: 15 ft,
   15 volunteer
NURSES: 30 ft, 8 volunteer

   TOTAL: 58 full-time, 5 part-time,
      25 volunteer

Cancer Patient Statistics:

BEDS: unrestricted
NO. IN-PATIENTS: 110
NO. OUT-PATIENTS: 53,000/yr

NEW PATIENTS: 1500
AVERAGE COST: $113.00

Library: 11,770 volumes, 4888 journals.

Tumor Registry.

Iowa: *Iowa City**

University of Iowa Hospitals and Clinics
Iowa City, Iowa 52241
(319) 356-2731

*Note: Complete information not available at time of publication.

Director: John W. Colloton

Admissions: W.D. Goddard

Affiliations: University of Iowa; Veterans Hospital.

Emphasis: Largest academic hospital in U.S. Comprehensive cancer treatment
with full chemotherapy services. Special care program for acute leukemia and a
pediatric unit. Granular site and matched platelet unit. Hematologic unit. One
thousand, one hundred unrestricted beds.

Equipment:

DIAGNOSTIC	THERAPEUTIC
CT whole body scanner	Cobalt 60
CT head scanner	Linear accelerators (4meV and 18meV)
Angiography	Radium
Mammography	Superficial X-ray
Nuclear medicine	Simulator
	Dosimetry
	Laminar flow unit

Cancer Library.

Tumor Registry.

Kansas: *Kansas City*

University of Kansas Medical Center
Mid-America Cancer Center Program
College of Health Sciences and Hospital
Rainbow Blvd. at 39th St.
Kansas City, Kansas 66103
(913) 588-5700

Director: James T. Lowman, M.D.

Affiliations: University of Kansas (Lawrence campus); Kansas State University;
Midwest Research Institute, Kansas City, Missouri.

Emphasis: Comprehensive cancer program headquartered in a tertiary care teaching hospital with a full range of medical specialties and services. Center draws
membership from faculty/staff of Medical Center, Hospital, and affiliated institutions, utilizing their services on matters of cancer control, research, education, and patient care.

Equipment:

DIAGNOSTIC

Full range of laboratory and radiology equipment including low-dose mammography, CTM breast scanner, and thermography

THERAPEUTIC

Full range of equipment

Cancer Personnel (Center staff):

M.D. AND M.D./Ph.D.: 2 ft, 2 pt
Ph.D.: 2 ft, 5 pt

TOTAL: 17 full-time, 9 part-time, 1 volunteer

TECHNICAL PERSONNEL: 10 ft, 1 volunteer
NURSES: 3 ft, 2 pt

Cancer Patient Statistics:

BEDS: (assigned to hospital beds)
NO. IN-PATIENTS: average 60
AVERAGE STAY: 7.8

NEW PATIENTS: 1319
AVERAGE COST: $85.00

Cancer Center Library: 350 volumes.

Tumor Registry.

Professional Education: Accredited programs in clinical, surgical, pediatric, gynecologic, and radiation oncology.

Louisiana: *New Orleans*

Charity Hospital of Louisiana at New Orleans
1532 Tulane Ave.
New Orleans, Louisiana 70140
(504) 568–2311

Administrator: Elliott C. Roberts, Sr.

Affiliations: Part of Louisiana State University Medical School in New Orleans; Tulane University School of Medicine.

Emphasis: Principal teaching hospital for both medical schools. Extensive chemotherapy and perfusion programs. Tumor embolization service. Leukemia treatment and head and neck therapy. Twenty M.D./Ph.D.s on staff.

Equipment:

DIAGNOSTIC

Mammography
Arteriography
CAT total body scanner

THERAPEUTIC

Linear accelerator
Cobalt
Orthovoltage X-ray

DIAGNOSTIC	THERAPEUTIC
Ultrasound	Superficial X-ray
Nuclear medicine	Conventional radiotherapy equipment

Cancer Patient Statistics:

BEDS: 51	NEW PATIENTS: 900
NO. OUT-PATIENTS: 14,000	AVERAGE COST: $105.00

Medical Schools' Libraries.

Tumor Registry.

Maryland: *Baltimore**

University of Maryland Hospital
22 S. Greene St.
Baltimore, Maryland 20201
(301) 528-6975

Director: Bruce G. McFadden

Admissions: John Smalley

Emphasis: A multidisciplinary approach to cancer treatment and rehabilitation. Total cancer care and treatment programs designed with review and psychosocial rehabilitation. Full range of diagnostic and therapeutic equipment. One thousand beds, unrestricted.

Library: Part of Health Sciences Library.

Tumor Registry.

Professional Education: Postgraduate education in surgical oncology, chemotherapy, radiology, diagnosis, and nuclear medicine with special visiting experts.

Maryland: *Bethesda*

National Naval Medical Center
Bethesda, Maryland 20014
(292) 295-0274

Director: RADM J.T. Horgan

Admissions: Capt. Q.E. Crews

Emphasis: Surgery, radiation therapy, chemotherapy, immunotherapy, physical therapy.

*Note: Complete information not available at time of publication.

Equipment:

DIAGNOSTIC
Mammography
Ultrasound
CAT scanner

THERAPEUTIC
Cobalt 60
Maxitron 250
Simulator

Cancer Personnel:

M.D. AND M.D./Ph.D.: 12
Ph.D.: 1
  TOTAL: 18

TECHNICAL PERSONNEL: 3
NURSES: 1

Cancer Patient Statistics:

NO. IN-PATIENTS: 1200
AVERAGE STAY: 14 days

NO. OUT-PATIENTS: 18,000
NEW PATIENTS: 425

Library: 40,000 volumes.

Tumor Registry.

Massachusetts: *Boston*

Beth Israel Hospital
330 Brookline Ave.
Boston, Massachusetts 02215
(617) 735-2000

Director: Mitchell T. Rabkin, M.D.

Affiliations: Harvard Medical School; Sidney Farber Cancer Center; Joint Center for Radiation Therapy, Harvard; Children's Hospital Medical Center.

Emphasis: Multidisciplinary facility for hematology, oncology, and treatment of solid tumors. Surgical Department emphasis on gastroenterologic and endocrine surgery. Kidney Transplant Unit in renal malignancies.

Equipment:

DIAGNOSTIC
Mammography
Nuclear medicine
CT head scanner (Sidney Farber
  Cancer Center)
Angiography
Ultrasound
Gamma camera
Thermography

THERAPEUTIC
6meV linear accelerator
Orthovoltage X-ray
Dosimetry
Supervoltage X-ray
Cobalt
Betatron
Cesium

Cancer Personnel:

> M.D. AND M.D./Ph.D.: 21 oncologic
> specialists on staff

Cancer Patient Statistics:

> BEDS: 432 (unrestricted)

Cancer Library.

Tumor Registry.

Professional Education: Major teaching hospital for Harvard Medical School. Residency programs in all subspecialties. Full range of seminar programs for local physicians.

Massachusetts: *Boston*

Children's Hospital Medical Center
300 Longwood Ave.
Boston, Massachusetts 02115
(617) 734-6000

President: David Werner

Admissions: Terrence Ford

Affiliation: Harvard Medical School.

Emphasis: Joint program in hematology and oncology with Sidney Farber Cancer Center. Act as in-patient hospital for child care cases. Specializes in diagnosis and treatment of pediatric cancer.

Equipment:

DIAGNOSTIC	THERAPEUTIC
Ultrasound	Complete radiation therapy depart-
Nuclear medicine	ment plus additional therapeutic
Polytome	equipment
Angiography	

Cancer Library.

Tumor Registry.

Professional Education: Teaching Hospital for Harvard Medical School; graduate degree program for radiologic technicians with Northeastern University. Continuing education in nursing. Regional seminars on pediatric and cardiatric specialties.

Massachusetts: *Boston*

New England Deaconess Hospital
185 Pilgrim Rd.
Boston, Massachusetts 02215
(617) 734-7000

Scientific Director: William V. McDermott, M.D.

Affiliations: Harvard Medical School; Sidney Farber Cancer Center; Lahey Clinic
   Foundation.

Emphasis: Investigations in biochemistry (metabolic mechanisms of transplanted
   rodent tumors); electron microscopy (osteogenesis at the light and microscopic
   levels); experimental pathology (radiation carcinogenesis, quantitation of dose
   effect relationships, parabiosis); growth lab, host reactions (dedifferentiating
   effect of transplanted tumor in young rats); transplantation and immunology
   (introduction of specific immunologic enhancement to tissue allografts,
   immunologic detection of cancer of the bladder, immunologic detection of
   human breast cancer, BCG stimulation of mice bearing murine fibrosarcomas,
   immunology of experimental ovarian carcinoma in fibrosarcomas in mice). Clinical investigations include lymphocyte reactivity to tumor antigens, effects of
   hyperalimentation of immunocompetence in cancer patients, immunologic
   status of patients with breast cancer and melanoma, relationship between oral
   contraceptive use and breast cancer, epidemiologic aspects of cancer of the pancreas, the treatment of hepatocellular carcinoma with adreamycin, lymphangiography with radioiodinated monospecific heterologous Hodgkin antiserum in the
   diagnosis of Hodgkin disease, the efficacy of Bleomycin by prolonged arterial
   infusion in the treatment of advanced cancers as part of a national oncology
   task force, normal and pathologic physiology of tumor markers produced by the
   liver, biliary tract, and pancreas in benign and malignant digestive diseases, in-
   appropriate immunoregulatory sialoglobulins in cancer, the effectiveness of
   various chemotherapeutic regimens in the treatment of acute myelogenous leukemia under the aegis of the national cooperative study.

Equipment:

DIAGNOSTIC	THERAPEUTIC
Conventional range of diagnostic equipment	4meV linear accelerator
	12meV linear accelerator
	Dynamic treatment couch

Cancer Personnel:

M.D. AND M.D./Ph.D.: 41	TECHNICAL PERSONNEL: 123
Ph.D.: 21	NURSES: 85
TOTAL: 270	

Cancer Patient Statistics:

BEDS: 150   NO. OUT-PATIENTS: 6633 (visits)

NO. IN-PATIENTS: 4309 NEW PATIENTS: 1100
AVERAGE STAY: 14.9

Cancer Library: 1700 volumes, 54 periodicals.

Tumor Registry.

Professional Education: Residency and internship programs. Pap screening test collaborative effort between American Cancer Society (Massachusetts Division) and Department of Pathology.

Massachusetts: *Boston*

Peter Bent Brigham Hospital
721 Huntington Ave.
Boston, Massachusetts 02115
(617) 732–6000

Director: William Hassan, M.D.

Admissions: Sylvia Hanrahan

Affiliations: Harvard Medical School; Sidney Farber Cancer Center; Children's Hospital Medical Center; Massachusetts General Hospital; Beth Israel Hospital; New England Deaconess Hospital; Joslin Diabetes Foundation.

Emphasis: Major facility with comprehensive chemotherapy and radiation therapy departments. NCI funded on joint programs with Sidney Farber Cancer Center.

Equipment:

DIAGNOSTIC	THERAPEUTIC
Mammography	12meV linear accelerator
CAT body scanner	Cobalt
CAT head scanner	Cesium
Nuclear medicine	Dosimetry
Angiography	Orthovoltage X-ray
Ultrasound	Supervoltage X-ray
Gamma camera	

Cancer Personnel:

M.D. AND M.D./Ph.D.: 35–40 TECHNICAL PERSONNEL: 100
Ph.D.: 12

Cancer Patient Statistics:

BEDS: 768

Cancer Library: Countway Library, Harvard Medical School.

Tumor Registry.

Professional Education: Seminars on subspecialties and postgraduate seminars on all major specialties and subspecialties.

Massachusetts: *Boston*

Tufts-New England Medical Center Cancer Center
171 Harrison Ave.
Boston, Massachusetts 02111
(617) 956–5406

Director: Douglas J. Marchant, M.D.

Admissions: William Costello

Affiliation: Tufts University School of Medicine.

Emphasis: Gynecologic and pediatric oncology. Multidisciplinary treatment and Rehabilitation Institute and Psycho-Social Clinics. New England Network Demonstration Project Breast Cancer.

Equipment:

DIAGNOSTIC	THERAPEUTIC
Conventional X-ray equipment	High voltage radiation therapy
Arteriography	Cobalt 60
CAT scanners	Betatron
Mammography	Superficial X-ray
Nuclear medicine	Radium
Ultrasound	

Tumor Registry.

Massachusetts: *Boston*

University Hospital, Boston University Cancer Research Center
75 E. Newton St.
Boston, Massachusetts 02118
(617) 247–5000

Directors: John Betjemann, S. Cooperband, M.D.

Affiliation: Boston University Medical School.

Emphasis: All areas of specialty with the exception of pediatric oncology. Rehabilitation specialty in voice and ostomy treatment. Development of a laser cystoscope for treatment of bladder cancer and new drug regimen for treatment of lung cancer. Cancer program approved by American College of Surgeons.

Equipment:

DIAGNOSTIC

All routine procedures
Colonoscope
CAT scanner
Immunodiagnosis
Radioisotopes

THERAPEUTIC

All routine procedures
Leukophoresis
Laminar flow beds
Betatron
Cobalt

Cancer Personnel:

M.D. AND M.D./Ph.D.: 28 ft, 19 pt
Ph.D.: 7 ft, 16 pt
   TOTAL: 124 full-time, 47 part-time

TECHNICAL PERSONNEL: 44 ft, 12 pt
NURSES: 45 ft

Cancer Patient Statistics:

BEDS: 70
NO. IN-PATIENTS: 1589
AVERAGE STAY: 14

NO. OUT-PATIENTS: 18,609
NEW PATIENTS: 800
AVERAGE COST: $163.00

Library: 78,500 volumes.

Tumor Registry.

Massachusetts: *Walpole*

Pondville Hospital
Box 111
Walpole, Massachusetts 02081
(617) 668–0385

Director: James E. Cassidy

Admissions: Ronald Messer, M.D.

Affiliations: Tufts-New England Medical Center; Boston University Medical School; Massachusetts General Hospital; University of Massachusetts, Medical School.

Emphasis: Comprehensive treatment with specialties in surgery, radiotherapy, chemotherapy, and immunotherapy treatment. Cancer research and rehabilitation program.

Equipment:

DIAGNOSTIC

Siemen special procedure unit
Siemen multiplanograph
Fluoroscopy units

THERAPEUTIC

Linear accelerator
45meV betatron
Superficial X-ray

Cancer Personnel:

M.D. AND M.D./Ph.D.: 12 ft, 60 pt
Ph.D.: 1 ft

TECHNICAL PERSONNEL: 41 ft, 5 pt,
5 volunteer

NURSES: 90 ft, 28 pt, 5 volunteer

TOTAL: 144 full-time, 93 part-time,
10 volunteer

Cancer Patient Statistics:

BEDS: 104
NO. IN-PATIENTS: 1276
AVERAGE STAY: 18

NO. OUT-PATIENTS: 25,000
NEW PATIENTS: 915
AVERAGE COST: $211.90

Library: 3000 volumes.

Tumor Registry.

Michigan: *Ann Arbor*

St. Joseph Mercy Hospital
5301 East Huron River Drive
Ann Arbor, Michigan 48106
(313) 572-3456

Executive Director: Robert Laverty

Affiliation: University of Michigan.

Equipment:

DIAGNOSTIC
CAT body scanner
Mammography
Nuclear medicine
Angiography
Ultrasound
Gamma camera
Fluoroscope
Endoscope
Bronchoscope

THERAPEUTIC*
4meV linear accelerator

Cancer Library.

Tumor Registry.

*Many patients are referred, on an individual basis, to the University of Michigan.

Michigan: *Dearborn*

Oakwood Hospital
18101 Oakwood Blvd.
Dearborn, Michigan 48124
(313) 336–3000

Director: Gerald Fitzgerald

Admissions: Genevieve Phelps

Affiliations: Metropolitan Detroit Cancer Control Program; University of Michigan; Wayne State University; Madonna College; Michigan Cancer Foundation.

Emphasis: Oncology-hematology, chemotherapy, and radiotherapy. Self-Help Living with Cancer Group. Hyperlipid therapy as an adjuvant to therapy. Multidisciplinary conferences and participation in Metropolitan Detroit Cancer Control Program (five-year research project).

Equipment:

DIAGNOSTIC	THERAPEUTIC
CAT scanner	Cobalt 60
Mammography	Superficial X-ray
Nuclear medicine	Linear accelerator
Radiochemistry: blood and plasma volume, RBC survival	Cesium

Cancer Personnel:

M.D. AND M.D./Ph.D.:   1 ft, 2 pt, 1 volunteer   NURSES: 9 ft, 3 pt
      TOTAL: 10 full-time, 5 part-time, 1 volunteer

Cancer Patient Statistics:

BEDS: 15	NO. OUT-PATIENTS: 11,673
NO. IN-PATIENTS: 825	NEW PATIENTS: 448
AVERAGE STAY: 15.2	AVERAGE COST: $120.00

Library: 13,000 volumes.

Tumor Registry.

Michigan: *Detroit*

Henry Ford Hospital
2799 West Grand Blvd.
Detroit, Michigan 48202
(313) 876–1846

Chief, Division of Oncology: Robert W. Talley, M.D.

Emphasis: Experimental chemotherapy—12 transplantable tumor lines. Studies in multiple drugs, tissue culture of primary human tumors, chemotherapy in tissue culture, immunology of murine tumors, virus isolation in selected tumors, biochemistry of selected human neoplasms, electron microscopy of human and murine neoplasms, and scanning electron microscopy of tissue cultures. Activities in karyotyping human malignant neoplasms, fixed enzyme chemotherapy, radiation-induced rodent mammary tumors, radiation biology of C3H mammary tumors, primary surgical therapy of any human neoplasm, and curative and palliative radiotherapy of any human neoplasm. Offers ostomy advice, facial prosthesis, physical medicine for amputees, social service for cancer patients, combination radiotherapy of human neoplasms, immunologic therapy of selected human neoplasms, and hormonal therapy for breast cancer. Basic research in identification of human tumor antigens, identification of hormonal bending properties in breast and prostatic cancer, and genetic studies of selected human neoplasms. Laboratory tests available with radiologic exams and xeroradiography.

Equipment: All conventional diagnostic and therapeutic equipment.

Cancer Personnel:

M.D. AND M.D./Ph.D.: 150	TECHNICAL PERSONNEL: 50
Ph.D.: 20	NURSES: 300
TOTAL: 520	

Cancer Patient Statistics:

BEDS: 150	NEW PATIENTS: 1350
AVERAGE STAY: 17	

Cancer Library: 3307 volumes, 1521 periodicals.

Tumor Registry.

Professional Education: Medical and surgical oncology training in all applicable specialties for Medical House Officers. Tumor Conference, Gynecology Tumor Conference, G.U. Tumor Conference and Radiotherapy-Oncology Conference monthly. Oncology Research Conference, Head and Neck Tumor Conference, Hematology and Oncology Clinic Conference weekly.

Michigan: *Flint*

Hurley Medical Center
6th and Begole St.
Flint, Michigan 48502
(313) 766-0000

Director: Richard C. Schripsema

Admissions: James Smith

Affiliations: M.S.U. Comprehensive Cancer Center.

Emphasis: Radiation therapy, medical oncology–O.P., chemotherapy, surgical oncology. Full ambulatory diagnostic and treatment capability.

Equipment:

DIAGNOSTIC	THERAPEUTIC
CAT scanner	Linear accelerator
Ultrasound	Cobalt
Nuclear medicine	Superficial X-ray
Fiberoptic endoscopy	

Cancer Personnel:

M.D. AND M.D./Ph.D.:   3 ft, 11 pt, 7 volunteer
Ph.D.:   1 ft, 1 pt
   TOTAL: 63 full-time, 27 part-time, 7 volunteer

TECHNICAL PERSONNEL: 33 ft, 6 pt
NURSES: 26 ft, 9 pt

Cancer Patient Statistics:

BEDS: 420
NO. IN-PATIENTS: 760
AVERAGE STAY: 18.7

NO. OUT-PATIENTS: 10,500
NEW PATIENTS: 572
AVERAGE COST: $134.00

Library: 5234 volumes, 417 journals.

Tumor Registry.

Michigan: *Grand Rapids*

Grand Rapids Clinical Oncology Program
   Blodgett Memorial Medical Center
   Butterworth Hospital
   St. Mary's Hospital
100 Michigan N.E.
Grand Rapids, Michigan 49503
(616) 774–1230

Director: Thomas C. Tucker

Affiliations: A community cancer center for all local acute care hospitals. It includes Ferguson-Droste-Ferguson Hospital (colon/rectum specialty) and Grand Rapids Osteopathic Hospital.

Emphasis: The Grand Rapids Clinical Oncology Program, funded by the National

Cancer Institute as a Model Community Cancer Center, serves the twelve-county Grand Rapids area. It guides the management of cancer patients through 14 city-wide, multidisciplinary, multi-institutional site committees (brain, breast, bone, colon and rectum, endocrine gynecologic, head and neck, hematologic, lung, pediatric solid tumors, skin, soft tissue sarcomas, upper digestive system, and urogenital). 118 physicians serve on one or more of the site committees and see 70% to 80% of all cancer patients managed in the consortium hospitals. Participating physicians have designed 45 site-specific tumor models, approved by a peer review process and the National Cancer Institute. Sophisticated care units are available in all hospitals and annual lifetime follow-up procedures are conducted on all patients. Special cancer problems are treated through a national referral program and psychosocial rehabilitation programs are available for patients and families.

Equipment: *

DIAGNOSTIC	THERAPEUTIC
Rectilinear and scintillation cameras	Linear accelerators
CAT scanners	Varian Clinic IV
Ultrasound	Superficial X-ray
	Isotopes

Cancer Personnel:

M.D. AND M.D./Ph.D.: 512	TECHNICAL PERSONNEL: 100 approx.
Ph.D.: 2	NURSES: 2000 approx.
TOTAL: 2514	

Cancer Patient Statistics:

BEDS: 1661	NO. OUT-PATIENTS: 5632
NO. IN-PATIENTS: 100 (treated per day)	NEW PATIENTS: 2500
AVERAGE STAY: 8.7	

Library: 10,000 (Blodgett).

Tumor Registry: Computerized for all participating hospitals.

Professional Education: Abstracts from 4500 journals, texts, and so forth reviewed monthly for information applicable to program. Experts in various disciplines brought to community for educational programs and consultation.

Michigan: *Pontiac*

St. Joseph Mercy Hospital
900 Woodward Ave.
Pontiac, Michigan 48053
(313) 858-3000

*Sophisticated range of equipment available at the consortium hospitals.

Administrator: Michael R. Schwartz

Admissions: Sister Mary Juliana Gust R.S.M.

Affiliations: University of Michigan; Wayne State University; Oakland University; Oakland Community College; Base for Pontiac Unit Mercy School of Nursing.

Emphasis: General cancer care with emphasis on chemotherapy. Cancer registry for all patients. Closed-circuit television presents films on cancer prevention for patients. Colostomy nurse and two oncologists on staff. Reach To Recovery Program. Psychosocial support. Access to investigational drugs from NCI.

Equipment:

DIAGNOSTIC	THERAPEUTIC
Nuclear medicine	Cesium-137
CAT scanner	
Gamma camera	
Scintillation unit	
Angiography	
Mammography	
Ultrasound	

Cancer Patient Statistics:

BEDS: 500 total (unrestricted)	NEW PATIENTS: 39
NO. IN-PATIENTS: 620	AVERAGE COST: $200.00
AVERAGE STAY: 12.2	

Cancer Library.

Tumor Registry.

Professional Education: Continuing Education seminars on chemotherapeutic agents. Training in all aspects of psychosocial support programs.

Minnesota: *Minneapolis*

Masonic Memorial Cancer Center
University of Minnesota, Health Sciences Center
University of Minnesota
Minneapolis, Minnesota 55455
(612) 373-4303

Director of Health Science Affairs: Lyle French

Affiliations: Minneapolis Veterans' Administration Hospital; St. Paul Ramsey Hospital; Hennepin County Hospital.

Emphasis: Medical oncology, surgery, therapeutic radiology, pediatric oncology, pathology, laboratory medicine, gynecology, otolaryngology. Cancer Detection Center. Research in role of estrogen receptors in breast cancer, immunotherapy, viral research, bone marrow transplantation, and new chemicals.

Equipment:

DIAGNOSTIC
CAT scanner
Echography
Radioactive isotopes
Pathology laboratory
Colonoscopy
Endoscopy

THERAPEUTIC
Linear accelerator
Cobalt

Cancer Patient Statistics:

BEDS: 608
AVERAGE STAY: 8 days

NO. OUT-PATIENTS: 53,332
NEW PATIENTS: 1316

Library: 255,195 volumes.

Tumor Registry.

Mississippi: *Jackson**

The University Hospital at the University of Mississippi Medical Center
2500 N. State St.
Jackson, Mississippi 39216
(601) 968-3500

Vice-Chancellor for Health Affairs: Norman C. Nelsen, M.D.

Affiliation: University of Mississippi.

Cancer Library.

Tumor Registry.

Missouri: *Columbia*

Ellis Fischel State Cancer Hospital
115 Business Loop, 70 West
Columbia, Missouri 65201
(314) 449-2711

Director: Virgil T. Yates

Affiliation: University of Missouri, Washington University, Missouri Division of Health.

*Note: Complete information not available at time of publication.

Emphasis: Specializes in skin, breast, and lung cancers. Clinical research in breast cancer detection. Maxillofacial rehabilitation.

Equipment:

DIAGNOSTIC
X-ray units
Mammography (2)
Thermography

THERAPEUTIC
Linear accelerator
Cobalt 60 (2)
Orthovoltage X-ray
Simulator
Radium
Iridium
Isotopes

Cancer Personnel:

M.D. AND M.D./Ph.D.: 13
Ph.D.: 2
TOTAL: 92

TECHNICAL PERSONNEL: 20
NURSES: 57

Cancer Patient Statistics:

BEDS: 113
NO. IN-PATIENTS: 2036
AVERAGE STAY: 17

NO. OUT-PATIENTS: 10,621
AVERAGE COST: $162.00

Library: 6500 volumes, 200 periodicals.

Tumor Registry.

Professional Education: Postgraduate training in radiology, surgery, pathology, and medical physics.

Missouri: *Kansas City**

St. Luke's Hospital of Kansas City
Wornall Rd. and 44th St.
Kansas City, Missouri 64111
(816) 932–2000

Executive Director: Charles C. Lindstrom.

Admissions: Irene Welch

Emphasis: General cancer care including chemotherapy and radiotherapy. Cancer detection program.

Cancer Library.

Tumor Registry.

*Note: Complete information not available at time of publication.

Missouri: *St. Louis*

Barnes Hospital
Barnes Hospital Plaza
St. Louis, Missouri 63110
(314) 454-2000

President: Robert E. Frank

Affiliations: Washington University School of Medicine; Mallinckrodt Institute of
Radiology; St. Louis Children's Hospital.

Emphasis: Radiation oncology, medicine, surgery, otolaryngology, and gynecology are areas of specialization.

Equipment:

DIAGNOSTIC	THERAPEUTIC
Conventional X-ray equipment	Cobalt 60
	Betatron
	Linear accelerators
	Radioactive sources, iridium-192, californium-252
	Hyperthermia

Cancer Personnel:

M.D. AND M.D./Ph.D.:   25 ft, 5 pt   TECHNICAL PERSONNEL: 75
Ph.D.:   28
   TOTAL: 128 full-time, 5 part-time

Tumor Registry: Radiation oncology, otolaryngology, and gynecology in Mallinckrodt Institute.

Missouri: *St. Louis*

St. Mary's Health Center
6420 Clayton Rd.
St. Louis, Missouri 63117
(314) 644-3000

Director: Sister Betty Brucker, S.S.M.

Admissions: Gerald Bermann

Affiliation: St. Louis University.

Emphasis: Basic cancer and clinical research with rehabilitation facility.

Equipment:

DIAGNOSTIC
CAT scanner
Ultrasound
Conventional X-ray equipment

THERAPEUTIC
Superficial X-ray
Deep therapy
Cobalt
Computer planning accessibility

Cancer Personnel:

M.D. AND M.D./Ph.D.: 3 pt
Ph.D.: 1 ft
   TOTAL: 6 full-time, 5 part-time

TECHNICAL PERSONNEL: 3 ft
NURSES: 2 ft, 2 pt

Cancer Patient Statistics:

BEDS: 200
NEW PATIENTS: 900

AVERAGE COST: $85.00

Library: 10,367 volumes and journals.

Tumor Registry.

Nebraska: *Omaha*

Clinical Cancer Center, University of Nebraska Hospital and Clinics
University of Nebraska Medical Center
42nd and Dewey Ave.
Omaha, Nebraska 68105
(402) 541–4802

Director: John F. Foley, M.D.

Emphasis: Clinical research in hyperthermia, surgery, radiation, chemotherapy.

Equipment:

DIAGNOSTIC
CAT scanner
Ultrasound
Radioactive isotopes

THERAPEUTIC
Hyperthermia
Electron beam
Conventional X-ray

Cancer Personnel:

M.D. AND M.D./Ph.D.: 8 ft, 3 pt
TECHNICAL PERSONNEL: 8 ft

NURSES: 3 ft

Cancer Patient Statistics:

BEDS: 50
NO. IN-PATIENTS: 716

NO. OUT-PATIENTS: 5362 (oncology),
   10,920 (radiation)

AVERAGE STAY: 10   NEW PATIENTS: 612
                                          AVERAGE COST: $84.00

Library: 157,000 volumes in campus-wide Library of Medicine.

Tumor Registry.

New Hampshire: *Hanover*

Mary Hitchcock Memorial Hospital
2 Maynard St.
Hanover, New Hampshire 03755
(603) 643–4000

Director: James W. Varnum

Admissions: Annelies Ostler

Affiliations: Dartmouth Medical School; Veterans' Administration Hospital in
   White River Junction; Hitchcock Medical Center (Dartmouth).

Emphasis: Comprehensive cancer treatment. First patient support programs.
   Norris-Cotton Cancer Center. Also part of New Hampshire Breast Cancer Project.
   Recipient of grants for cancer control. Chemotherapy and radiotherapy facilities.
   Comprehensive rehabilitation program.

Equipment:

DIAGNOSTIC   THERAPEUTIC
Standard diagnostic equipment   Standard therapeutic equipment

Cancer Patient Statistics:

BEDS: 420   NO. OUT-PATIENTS: 9195
NO. IN-PATIENTS: 2824   NEW PATIENTS: 700
AVERAGE STAY: 12

Cancer Library.

Tumor Registry.

New Jersey: *Livingston*

St. Barnabas Medical Center
Old Short Hills Rd.
Livingston, New Jersey 07039
(201) 533–5000

Director: John D. Phillips, M.H.A.

Admissions: Doris Bardusch

Affiliation: Memorial Sloan-Kettering Cancer Center Consortium.

Emphasis: Comprehensive cancer treatment program with specialties in rehabilitation and research.

Equipment:

DIAGNOSTIC
Endoscope
Radioisotopes
Anatomic/clinical pathology
Conventional X-ray equipment

THERAPEUTIC
Orthovoltage X-ray
Cobalt 60
Linear accelerator
Hyperbaric unit

Cancer Patient Statistics:

BEDS: 735 (unrestricted)
NO. IN-PATIENTS: 4400
AVERAGE STAY: 16

NO. OUT-PATIENTS: 23,893
NEW PATIENTS: 1400
AVERAGE COST: $120.00

Library: 7000 volumes.

Tumor Registry.

New Jersey: *Long Branch*

Monmouth Medical Center
300 Second Ave.
Long Branch, New Jersey 07740
(201) 222-5200

Executive Director: Felix Pilla

Admissions: Mary Pickett

Affiliation: The Hahnemann Medical College.

Emphasis: Full range of treatment with emphasis on radiotherapy and chemotherapy. Offers major Rehabilitation Department.

Equipment:

DIAGNOSTIC
CAT body scanner
Nuclear medicine
Ultrasound
Gamma camera
Angiography
Mammography

THERAPEUTIC
6meV linear accelerator
Orthovoltage X-ray
Superficial X-ray
2meV Van de Graaff generator

Cancer Patient Statistics:

BEDS: 510 (unrestricted)   NEW PATIENTS: 350
NO. OUT-PATIENTS: 4150

Cancer Library.

Tumor Registry.

Professional Education: Accredited continuing education program with Hahnemann Medical College. Community health education program and monthly
tumor board.

New Mexico: *Albuquerque*

University of New Mexico Cancer Research and Treatment Center
900 Camino de Salud N.E.
Albuquerque, New Mexico 87131
(505) 277–2151

Director: Martin Kligerman, M.D.

Emphasis: Comprehensive treatment including chemotherapy, radiotherapy, and
immunotherapy. Specializes in radiation therapy, research in radiation therapy.
M.D./Ph.D. staff of 22.

Equipment:

DIAGNOSTIC	THERAPEUTIC
Xeromammography	Cobalt 60
Rectilinear magna-scanner	Clinac 18
Dyna camera	Orthovoltage X-ray
Ultrasound	Simulator
Angiography	Cesium/radium
Thermography	

Tumor Registry.

New York: *Bronx*

Misericordia Hospital Medical Center
600 E. 233rd St.
Bronx, New York 10466
(212) 653–3000

Director: Frank Cicero, M.D.

Affiliation: New York Medical College.

Emphasis: Comprehensive treatment including chemotherapy, surgery, and radio-therapy. Thirty full-time staff.

Equipment:

DIAGNOSTIC	THERAPEUTIC
Conventional X-ray equipment	Cobalt 60
Nuclear medicine	Cesium
Ultrasound	Orthovoltage X-ray
Mammography	Superficial X-ray

Cancer Patient Statistics:

BEDS: 386 (unrestricted)   NEW PATIENTS: 450

Library: 50 volumes.

Tumor Registry.

New York: *Bronx*

Montefiore Hospital and Medical Center
111 E. 210th St.
Bronx, New York 10467
(212) 430–2000

Director: D. Kindig, M.D.

Admissions: David Doretsky

Affiliations: Albert Einstein College of Medicine; Beth Abraham Hospital; Martin Luther King Health Center; North Central Bronx Hospital.

Emphasis: Comprehensive treatment including gynecologic and head and neck oncology.

Equipment:

DIAGNOSTIC	THERAPEUTIC
Complete X-ray dept.	Betatron
Mammography	Linear accelerator
Angiography	Cobalt 60
Sonography	Cesium
Nuclear medicine	
Gamma camera	
Scintillation camera	
CAT scanner	

Cancer Personnel:

> M.D. AND M.D./Ph.D.: 15   NURSES: 31
> TECHNICAL PERSONNEL: 6
>   TOTAL: 52

Cancer Patient Statistics:

> BEDS: 36 (oncology unit)   NO. OUT-PATIENTS: 2121+
> NO. IN-PATIENTS: 597   NEW PATIENTS: 1740
> AVERAGE STAY: 20.3

Cancer Library.

Tumor Registry.

New York: *Brooklyn*

Methodist Hospital of Brooklyn
Crown St. and Albany Ave.
Brooklyn, New York 11213
(212) 780–3000

Director: Donald Rece

Affiliation: SUNY Downstate Medical Center.

Emphasis: Special grant for breast research. Other specialties include head and neck, G.I., and G.U. cancers and lymphomas.

Equipment:

> DIAGNOSTIC   THERAPEUTIC
> Full range of equipment   Linear accelerator
>   Cobalt
>   Simulators
>   Complete radiation therapy

Cancer Personnel:

> M.D. AND M.D./Ph.D.: 50–60   TECHNICAL PERSONNEL: 120
> Ph.D.: 3

Cancer Patient Statistics:
> BEDS: 150   NEW PATIENTS: 700

Cancer Library.

Tumor Registry.

New York: *Brooklyn*

SUNY Downstate Medical Center
Kings County Hospital Center
451 Clarkson Ave.
Brooklyn, New York 11203
(212) 270-1000

Directors: Bernard Gardner, M.D., Prof. of Surgery
James Nelson, M.D., Prof. of Obs. and Gyn.
Julian Rosenthal, M.D., Asst. Prof. of Medicine

Affiliation: State University of New York.

Emphasis: Program areas in biophysics (nuclear magnetic resonance in the diagnosis and detection of cancer); biochemistry (isolation and characterization of
the serum amyloid precursor from patients with neoplastic diseases); virology
(studies of interferon in neoplastic diseases); experimental immunology (studies
of neoplastic cell neoantigens, studies and characterization of the active component of BCG in its nonspecific stimulation of cellular immune response,
studies of immunoglobulin mutants in neoplastic diseases). A full range of diagnostic, surgical, radiotherapeutic, chemotherapeutic, and immunotherapeutic
facilities, as well as physical, occupational, and social rehabilitation services.
Multidisciplinary approaches to treatment are emphasized and developed by five
tumor boards meeting weekly. Tumors of all sites are treated with special competence in breast cancer, various hematologic malignancies, multiple myeloma,
leukemia, lymphoma—including Hodgkin disease, lung tumors, and gastrointestinal tumors. Active psychiatric and social services participate in the
management of cancer patients. Research areas include studies of the immune
response in patients with lymphoma, myeloma, and chronic myelocytic leukemia; radiotherapy of prostatic carcinoma and of the non-Hodgkin lymphoma;
approaches in the surgical and radiotherapeutic treatment of gynecologic
tumors; prospective combination therapy of metastasizing lung carcinoma;
immunotherapeutic studies with white cell antigens and MER; radioimmunoassay of hormone levels and of a serum component monitoring disease activity
in lymphoma and solid tumors.

Equipment:

DIAGNOSTIC	THERAPEUTIC
Comprehensive range of diagnostic equipment	4meV linear accelerator
	3meV telecobalt unit
	Cesium
	Superficial X-ray
	Isotopes

Cancer Personnel:

M.D. AND M.D./Ph.D.: 25 ft, 8 pt, 2 volunteer	NURSES: 23 ft, 2 pt

Ph.D.: 11 ft
  TOTAL: 59 full-time, 10 part-time,
    2 volunteer

Cancer Patient Statistics:

BEDS: 275
AVERAGE STAY: 40

NO. OUT-PATIENTS: 6240 (visits)
NEW PATIENTS: 1550

Cancer Library: 5000 volumes, 150 periodicals.

Tumor Registry.

Professional Education: All cancer units offer training courses for staff and general practitioners, radiotherapy and clinical oncology courses for medical students, and postgraduate training programs in medical, surgical, and gynecologic oncology and radiotherapy. Medical seminars with topics covering recent information concerning various neoplastic diseases held weekly. Postgraduate trainees and medical students participate in daily multidisciplinary tumor boards. The Breast Cancer Unit operates an early detection program using computer analysis and maintains demonstration facilities in five local hospitals.

New York: *Brooklyn*

Long Island College Hospital
340 Henry St.
Brooklyn, New York 11201
(212) 780–1717

President: Harold Light

Admissions: Carol Maher

Affiliation: SUNY Downstate Medical Center.

Equipment:

DIAGNOSTIC
Mammography
Nuclear medicine
Head scanner
Angiography
Ultrasound
Gamma camera
Fluoroscope
Endoscope
Bronchoscope

THERAPEUTIC
Cobalt
Cesium
Dosimetry
Orthovoltage X-ray
Superficial X-ray
Simulation (scanner)
Hyperthermia

Cancer Patient Statistics:

BEDS: 567 (unrestricted)   NEW PATIENTS: 400
IN- AND OUT-PATIENTS: 11,500
   (treatments)

Cancer Library.

Tumor Registry.

Professional Education: Residency program in all subspecialties and Fellowship programs. Conferences on all subspecialties held daily and/or weekly.

New York: *East Meadow*

Nassau County Medical Center
2201 Hempstead Turnpike
East Meadow, New York 11554
(516) 542-0123

Director: Donald H. Eisenberg

Admissions: William Mullan

Affiliations: Clinical Campus SUNY at Stonybrook and 34 additional teaching institutions in New York metropolitan area.

Emphasis: Largest facility for nuclear medicine and radiotherapy on Long Island, New York. Blood bank with platelet unit for leukemia treatment. Recipient of NCI grant for detection and treatment of cancer. 1152 chemotherapy treatments in 1977.

Equipment:

DIAGNOSTIC	THERAPEUTIC
Nuclear medicine	Cobalt 60
CT whole body scanner	Linear accelerator
Scintillation camera	Isotopes
Mammography	Betatron
Thermography	
Ultrasound	

Cancer Library.

Tumor Registry.

Professional Education: Continuing education courses. Daily seminars in all subspecialties for Long Island physicians and dentists. Ongoing graduate instruction.

New York: *Mineola**

Nassau Hospital
259 First St.
Mineola, New York 11501
(516) 663–0333

Emphasis: Comprehensive cancer treatment with chemotherapy and radiation
facilities.

Equipment:

DIAGNOSTIC
Conventional X-ray equipment
Nuclear medicine

THERAPEUTIC
Cobalt 60 (rotating and stationary)
Orthovoltage X-ray
Cesium

New York: *Manhasset*

North Shore University Hospital
300 Community Drive
Manhasset, New York 11030
(516) 562–0100

Executive Vice-President: Dennis F. Buckley

Admissions: Helen Connelly

Affiliations: Cornell University Medical College; New York Hospital;
Memorial Sloan-Kettering Hospital

Emphasis: Major oncology and hematology departments with special emphasis
on the treatment of leukemia.

Equipment:

DIAGNOSTIC
Mammography
Nuclear medicine
CAT body scanner
CT head scanner
Angiography
Ultrasound

THERAPEUTIC
Cesium
Supervoltage X-ray
Superficial X-ray

Cancer Library: 13,500 volumes.

Tumor Registry.

Note: Complete information not available at time of publication.

New York: *New Hyde Park*

Long Island Jewish-Hillside Medical Center
New Hyde Park, New York 11040
(212) 470-2000

Director: Robert K. Match, M.D.

Admissions: Roslyn Fink

Affiliations: Downstate Medical Center at SUNY Stonybrook; Queens Hospital
Center.

Emphasis: Comprehensive pathology laboratories. Surgical oncology in hematologic, pediatric, colon and rectal, head and neck, and thoracic cancers. All treatment modalities, rehabilitation medicine, plastic surgery, speech and physical therapies. Research in immunopathology and human genetics.

Equipment:

DIAGNOSTIC	THERAPEUTIC
Nuclear medicine	Cobalt 60
Electron microscope	Orthovoltage X-ray
CAT body scanner	Superficial X-ray
Tomography	
Spectrometers	

Cancer Library.

Tumor Registry.

Professional Education: Continuing education for physicians, nurses, and lay
community.

New York: *New York*

Cancer Center, Columbia University
701 W. 168th St.
New York, New York 10032
(212) 694-6904

Director: Paul A. Marks, M.D.

Affiliations: Presbyterian Hospital; St. Luke's Hospital; Harlem, Roosevelt,
Overlook Hospitals; New Jersey Cancer Control Network.

Emphasis: Comprehensive cancer treatment and rehabilitation service with research
program.

Equipment:

DIAGNOSTIC
Angiography
Lymphangiography
Mammography
Thermography
Specimen radiography
Ultrasound
Tomography
EMI brain scanner
EMI total body scanner

THERAPEUTIC
Cobalt 60
Linear accelerator
Betatron
Radium
Orthovoltage X-ray
Superficial X-ray
Megavoltage X-ray
Supervoltage X-ray

Cancer Patient Statistics:

BEDS: unrestricted in Center,
22 specialized
NO. IN-PATIENTS: 6242
AVERAGE STAY: 12

NO. OUT-PATIENTS: 927
NEW PATIENTS: 3186
AVERAGE COST: $190.00

Tumor Registry: Reports to New York State tumor registry.

New York: *New York*

Mount Sinai Medical Center
5th Ave. and 100th St.
New York, New York 10009
(212) 650-6500

Director of Oncology: James F. Holland

Affiliation: Mount Sinai School of Medicine.

Emphasis: Full-range program in surgery, radiation, and chemotherapy. Orthopedic rehabilitation and specialization in chemoimmunotherapy for acute leukemia. 16,177 radiotherapy visits in 1977.

Equipment:

DIAGNOSTIC
Full range of nuclear medicine
and diagnostic equipment

THERAPEUTIC
Complete radiotherapy department
including
Betatron
Laminar flow rooms
Linear accelerator
Microneurosurgery
Cobalt

Cancer Personnel:

M.D. AND M.D./Ph.D.:   6 ft, 3 pt,
   6 volunteer
Ph.D.:   5 ft
   TOTAL: 91 full-time,
      3 part-time, 6 volunteer

TECHNICAL PERSONNEL: 60 ft
NURSES: 20 ft

Cancer Library.

Tumor Registry.

New York: *New York*

The New York Hospital
525 East 68th St.
New York, New York 10021
(212) 472–5454

Director: David Thompson, M.D.

Acting Admissions Director: Mrs. Mary Richardson

Affiliations: Memorial Sloan-Kettering Cancer Center; Hospital for Special
Surgery; North Shore University Hospital, Manhasset; Burke Rehabilitation
Center, White Plains.

Equipment:

DIAGNOSTIC
CAT body scanner
CTT brain scanner (2)
Nuclear medicine
Mammography
Angiography
Ultrasound
Gamma camera

THERAPEUTIC
Full range of equipment

Cancer Patient Statistics:

BEDS: 1031 (unrestricted)

Cancer Library.

Tumor Registry.

New York: *New York*

New York University Medical Center
   Institute of Rehabilitation Medicine
400 East 34th St.
New York, New York 10016
550 First Ave.
New York, New York 10016

University Hospital
560 First Ave.
New York, New York 10016

Provost: Ivan Bennett, M.D.

Admissions: Richard Alvenzo, University Hospital

Affiliations: Veterans' Administration Hospital; Bellevue Hospital Center; Booth Memorial Medical Center; Brookdale Hospital Medical Center; Goldwater Memorial Hospital; Gouverneur Hospital; New York Infirmary.

Emphasis: A leading research center as well as a teaching institution and treatment facility. Cancer-related research has been undertaken to identify potentially dangerous substances in the environment. Efforts concentrate on ways to prevent harmful effects of pollutants: to learn more about the mechanisms that govern cell division and control their excessive growth and to perfect immunologic methods to increase the body's resistance to the growth of tumor cells.

Equipment:

DIAGNOSTIC	THERAPEUTIC
Nuclear medicine	4meV linear accelerator
Mammography	Simulator
CAT body scanner	Cobalt
CT head scanner	Treatment plan computer
Generators (3)	Dosimetry
Conventional X-ray equipment	Superficial X-ray
Ultrasound	Ionization chamber
Polytome	
Angiography	
Maximus 1000 (2)	
Gamma camera	
Mimer III	

Cancer Personnel (Nuclear Medicine Only):

M.D. AND M.D./Ph.D.:   10   TECHNICAL PERSONNEL: 6
Ph.D.:   6

Cancer Patient Statistics:

BEDS: 629 (Univ. Hosp.),
152 (Inst. of Rehab.)
NO. IN-PATIENTS: 3000

NO. OUT-PATIENTS: 5700 (Univ. Hosp.)
NEW PATIENTS: 495

Cancer Library: 119,774 volumes.

Tumor Registry.

Professional Education: Postgraduate studies in all subspecialties. Residency in radiation oncology. Clinical instruction for technicians on ongoing basis.

New York: *New York*

St. Vincent's Hospital and Medical Center
153 West 11 Street
New York, New York 10011
(212) 620-1234

Director: Evelyn Schneider

Affiliation: New York University School of Medicine.

Emphasis: Morphology of leucocytes in cancer patients. Radiobiology, kinetics of cellular radiation. Studies of nutrition in patients with cancer and studies in Hodgkin disease. Complete chemotherapy program treating colorectal cancer and solid tumors with immunotherapy for melanoma and combined therapies for lung cancer. Screening for breast, colorectal, and lung cancer. Active in-patient and out-patient programs.

Equipment:

DIAGNOSTIC
Complete range of diagnostic
    equipment

THERAPEUTIC
Linear accelerator
Comprehensive radiotherapy
    equipment including
    cobalt

Cancer Personnel:

M.D. AND M.D./Ph.D.: 24 ft, 48 pt

Tumor Registry.

Professional Education: Tumor Board, Lung Pathology Tumor Conference and Lymphoma Conference meet weekly. Radiotherapy Conference meets twice weekly.

New York: *Queens*

Queens Hospital Center
82–68 164th St.
Jamaica, New York 11432
(212) 990–3377

Director: Lawrence Duncan

Admissions: Lawrence Blum

Affiliations: Long Island Jewish Hospital, New Hyde Park; Hillside Medical Center, Queens; Capitol Medical Center, Queens.

Emphasis: Conventional diagnostic and therapeutic treatments available.

Cancer Library.

Tumor Registry.

New York: *Syracuse*

Crouse-Irving Memorial Hospital
736 Irving Ave.
Syracuse, New York 13210
(315) 424–6611

President: David Beers

Admissions: Marion LaForty

Affiliation: Upstate Medical Center.

Emphasis: Development of an out-patient infusion center for chemotherapy treatment. Equipped with ultrasound, CT brain scanner, and nuclear medicine for diagnostic treatment. More than 400 beds available for cancer patients.

New York: *Syracuse*

University Hospital of Upstate Medical Center
750 E. Adams St.
Syracuse, New York 13210
(315) 473–5540

Director: Thomas Campbell

Emphasis: Surgery radio- and chemotherapy research. Pediatric hematology.

Equipment:

DIAGNOSTIC	THERAPEUTIC
Delta scanner	Linear accelerator
Ultrasound	Cobalt 60
Thermography	Radium
Mammography	Isotopes
Nuclear medicine	

Tumor Registry.

Ohio: *Akron*

Akron City Hospital
525 East Market St.
Akron, Ohio 44309
(216) 375–3107

Executive Director: Albert F. Gilbert

Admissions: Christine Green

Affiliations: Northeastern Ohio Universities College of Medicine; The Ohio State University College of Medicine

Emphasis: Specializes in radiation oncology. Invasive radiologist available.

Equipment:

DIAGNOSTIC	THERAPEUTIC
Conventional X-ray equipment	Linear accelerator
CAT body scanner	Cobalt 60
Picker prototype scanner	Superficial X-ray

Cancer Personnel:

M.D. AND M.D./Ph.D.:   5 ft,
    6 volunteer
Ph.D.:   1 ft, 1 volunteer
    TOTAL: 15 full-time, 7 part-
    time, 7 volunteer

TECHNICAL PERSONNEL: 1 ft, 1 pt
NURSES: 8 ft, 6 pt

Cancer Patient Statistics:

BEDS: 13
NO. IN-PATIENTS: 1769
AVERAGE STAY: 3–5

NO. OUT-PATIENTS: 720
NEW PATIENTS: 1047
AVERAGE COST: $94.50

Cancer Library: 35 volumes.

Tumor Registry.

Ohio: *Cincinnati**

University of Cincinnati Medical Center
234 Goodman St.
Cincinnati, Ohio 45267
(513) 872-3100

Director: Vito Rollo

Emphasis: Comprehensive treatment with a breast cancer detection clinic and tumor, oncologic, gynecologic, and ear, nose, and throat clinics.

Equipment:

DIAGNOSTIC	THERAPEUTIC
Tomography	Cesium
CAT scanner	Radium
Nuclear medicine	Superficial X-ray
Brain scanner	Theratron 80
Gamma camera	Linear accelerator
Scintillation camera	Cobalt 60
Ultrasound	Simulator
	Orthovoltage X-ray
	Beta applicator
	Strontium 90

Tumor Registry.

Ohio: *Cleveland*

Cleveland Metropolitan General Hospital
3395 Scranton Rd.
Cleveland, Ohio 44109
(216) 398-6000

Director: Glenn E. Potter

Admissions: Joan Ragulen

Affiliation: Case Western Reserve University.

Emphasis: Specializes in surgical oncology and hepatic artery profusion process. Chemical research in surgical adjuvant breast program. Research in blood cells, and in tumor cell growth and differential in tissue cultures. Physical rehabilitation program.

*Note: Complete information not available at time of publication.

Equipment:

DIAGNOSTIC
CT scanner
Nuclear medicine
Gamma camera
Tomography
Scintillation camera
Mammography
Ultrasound (available in outside
    facility)
Angiography

THERAPEUTIC
Cobalt
Orthovoltage X-ray
Linear accelerator (available in outside
    facility)
Dosimetry

Cancer Personnel:

M.D. AND M.D./Ph.D.:   6

NURSES: 4

Cancer Patient Statistics:

BEDS: 528 total (unrestricted)

NO. OUT-PATIENTS: 1900

Cancer Library.

Tumor Registry.

Ohio: *Dayton*

Miami Valley Hospital
One Wyoming St.
Dayton, Ohio 45409
(513) 223–6192

Director: Luther W. Goehring

Admissions: Howard Cotterman

Affiliations: Wright State University School of Medicine; University of Dayton; Sinclair Community College.

Emphasis: Oncology Unit and Regional Radiation Therapy Center. Holds Annual Cancer Symposium. Tumor Board and other oncology-related topics.

Equipment:

DIAGNOSTIC
CAT scanner
Ultrasound
Radioisotope scanner

THERAPEUTIC
Betatron
Linear accelerator

Cancer Personnel:

M.D. AND M.D./Ph.D.: 9 ft, 7 pt
Ph.D.: 1 ft

TECHNICAL PERSONNEL: 15 ft,
5 volunteer
NURSES: 8 ft

TOTAL: 33 full-time, 7 part-
time, 5 volunteer

Cancer Patient Statistics:

BEDS: 27
NO. IN-PATIENTS: 65–70
AVERAGE STAY: 12–15

NO. OUT-PATIENTS: 100,000
NEW PATIENTS: 1282
AVERAGE COST: $200.00

Library: 1000 volumes.

Tumor Registry.

Oregon: *Portland*

Emanuel Hospital
2801 N. Gantenbein Ave.
Portland, Oregon 97227
(503) 280–3200

Director: Hugo Uhland, M.D., Director of Medical Affairs

Admissions: Leroy Groshong, M.D.

Affiliation: Medical School Hospital, University of Oregon.

Emphasis: Cancer rehabilitation for patients with metastatic cancer and for those with prostheses. Surgery, chemotherapy, and radiotherapy. Clinical research in treatment protocols.

Equipment:

DIAGNOSTIC
CT whole body scanner
Tomography
Polytome
Fluoroscope
Angiography

THERAPEUTIC
Linear accelerator
Cobalt 60
Simulator
Superficial X-ray
Cesium 137
Iridium 192
Iodine 125 seeds

Cancer Personnel:

M.D. AND M.D./Ph.D.: 85
Ph.D.: 2

NURSES: 22

Cancer Patient Statistics:

BEDS: 20   NEW PATIENTS: 706
NO. IN-PATIENTS: 1108   AVERAGE COST: $120.00
AVERAGE STAY: 11

Library: 35 volumes and journals.

Tumor Registry.

Professional Education: Resident training in gynecologic oncology.

Oregon: *Portland*

University of Oregon Health Sciences Center
University Hospital
3181 S.W. Sam Jackson Park Rd.
Portland, Oregon 97201
(503) 225–8311

Director: Donald G. Kassebaum, M.D.

Affiliation: Includes Doernbecher Memorial Hospital for Children.

Emphasis: Includes general out-patient clinic. Only children's hospital in state and only academic hospital in state. Specialties in bladder cancer study and prostatic cancer research. Estrogen receptive lab for breast and prostatic cancers to determine treatment process.

Equipment:

DIAGNOSTIC   THERAPEUTIC
Mammography   25 meV betatron
Nuclear medicine   Cobalt
CAT body scanner   Radium
CT head scanner   Dosimetry
Angiography   Orthovoltage X-ray
Gamma camera   Supervoltage X-ray
Fluoroscope   Superficial X-ray
Endoscope   Simulator
Bronchoscope
Electron microscope (off site)
Ultrasound
Xerography

Cancer Library.

Tumor Registry.

Pennsylvania: *Danville*

Geisinger Medical Center
North Academy Ave.
Danville, Pennsylvania 17821
(717) 275-6211

President: Henry L. Hood, M.D.

Medical Director: Harry C. Stamey, M.D.

Affiliations: Fox Chase Comprehensive Cancer Center; Cornell and PSU Medical Schools.

Emphasis: Tertiary care in all major specialties with full range of cancer rehabilitation and research facilities. Hematology/Oncology Unit.

Equipment:

DIAGNOSTIC
Head/body CAT scanners
Ultrasound
Nuclear medicine
Xeromammography

THERAPEUTIC
4meV linear accelerator
Cobalt 60
250kVP orthovoltage X-ray
Computer for dosimetry

Cancer Personnel:

M.D. AND M.D./Ph.D.: 12 ft
Ph.D: 1 ft
   TOTAL: 56 full-time, 5 part-time

TECHNICAL PERSONNEL: 5 ft
NURSES: 38 ft, 5 pt

Cancer Patient Statistics:

BEDS: 40
NO. IN-PATIENTS: 38
AVERAGE STAY: 8.1

NO. OUT-PATIENTS: 321,078
NEW PATIENTS: 1493
AVERAGE COST: $118.00

Cancer Library: 20,175 volumes.

Tumor Registry.

Pennsylvania: *Philadelphia*

Albert Einstein Medical Center, Northern Division
York and Tabor Rds.
Philadelphia, Pennsylvania 19141
(215) 329-0700

President: Raymond Alexander

Admissions: Alan E. Davis

Affiliation: Temple University School of Medicine; Philadelphia Geriatric Center.

Emphasis: Pioneering work in mammography radiotherapy with Dr. Harold Isard.
Part of Radiotherapy Oncology Group, the only non-university hospital in group.
Dr. Herman Freedman leader in immunotherapy research.

Equipment:

DIAGNOSTIC
Full range of equipment
CAT scanner
Mammography

THERAPEUTIC
4meV linear accelerator
Cesium
250kVP orthovoltage X-ray
Superficial X-ray
Simulator
Radium
Computer dosimetry

Cancer Personnel:

M.D. AND M.D./Ph.D.:   46
Ph.D: 2

TECHNICAL PERSONNEL: 18

Cancer Patient Statistics:

BEDS: 650

Cancer Library.

Tumor Registry.

Pennsylvania: *Philadelphia*

Hahnemann Medical College and Hospital
230 North Broad St.
Philadelphia, Pennsylvania 19102
(215) 448–8409

Chairman: Luther W. Brady, M.D., Prof.

Emphasis: Radiopharmaceutical development. Cancer biology and immunology.
Head and neck cancer demonstration project. Radiation therapy network in
region. Evaluation of electron radiography. Four programs of national clinical
cooperative trials.

Cancer Personnel:

M.D. AND M.D./Ph.D.:   19 ft, 13
    volunteer
TECHNICAL PERSONNEL: 5 ft, 2 pt

NURSES: 2 ft

Cancer Library: Access to Medical College Library.

Tumor Registry.

Professional Education: Training of residents in radiation therapy and nuclear medicine and instruction for medical students, nurses, and technologists. Continuing education seminars for physicians.

Pennsylvania: *Philadelphia*

Mercy Catholic Medical Center
Mailing address:
 Box 19709
 Philadelphia, Pennsylvania 19143
 (215) 747-7600
Fitzgerald Mercy Division
 Lansdowne Ave. and Baily Rd.
 Darby, Pennsylvania 19023
 (215) 586-5020
Misericordia Division
 5301 Cedar Ave.
 Philadelphia, Pennsylvania 19143

President: Sister Marie Lenahan

Vice-President: Plato A. Marinakos

Emphasis: Clinical program combining high-dose chemotherapy and radiation.

Equipment:

DIAGNOSTIC	THERAPEUTIC
Mammography	4meV linear accelerator
Nuclear medicine	Cobalt units (3)
CAT body scanner	Radium
Angiography	Dosimetry
Ultrasound	Orthovoltage X-ray
Gamma camera (2)	Supervoltage X-ray
Fluoroscope	Superficial X-ray
Endoscope	
Bronchoscope	
Xerography	

Cancer Personnel:

M.D. AND M.D./Ph.D.: 10	TECHNICAL PERSONNEL: 11
Ph.D.: 2	

Cancer Patient Statistics:

PATIENTS: 9,000 treatments/yr.　　NEW PATIENTS: 632 (consultation)
(radiation therapy)

Cancer Library.

Tumor Registry.

Professional Education: Six conferences a year on all subspecialties. Monthly
gynecologic cancer conferences and surgical conferences.

Pennsylvania: *Philadelphia*

Temple University Hospital
3401 N. Broad St.
Philadelphia, Pennsylvania 19140
(215) 221–2000

Administrator: Edward H. Nordian

Affiliation: Temple University.

Emphasis: Specializes in skin disease; cancer research and evaluation facilities for
oral cancer. Dermatology Department one of few in world concentrating on
skin diseases with outstanding diagnostic and treatment facilities. Leading
research institute in chemical carcinogenesis. Full range of diagnostic and
therapeutic equipment. 540 unrestricted beds.

Cancer Personnel (Skin and Cancer Hospital):

M.D. AND M.D./Ph.D.: 7 ft, 14 pt　　TECHNICAL PERSONNEL: 40 ft
Ph.D.: 7 ft

Library: 53,778 books and journals.

Tumor Registry: Head and neck.

Professional Education: Continuing seminars in all subspecialties.

Pennsylvania: *Philadelphia*

Thomas Jefferson University Hospital
11th and Walnut Sts.
Philadelphia, Pennsylvania 19107
(215) 829–6000

Director: Francis J. Sweeney, Jr., M.D.

Admissions: Waldren Bailey

Affiliation: Thomas Jefferson University (College of Allied Health Sciences, College of Graduate Studies, Jefferson Medical College).

Emphasis: Emphasis on nuclear medicine and radiation therapy.

Equipment:

DIAGNOSTIC
Mammography
Nuclear medicine
ACTA body scanner
Angiography
Ultrasound
Gamma camera

THERAPEUTIC
Linear accelerator
Cobalt
Betatron
Cesium
Radium
Dosimetry
Orthovoltage X-ray
Supervoltage X-ray
Superficial X-ray
Simulator

Cancer Patient Statistics:

BEDS: 687 (unrestricted)
NO. IN-PATIENTS: 1493

NO. OUT-PATIENTS: 407 (radiation
   therapy only)
NEW PATIENTS: 1453

Cancer Library.

Tumor Registry.

Professional Education: Residency program and Fellowship program in radiation therapy. Weekly tumor conferences. Lecture Bureau Program with visiting educators.

Pennsylvania: *Philadelphia*

University of Pennsylvania Cancer Center
578 Maloney Bldg.
Hospital of the University of Pennsylvania
3400 Spruce St.
Philadelphia, Pennsylvania 19104
(215) 662–3910

Director: Richard A. Cooper, M.D.

Admissions: S. Betty Treichel

Affiliations: Presbyterian, Veterans' Administration, Pennsylvania Graduate Hospitals; Institute for Cancer Research.

Emphasis: Medical and gynecologic oncology, radiation therapy, fundamental science, education, and training, cancer control, epidemiology, and biostatistics. Specializes in immunobiology and cell biology. Psychosocial rehabilitation.

Equipment:

DIAGNOSTIC
Mammography
Conventional X-ray equipment

THERAPEUTIC
Jobst machine
Conventional X-ray equipment

Cancer Personnel:

M.D. AND M.D./Ph.D.: 85 pt

Cancer Patient Statistics:

BEDS: 731
NO. IN-PATIENTS: 1946
AVERAGE STAY: 15.8 days

NO. OUT-PATIENTS: 1600
NEW PATIENTS: 1704
AVERAGE COST: $203.00

Library: 75,000 volumes.

Tumor Registry.

Pennsylvania: *Pittsburgh*

Mercy Hospital of Pittsburgh
1400 Locust St.
Pittsburgh, Pennsylvania 15219
(412) 232-8111

Executive Director: Sister M. Ferdinand Clark, RSM

Admissions: Sister Barbara Hudson

Affiliations: Duquesne University; University of Pittsburgh; McKeesport Hospital.

Emphasis: Specialized oncology floor with combined multidisciplinary approach. Nuclear Pathology Laboratory specializes in research with clinical oncologic implications. Share facilities and computers with McKeesport Hospital.

Equipment:

DIAGNOSTIC
Mammography
Nuclear medicine
CAT head/body scanners
Angiography
Ultrasound
Gamma camera

THERAPEUTIC
4meV linear accelerator
Cobalt 60
Cesium
Computerized dosimetry
Orthovoltage X-ray

Cancer Personnel:

M.D. AND M.D./Ph.D.: 25
Ph.D.: 3
   TOTAL: 55

TECHNICAL PERSONNEL: 12
NURSES: 15

Cancer Patient Statistics:

BEDS: 20
IN- AND OUT-PATIENTS: 600
(radiation therapy only)

NEW PATIENTS: 490 (radiation therapy only)

Cancer Library.

Tumor Registry.

Professional Education: Tumor Board meets weekly. Monthly seminars on all subspecialties for interns, residents, and staff members.

Pennsylvania: *Pittsburgh*

St. Francis General Hospital
45th St.
Pittsburgh, Pennsylvania 15201
(412) 622–4343

Executive Director: Sister M. Sylvia Schuler

Admissions: Sister M. Georgeann Oehling

Emphasis: Radiation therapy.

Equipment:

DIAGNOSTIC
Anger cameras
Magna-scanner
Ultrasound
CAT scanners

THERAPEUTIC
25meV betatron
Cobalt 60
Complete radium facilities

Cancer Personnel:

M.D. AND M.D./Ph.D.: 10 ft, 2 pt
Ph.D.: 1 ft, 1 pt
   TOTAL: 26 full-time, 4 part-time

TECHNICAL PERSONNEL: 7 ft, 1 pt
NURSES: 8 ft

Cancer Patient Statistics:

BEDS: unrestricted
NO. IN-PATIENTS: 545
AVERAGE STAY: 15

NO. OUT-PATIENTS: 14,297
NEW PATIENTS: 1007
AVERAGE COST: $139.00

Library: 8,000 volumes.

Tumor Registry.

Pennsylvania: *Pittsburgh*

Western Pennsylvania Hospital
4800 Friendship Ave.
Pittsburgh, Pennsylvania 15224
(412) 682–4200

Executive Vice-President: James I. McGuire

Admissions: Ruth Fitzgerald

Affiliation: University of Pittsburgh.

Emphasis: Extensive chemotherapy program.

Equipment:

DIAGNOSTIC	THERAPEUTIC
Mammography	Linear accelerator
Nuclear medicine	Cobalt
CAT head and body scanner	Cesium
Angiography	Radium
Ultrasound	Dosimetry
Gamma camera	Orthovoltage X-ray
	Superficial X-ray
	Simulator

Cancer Personnel:

M.D. AND M.D./Ph.D.: approx. 50	TECHNICAL PERSONNEL: 12
Ph.D.: 3	

Cancer Patient Statistics:

BEDS: 650 (unrestricted)

Cancer Library.

Tumor Registry.

Professional Education: Continuing education programs in all subspecialties.
Undergraduate teaching hospital for University of Pittsburgh.

Rhode Island: *Providence*

Rhode Island Hospital
593 Eddy St.
Providence, Rhode Island 02902
(401) 277–4000

President: Lloyd L. Hughes

Admissions: Dorothy M. Davis

Affiliation: Brown University Medical School.

Emphasis: Adult and pediatric treatment and rehabilitation center. Development of head and neck protocol and computerized three-dimensional treatment planning program.

Equipment:

DIAGNOSTIC	THERAPEUTIC
CAT scanner	18meV linear accelerators
Tomography	Dosimetry
Ultrasound	Simulator
	Cobalt 60

Cancer Personnel:

M.D. AND M.D./Ph.D.:   14 ft, 4 pt   TECHNICAL PERSONNEL: 20 ft
Ph.D.:   6 ft   NURSES: 5 ft
    TOTAL: 45 full-time, 4 part-time

Cancer Patient Statistics:

NO. OUT-PATIENTS: 27,753   AVERAGE COST: $137.00
NEW PATIENTS: 1587

Tumor Registry.

South Carolina: *Charleston*

Medical University, Hospital of South Carolina
171 Ashley Ave.
Charleston, South Carolina 29403
(803) 792–3131

Director: William A. McLees

Admissions: Fred Latham

Affiliation: Medical University of South Carolina.

Emphasis: Full cancer center with emphasis on gynecologic, surgical, pediatric, and hematologic oncology. Pap Mobile travels around eastern third of state giving pap smears.

Equipment:

DIAGNOSTIC
CAT scanner
Ultrasound
Nuclear medicine

THERAPEUTIC
Orthovoltage X-ray
Superficial X-ray
Cobalt unit
Linear accelerator
Radium

Cancer Patient Statistics:

NO. OUT-PATIENTS: 13,000   NEW PATIENTS: 750/yr.

Cancer Library.

Tumor Registry.

Tennessee: *Memphis*

Methodist Hospital
1265 Union Ave.
Memphis, Tennessee 38104
(901) 726-7000

Executive Director: John J. Laverty

Admissions: Robert Burton

Affiliation: University of Tennessee.

Emphasis: Cardiovascular oncology. Multidisciplinary research, treatment, and rehabilitation programs.

Equipment:

DIAGNOSTIC
Whole body scanner
Electron microscope
CAT scanner

THERAPEUTIC
Betatron
Cobalt 60
Superficial X-ray

Cancer Personnel:

M.D. AND M.D./Ph.D.: 2   TECHNICAL PERSONNEL: 3
Ph.D.: 2   NURSES: 17
   TOTAL: 24

Cancer Patient Statistics:

BEDS: 36
NO. IN-PATIENTS: 3146
AVERAGE STAY: 11

NO. OUT-PATIENTS: 13,789
NEW PATIENTS: 1539
AVERAGE COST: $97.50

Cancer Library.

Tumor Registry.

Professional Education: Annual cancer update seminars.

Tennessee: *Nashville*

Vanderbilt University Medical Center
1161 21st Avenue South
Nashville, Tennessee 37232
(615) 322–7311

Vice-President, Medical Affairs: Vernon E. Wilson

Admissions: James Baxendale

Affiliations: Vanderbilt University School of Medicine; Veterans' Administration Hospital; Metropolitan-Nashville General Hospital; St. Thomas Hospital.

Emphasis: Combined therapy approach: chemotherapy, radiotherapy, immuno-therapy, and surgery. Pediatric cancers and leukemia. Research on pre-malignancy in breast cancer. Clinical programs in medical oncology, adult hematology, pediatric hematology/oncology, radiation and surgical oncology, and diagnostic pathology. Out-patient oncology/hematology clinic capable of handling 1200 patients per month. Designated Breast Cancer Detection Center.

Equipment:

DIAGNOSTIC
CT whole body scanner
Scintillation camera
Brain scanner
Nuclear medicine

THERAPEUTIC
Cobalt 60
Linear accelerator

Cancer Library.

Tumor Registry.

Texas: *Dallas*

Charles A. Sammons Cancer Center
Baylor University Medical Center
3500 Gaston Ave.
Dallas, Texas 75246
(214) 820–3473

Director: Marvin J. Stone, M.D.

Affiliations: Southwest Oncology Group; Association of Community Radiation
   Therapy Centers.

Emphasis: Sixth largest voluntary medical complex in U.S.A. Specializes in
   medical oncology/hematology, radiation and surgical oncology.

Equipment:

DIAGNOSTIC	THERAPEUTIC
EMI total body scanner	Linear accelerators
EMI head scanner	Cobalt 60
Sonography	Simulator
Vascular radiographic equipment	Conventional X-ray equipment

Cancer Personnel:

M.D. AND M.D./Ph.D.:   92   NURSES: 9
TECHNICAL PERSONNEL: 8
   TOTAL: 109

Cancer Patient Statistics:

BEDS: 1275   NO. OUT-PATIENTS: 58,966
NO. IN-PATIENTS: 3344   NEW PATIENTS: 2200
AVERAGE STAY: 8.47   AVERAGE COST: $79.00

Library: 25,000 volumes.

Tumor Registry.

Texas: *Dallas*

Methodist Central Hospital
301 W. Colorado St.
Dallas, Texas 75222
(214) 946–8181

Executive Vice-President: William E. Parisi

Admissions: Robert Carson

Affiliation: Southwestern Medical School.

Emphasis: Comprehensive cancer treatment with specialization in chemotherapy.

Equipment:

DIAGNOSTIC
Fluoroscope
Gamma camera
CT head scanner
Angiography
Polytome
Xerography
Mammography
Sonography
Nuclear medicine

THERAPEUTIC
Cobalt
Iodine
Radium implants
Dosimetry

Cancer Personnel:

M.D. AND M.D./Ph.D.:   6

TECHNICAL PERSONNEL: 1

Cancer Patient Statistics:

BEDS: 508 total (7% for cancer treatment)

Cancer Library.

Tumor Registry.

Texas: *Dallas*

St. Paul's Hospital
5909 Harry Hines Blvd.
Dallas, Texas 75235
(214) 689-2000

Cancer Committee Chairman: Dr. William L. Crofford

Admissions: Tom Gilbert

Affiliations: M.D. Anderson Hospital and Tumor Institute, Houston; Southwestern Medical School.

Emphasis: Radiation oncology, surgery, cancer chemotherapy, and rehabilitation center.

Equipment:

DIAGNOSTIC
EMI head scanner

THERAPEUTIC
4meV linear accelerator

DIAGNOSTIC	THERAPEUTIC
EMI whole body scanner	Simulator
Conventional X-ray equipment	Conventional X-ray equipment

Cancer Personnel:

M.D. AND M.D./Ph.D.:   30 ft, 200 pt
Ph.D.:   1 ft

Cancer Patient Statistics:

BEDS: 34
NO. IN-PATIENTS: 1241/yr
AVERAGE STAY: 10 days

NO. OUT-PATIENTS: 14,948 (radiation oncology)
NEW PATIENTS: 900/yr
AVERAGE COST: $198.00

Library: 5600 volumes.

Tumor Registry.

Texas: *Fort Sam Houston*

Brooke Army Medical Center
Oncology Service
Box 517, Beach Pavilion
Fort Sam Houston, Texas 78234
(512) 221–4287/6504

Director: Joseph D. McCracken, M.D., LTC, MC

Affiliation: Southwest Oncology Group.

Emphasis: Care restricted to eligible military patients. Specializes in medical radiation, surgical, and gynecologic oncology.

Equipment:

DIAGNOSTIC	THERAPEUTIC
Nuclear medicine	Cobalt 60
Sonography	Radiation therapy unit
Mammography	Leukopheresis
	Plateletpheresis
	Laminar flow isolation facility

Cancer Personnel:

M.D. AND M.D./Ph.D.:   10
Ph.D.:   1
   TOTAL: 19

TECHNICAL PERSONNEL: 7
NURSES: 1

Cancer Patient Statistics:

BEDS: 25   NO. OUT-PATIENTS: 7461
NO. IN-PATIENTS: 2739   NEW PATIENTS: 480
AVERAGE STAY: 7–14

Library: 34,000 volumes.

Tumor Registry.

Texas: *Galveston*

University of Texas Medical Branch Hospitals
Eighth and Mechanic St.
Galveston, Texas 77550
(713) 765–1011

President: William C. Levin

Assistant Vice-President: John Paul Poretto, Hospital Affairs

Affiliation: Component of University of Texas.

Emphasis: Comprehensive Oncology Department with emphasis on general acute care. Designated by NCI as Specialized Cancer Center. Research conducted in development of enzymes that may have anticancer properties and environmental carcinogenesis. Large program in immunology consisting of development of various modalities.

Equipment:

DIAGNOSTIC	THERAPEUTIC
Atomic absorption spectrometer	Cyclotron (applied for with M.D.
X-ray spectrometer	Anderson as a consortium)
Thermography	18meV linear accelerator
Mammography	Cobalt
CAT body scanner	Betatron
CT head scanner	Cesium
Angiography	Radium
Ultrasound	Iridium
Gamma camera	Dosimetry
Fluoroscope	Orthovoltage X-ray
Endoscope	Superficial X-ray
Bronchoscope	Supervoltage X-ray
Electron microscope (2)	Simulator

Cancer Patient Statistics:

BEDS: 1200 (unrestricted)

Cancer Library: University of Texas—one of largest medical libraries in the country.

Tumor Registry.

Professional Education: Institution connected with Medical School, Graduate School of Biomedical Sciences, Nursing School, and Allied Health Sciences School.

Texas: *Houston*

Ben Taub General Hospital
1502 Taub Loop
Houston, Texas 77030
(713) 797-1122

Administrator: Richard Durbin

Admissions: John Gore

Affiliations: Baylor College of Medicine.

Emphasis: Comprehensive cancer treatment with Nuclear Medical Department and full range of radiotherapy and chemotherapy services. Major teaching hospital of Baylor College of Medicine which contains radiotherapy facility.

Equipment:

DIAGNOSTIC	THERAPEUTIC
Nuclear medicine	Radiotherapy equipment (Baylor)
Tomography	
Mammography	
Ultrasound	

Cancer Library.

Tumor Registry.

Professional Education: Program through Baylor College of Medicine.

Texas: *Houston*

St. Joseph Hospital
1919 La Branch St.
Houston, Texas 77002
(713) 757-1000

Administrator: Sister Mary Henrietta Murphy

Admissions: Willene Guttenberger

Affiliation: University of Texas Medical School at Houston

Emphasis: Hospital houses The Stehlin Foundation for Cancer Research, the activities of which are covered in Chapter 3, including the new "nude mice" stand-in program, hyperthermia, and blood perfusion. The only Breast Cancer Detection Center in Texas.

Equipment:

DIAGNOSTIC	THERAPEUTIC
CAT scanner	Linear accelerator
Radioisotope scanner	Cobalt 60
Conventional X-ray equipment	Conventional X-ray equipment

Cancer Library.

Tumor Registry.

Texas: *Houston*

St. Luke's Episcopal Hospital
6720 Bertner Ave.
Houston, Texas 77025
(713) 521–2011

Director: Newell E. France

Admissions: Ollivene Hickman, R.N.

Affiliations: Texas Children's Hospital; Baylor College of Medicine.

Emphasis: Specializes in hematology and oncology for children with out-patient and in-patient care program at Texas Children's Hospital. Radiology, hematology, and pathology services.

Equipment:

DIAGNOSTIC	THERAPEUTIC
Nuclear medicine	Radioisotopes
CAT scanner	Radium
Conventional X-ray equipment	

Cancer Library.

Tumor Registry.

Professional Education: Nursing in-service workshops and continuing medical education programs.

Texas: *Lackland*

Wilford Hall USAF Medical Center
Lackland AFB, Texas 78236
(512) 671–7420

Director: Col. Thomas R. Maloney, USAF, MC

Affiliation: Southwest Oncology Group.

Emphasis: Comprehensive treatment with specialties in leukemia and lymphoma. Patients restricted to qualified military personnel.

Equipment:

DIAGNOSTIC
Computerized tomography
Sonography
Conventional X-ray equipment

THERAPEUTIC
Aminco celltrifuge
Haemonetics Model 30 (blood cell separators)
Conventional X-ray equipment

Cancer Personnel:

M.D. AND M.D./Ph.D.:   8
Ph.D.:   1
TOTAL: 44

TECHNICAL PERSONNEL: 15
NURSES: 20

Cancer Patient Statistics:

BEDS: 100
NO. IN-PATIENTS: 1320
AVERAGE STAY: 12 weeks

NO. OUT-PATIENTS: 6941
NEW PATIENTS: 656+

Tumor Registry.

Texas: *Temple*

Scott and White Memorial Hospital
Scott Sherwood and Brindley Foundation
2401 S. 31st St.
Temple, Texas 76501
(817) 774–2111

President: Richard Haines, M.D.

Admissions: Luis Garcia

Affiliations: Texas A & M Medical School; Southwest Oncology Group.

Emphasis: Specializes in hematologic oncology, therapeutic radiology, and gynecologic oncology.

Equipment:

DIAGNOSTIC
Nuclear medicine
CAT scanner/head
Tomography
Angiography
Mammography
Ultrasound
Gamma camera

THERAPEUTIC
Radium
Cobalt 60
Linear accelerator
Orthovoltage X-ray
Simulator
Dosimetry
Megavoltage therapy
Supervoltage therapy

Cancer Library.

Tumor Registry.

Utah: *Salt Lake City*

L.D.S. (Latter Day Saints) Hospital
325 Eighth Ave.
Salt Lake City, Utah 84143
(801) 350–1100

Administrator: David B. Wirthlin

Admissions: LaRene Vaughn

Affiliations: Inter-Mountain Health Care, Inc.
University of Utah College of Medicine.

Emphasis: Radiation Center, principal facility in West. Comprehensive treatment with chemotherapy, immunotherapy, radiation and surgical oncology. Program in genetic research.

Equipment:

DIAGNOSTIC
Whole body scanner
Simulator
Mammography
Conventional X-ray equipment

THERAPEUTIC
Cobalt 60
Linear accelerator
Hyperbaric oxygen chamber

Cancer Personnel:

M.D. AND M.D./Ph.D.:   20
Ph.D.:   4
   TOTAL: 67

TECHNICAL PERSONNEL: 25
NURSES: 18

Cancer Patient Statistics:

BEDS: unrestricted (18-bed
   oncology unit)
NO. OUT-PATIENTS: 2613

NEW PATIENTS: 1100

Utah: *Salt Lake City*

University of Utah Hospital
50 No. Medical Dr.
Salt Lake City, Utah 84132
(801) 581–2258

Executive Director: John A. Reinertsen

Admissions: Hal Kelley

Affiliations: L.D.S. Hospital; V.A. Hospital; Primary Children's Hospital.

Emphasis: Establishment of Center for Cancer Genetic Studies. Specializes in cancer chemotherapy, radiotherapy, and surgery with emphasis on hematologic malignancy.

Equipment:

DIAGNOSTIC	THERAPEUTIC
Nuclear medicine	18meV linear accelerator
CAT scanners	Electron beam therapy
Serologic tumor markers	Conventional X-ray equipment

Cancer Personnel:

M.D. AND M.D./Ph.D.:	29	TECHNICAL PERSONNEL:	6
Ph.D.:	6	NURSES:	5
TOTAL:	46		

Cancer Patient Statistics:

BEDS:	75+	NO. OUT-PATIENTS:	5115
NO. IN-PATIENTS:	450	NEW PATIENTS:	1001
AVERAGE STAY:	10	AVERAGE COST:	$103.00

Tumor Registry.

Vermont: *Burlington**

Cancer Center Hospital of Vermont
Colchester Ave.
Burlington, Vermont 05401
(802) 656–2345

President: Herluf V. Olsen

Affiliations: University of Vermont College of Medicine; University of Vermont

*Note: Complete information not available at time of publication.

Nursing School; Fanny Allen Hospital, School of Nursing and School of Allied Health.

Cancer Library.

Tumor Registry.

Virginia: *Charlottesville*

University of Virginia Hospitals
Jefferson Park Ave.
Charlottesville, Virginia 22901
(804) 924-0211

Director: John F. Harlan, Jr.

Affiliations: Roanoke Memorial Hospital; Lynchburg General Hospital.

Emphasis: Pediatric oncology. Endocrine cancer program. Solid tumor therapy. Research in microbiology, combined modality treatment of experimental tumors in animals.

Equipment:

DIAGNOSTIC	THERAPEUTIC
CT scanner	Linear accelerators
Isotope detection unit	Cobalt 60
Conventional X-ray equipment	Orthovoltage X-ray
Gamma camera	

Cancer Personnel:

M.D. AND M.D./Ph.D.: 35	TECHNICAL PERSONNEL: 20
Ph.D.: 25	NURSES: 20
TOTAL: 100	

Cancer Library.

Tumor Registry.

Virginia: *Richmond**

Medical College of Virginia Hospitals of the Virginia Commonwealth University
1200 E. Broad St.
Richmond, Virginia 23298
(804) 770-2486

*Note: Complete information not available at time of publication.

Executive Director: Robert C. Kidd II

Admissions: Catherine Smith

Affiliations: McGuire V.A. Hospital in Richmond; Medical College of Virginia.

Emphasis: Comprehensive cancer treatment with a multidisciplinary research center. Tumor clinic: 15,000 visits/yr.; radiation facility: 18,000 visits. A medical center completely equipped for diagnostic and therapeutic services.

Professional Education: Continuing Education department.

Washington: *Seattle*

Swedish Hospital Medical Center
747 Summit Ave.
Seattle, Washington 98104
(206) 292-2121

Director: Allan Lobb, M.D.

Admissions: Gunvor Thilberg

Affiliation: Fred Hutchinson Cancer Research Center; Southwest and Northwest Oncological Groups.

Emphasis: Treatment in all adult malignancies. Lung, breast, colon, Hodgkin, and non-Hodgkin diseases and acute leukemia.

Equipment:

DIAGNOSTIC	THERAPEUTIC
Conventional X-ray equipment	Superficial X-ray
Mammography	Cobalt 60
Tomography	4meV linear accelerator
Ultrasound	Simulator
Nuclear medicine	Radium
	Cesium
	Iridium

Cancer Personnel:

M.D. AND M.D./Ph.D.: 10	NURSES: 4
TECHNICAL PERSONNEL: 5	
TOTAL: 19	

Tumor Registry.

Washington: *Seattle*

Virginia Mason Hospital
925 Seneca St.
Seattle, Washington 98101
(206) 624-1144

Administrator: Donald Olsen

Admissions: Linda Griffith

Affiliation: Fred Hutchinson Cancer Research Center; Northwest Oncology Group.

Emphasis: Multidisciplinary treatment and research hospital with specialization in prostrate cancer. Major referral center for northwest area patients. Member of National Prostatic Cancer Project, National Bladder Project, and National Breast Cancer Detection Project. NCI approved institution for experimental chemotherapy.

Equipment:

DIAGNOSTIC	THERAPEUTIC
Nuclear medicine	18meV linear accelerator
Gamma camera	4meV linear accelerator
Scintillation camera	Cobalt 60
Mammography	Orthovoltage X-ray
Xerography	Superficial X-ray
Thermography	Simulator
Ultrasound	Cesium
CT brain scanner	Radium

Cancer Personnel:

M.D. AND M.D./Ph.D.:	14	TECHNICAL PERSONNEL:	20
Ph.D.:	4	NURSES:	12
TOTAL:	50		

Cancer Library.

Tumor Registry.

Professional Education: Fourteen postgraduate training programs in all subspecialties of medicine and surgery. Annual Cancer Conference cosponsored with American Cancer Society for Pacific Northwest Area.

Washington: *Spokane*

Sacred Heart Medical Center
West 101 Eighth Ave.
Spokane, Washington 99204
(509) 455-3131

Director: Sister Peter Claver

Admissions: Jean Denbeigh

Emphasis: Full treatment modalities with specialization in chemotherapy. Regional cancer center for eastern Washington, northern Idaho and western Montana.

Equipment:

DIAGNOSTIC
Nuclear medicine
Gamma camera
CT scanner
Mammography
Xerography
Thermography
Ultrasound
Electron microscope

THERAPEUTIC
Linear accelerators (2)
Conventional X-ray equipment

Cancer Library.

Tumor Registry.

Professional Education: Four residency programs in conjunction with the University of Washington.

Wisconsin: *Milwaukee*

Milwaukee County Medical Complex
8700 West Wisconsin Ave.
Milwaukee, Wisconsin 53226
(414) 257–5936

Administrator: Marvin F. Neely, Jr.

Affiliations: Veterans Hospital; Milwaukee Psychiatric Hospital; Milwaukee Children's Hospital.

Emphasis: Full range of therapy and rehabilitation.

Equipment:

DIAGNOSTIC
CAT scanners
Ultrasound
Conventional X-ray equipment

THERAPEUTIC
Betatron
Linear accelerators
Cobalt 60
Conventional X-ray equipment

Cancer Personnel:

M.D. AND M.D./Ph.D.: 32 ft, 13
volunteer
Ph.D.: 5 ft, 16 volunteer
TOTAL: 112 full-time, 29
volunteer

TECHNICAL PERSONNEL: 75 ft

Cancer Patient Statistics:

BEDS: unrestricted
NO. IN-PATIENTS: 402
AVERAGE STAY: 9.2

NO. OUT-PATIENTS: 20,000
NEW PATIENTS: 854
AVERAGE COST: $140.00

Library: 36,000 volumes.

Tumor Registry.

LEADING CANCER TREATMENT
CENTERS THROUGHOUT THE WORLD

The statistics and descriptions contained in this section were compiled from information made available to us up to the date of publication. However, a number of the cancer centers included had not yet responded to our questionnaires; consequently, the statistical data shown for those institutions whose names are immediately followed with a single asterisk (*) is accurate as of 1973, and those with a double asterisk (**), as of 1974.

ARGENTINA

Buenos Aires: Angel H. Roffo Institute of Oncology
Buenos Aires Central Radiation Hospital

AUSTRALIA

Queensland: Queensland Radium Institute
Victoria: Cancer Institute, Peter MacCallum Hospital

BELGIUM

Bruxelles: Jules Bordet Institute
Ghent: Department of Radiotherapy and Nuclear Medicine

BRAZIL

Belo Horizonte: Borges da Costa Hospital
Curitiba-Parana: Erasto Gaertner Hospital
Porto Alegre: Santa Rita Hospital
Recife: Pernambuco Cancer Hospital

Rio de Janeiro: Brazilian National Cancer Institute
   Mario Kroeff Hospital
Sao Paulo: Central Institute, A.C. Camargo Hospital, A. Prudente Foundation

BULGARIA

Sofia: Bulgarian Oncological Research Institute

CANADA

Alberta: Cross Cancer Institute
British Columbia: British Columbia Cancer Institute
   Manitoba Cancer Treatment and Research Foundation
Ontario: Ontario Cancer Foundation, London Clinic
   The Ontario Cancer Institute
Quebec: Centre d'Oncologie, Hospital Notre-Dame
Saskatchewan: Allan Blair Memorial Clinic
   Saskatchewan Cancer Commission
   Saskatoon Cancer Clinic

CHILE

Santiago: Dr. C.P. Correa National Radium Institute

COLUMBIA

Bogota: Instituto Nacional de Cancerologia

CUBA

Habana: Cuban Institute of Oncology and Radiobiology

CZECHOSLOVAKIA

Bratislavia: Slovakia Oncological Institute
Prague: Institute of Radiotherapy

DENMARK

Aarhus: Department of Radiotherapy and Oncology
Copenhagen: Finsen Institute

EGYPT

Cairo: Cairo University Cancer Institute

ENGLAND

London: Charing Cross Hospital Medical Oncology and Radiotherapy Oncology
   Departments

Royal Marsden Hospital
Manchester: Christie Hospital and Holt Radium Institute and Paterson Labs.
Newcastle-Upon-Tyne: Cancer Research Campaign Oncological Center

FRANCE

Angers: Paul Papin Cancer Center
Bordeaux: Bergonié Foundation Regional Cancer Center
Dijon: George-François Leclerc Anti-Cancer Center
Lille: Oscar Lambret Center.
Lyon: Leon Berard Center
Marseilles: J. Paoli—I. Calmettes Institute
Montpellier: Montpellier Regional Cancer Center
Nantes: Nantes Cancer Center
Nice: Antoine-Lacassagne Center
Paris: Foundation Curie Institute du Radium
Rouen: Centre Regional de Lutte Contre le Cancer
Saint-Cloud: Rene Huguenin Center
Toulouse: Claudius Regaud Center
Vandoeuvre les Nancy: Alexis Vautrin Center
Villejuif: Gustave-Roussy Institute

GERMANY

Berlin-Buch: Central Institute for Cancer Research
Essen: West German Tumor Center

GREECE

Athens: Hellenic Anticancer Institute
Piraeus: Metaxas Memorial Cancer Hospital
Thessalonika: Theagenion Medical Institute

HONG KONG

Kowloon: M. & H.D. Institute of Radiology and Oncology

HUNGARY

Budapest: Hungarian National Institute of Oncology

INDIA

Ahmedabad: Gujarat Cancer and Research Institute
Bombay: Tata Memorial Center
Hyderabad: Mehdi Nawaz Jung Cancer Hospital and Radium Institute
Madras: Cancer Institute (W.I.A.)

IRAN

Tehran: Taj Pahlavi Cancer Institute

IRAQ

Baghdad: Institute of Radiology and Nuclear Medicine

IRELAND

Dublin: St. Anne's City Hospital for Diseases of the Skin and Cancer
St. Luke's Hospital Radiotherapy and Clinical Oncology Center

ISRAEL

Haifa: The Northern Israel Oncology Center, Ramban Medical Center

ITALY

Cagliari: Cagliari Oncological Hospital
Milan: National Cancer Institute of Milan
Naples: Senatore Pascale Foundation
Torino: Turin Oncological Institute

JAPAN

Nagoya: Aichi Cancer Center
Tokyo: Japanese Foundation for Cancer Research
National Cancer Center

KOREA

Seoul: Cancer Research Hospital and Korea Atomic Energy Research Institute

MEXICO

Mexico City: C.M.N. Oncological Hospital
National Cancer Institute

NETHERLANDS

Amsterdam: Netherlands Cancer Institute
Rotterdam: Dr. Daniel Den Hoed Clinic/Rotterdam Radiotherapy Institute

NORWAY

Oslo: Det Norske Radium Hospital
Norwegian National Hospital

PERU

Lima: Peruvian National Neoplastic Disease Institute

POLAND

Gliwice: Gliwice Institute of Oncology
Krakow: Krakow Institute of Oncology
Warsaw: Maria Sklodowska-Curie Memorial Institute of Oncology

PORTUGAL

Lisbon: Portuguese Institute of Oncology—Francisco Gentil

PUERTO RICO

Rio Piedras: I. Gonzales Martinex Oncologic Hospital
Santurce: Puerto Rico Cancer Control Program

ROMANIA

Bucharest: Oncological Institute
Cluj-Napoca: Cluj-Napoca Oncological Institute
Itasi: Jassy Radiological Clinic

SCOTLAND

Edinburgh: Radiotherapy Institute, Western General Hospital
Glasgow: West of Scotland Cancer Intelligence Unit

SOUTH AFRICA

Bloemfontein: O.F.S. Institute of Isotopes and Radiation
Cape Town: Radiotherapy Department, Groote Schuur Hospital
Johannesburg: Department of Radiation Therapy, Johannesburg General Hospital

SWEDEN

Goteburg: Institute for Radiotherapy
Lund: Lund University Radiotherapy Department
Stockholm:Radiumhemmet, Karolinska Institute

SWITZERLAND

Basel: University of Basel, Kantonsspital, Medical Center, Department of Oncology

TUNISIA

Tunis: Institute Salah Azaiz

Argentina: *Buenos Aires*

Angel H. Roffo Institute of Oncology*
Avenida San Martin 5481, Buenos Aires, Argentina
Tel: 50–7100

Director: Gualterio Cristiani, M.D.

Affiliation: International Union Against Cancer

Emphasis: Experimental cancer research in breast cancer and immunologic research. Treatment and rehabilitation in gynecologic and breast cancer. Reconstructive surgery, endocrinology, chemotherapy, and radiotherapy.

Equipment: Conventional diagnostic and radiotherapeutic equipment.

Cancer Personnel:

M.D. AND M.D./Ph.D.:   1 ft, 112 pt,   NURSES: 121 pt
   27 volunteer
TECHNICAL PERSONNEL: 47 pt
   TOTAL: 1 full-time, 280 part-
      time, 27 volunteer

Cancer Patient Statistics:

BEDS: 76   AVERAGE STAY: 14
NO. IN-PATIENTS: 1100   NO. OUT-PATIENTS: 40,761

Cancer Library: None.

Tumor Registry: None.

Professional Education: Oncology Chair, University of Buenos Aires.

Argentina: *Buenos Aires*

Buenos Aires Central Radiation Hospital**
Patricias Argentinas 750, Buenos Aires, Argentina
Tel.: 812–3972

Director: Jorge Serrano Fernandez

Emphasis: Surgery, radiotherapy, and chemotherapy with rehabilitation programs.

Equipment:

DIAGNOSTIC
Conventional X-ray equipment
Nuclear medicine

THERAPEUTIC
Cobalt 60
Cesium 137
Isotopes

Cancer Personnel:

M.D. AND M.D./Ph.D.:   6 ft, 63 pt   NURSES: 102 pt, 46 volunteer
TECHNICAL PERSONNEL: 74 pt
   TOTAL: 6 full-time, 239 part-time,
   46 volunteer

Cancer Patient Statistics:
BEDS: 150   NO. OUT-PATIENTS: 49,000
NO. IN-PATIENTS: 1720   NEW PATIENTS: 9600
AVERAGE STAY: 21

Library: 12,721 volumes, 12 periodicals.

Tumor Registry: None.

Professional Education: Training for nurses and radiologic technicians. Program in
general oncology and qualification courses for radiotherapists.

Australia: *Queensland*

Queensland Radium Institute*
Brisbane Base Hospital
Herston Road
Brisbane, Queensland 4029, Australia
Tel.: 52–0111

Director: Keith S. Mowatt, M.B., Ch.B.

Affiliation: North Brisbane Hospitals Board.

Emphasis: Treatment and rehabilitation with radiotherapy and chemotherapy.
Research in ovarian carcinoma with experimental immunotherapy. Clinical research in skin and mouth cancer.

Equipment:

DIAGNOSTIC
Conventional X-ray equipment

THERAPEUTIC
Linear accelerators (3)
Orthovoltage X-ray
Cobalt 60
Cesium
Isotopes

Cancer Personnel:

M.D. AND M.D./Ph.D.:   20 ft, 25 pt
Ph.D.:   9 ft
   TOTAL: 124 full-time, 31 part-
     time

TECHNICAL PERSONNEL: 82 ft
NURSES: 13 ft, 6 pt

Cancer Patient Statistics:

NO. IN-PATIENTS: 2088
AVERAGE STAY: 17

NO. OUT-PATIENTS: 24,400
NEW PATIENTS: 5323

Library: 500 volumes, 40 periodicals.

Tumor Registry: None.

Professional Education: Undergraduate education for medical, dental and veterinary students. Postgraduate training for radiotherapists.

Australia: *Victoria*

Cancer Institute, Peter MacCallum Hospital
481 Little Lonsdale St.
Melbourne, Victoria, 3000 Australia
Tel.: 602–1333

Director: Peter L.T. Ilbery, M.D.

Affiliation: University of Melbourne; University of Monash

Emphasis: Radiotherapy, chemotherapy, and reparative surgery. Introduction of
clinical trials and cancer therapy protocols in 15 special consultative cancer
clinics: head and neck, breast, lung, skin, pediatric, barotherapy, gynecology,
neurology, gastroenterology, genito-urinary, germinal tumor, sarcoma, lymphoma, reparative surgery, and melanoma.

Equipment:

DIAGNOSTIC
Radiography
Nucleography
High-pressure liquid
  chromatography

THERAPEUTIC
Linear accelerators (6)
Curietrons (6)
Celltrifuge

Cancer Personnel:

M.D. AND M.D./Ph.D.: 51 ft, 56 pt
Ph.D.: 15 ft
   TOTAL: 416 full-time, 146
     part-time

TECHNICAL PERSONNEL: 186 ft
NURSES: 164 ft, 90 pt

Cancer Patient Statistics:

BEDS: 180
NO. IN-PATIENTS: 4419
AVERAGE STAY: 9

NO. OUT-PATIENTS: 54,608
AVERAGE COST: $35.00
NEW PATIENTS: 6017

Library: 5280 volumes, 240 periodicals.

Tumor Registry: Selective.

Professional Education: Medical, scientific, technical, and nursing education.

Belgium: *Bruxelles*

Jules Bordet Institute*
1 rue Heger Bordet
1000 Bruxelles, Belgium
Tel.: 02/538 00 00

Affiliation: Universite Libre de Bruxelles.

Emphasis: Radiotherapy, chemotherapy, and endocrine therapy. Cervico-facial surgery and reconstruction. Research in cell kinetics, drug action, and hormone regulatory mechanism; high-energy irradiation, acute leukemia, breast, genitourinary, and digestive tract cancers.

Equipment:

DIAGNOSTIC
Conventional X-ray equipment
Electron microscope

THERAPEUTIC
Orthovoltage X-ray
Nuclear medicine

Cancer Personnel:

M.D. AND M.D./Ph.D.: 54
Ph.D.: 6
   TOTAL: 281

TECHNICAL PERSONNEL: 45
NURSES: 176

Cancer Patient Statistics:

BEDS: 99
NO. IN-PATIENTS: 1809
AVERAGE STAY: 16

NO. OUT-PATIENTS: 21,922
NEW PATIENTS: 1000

Library: 1200 volumes, 35 periodicals.

Tumor Registry: None.

Professional Education: Postgraduate and graduate training in internal medicine, oncology, radiation therapy, radiodiagnosis, pathology, pharmacology, and anesthesiology.

Belgium: *Ghent*

Department of Radiotherapy and Nuclear Medicine
University Hospital
De Pintelaan 135
9000 Ghent, Belgium
Tel.: (091) 22 57 41

Director: Professor A. De Schryver, M.D.

Affiliation: University of Ghent.

Emphasis: Radiotherapy, curietherapy, radioisotope, and chemotherapy. Research on breast cancer.

Equipment:

DIAGNOSTIC	THERAPEUTIC
Conventional X-ray equipment	Cobalt 60
Full range of radioisotope equipment	Linear accelerator
Scanning electron microscope	Betatron
	Contact therapy

Cancer Personnel:

M.D. AND M.D./Ph.D.: 14	TECHNICAL PERSONNEL: 30
Ph.D.: 5	NURSES: 16
TOTAL: 65	

Cancer Patient Statistics:

BEDS: 88	NO. OUT-PATIENTS: 12,030
NO. IN-PATIENTS: 1213	NEW PATIENTS: 952
AVERAGE STAY: 18	

Library: 1760 volumes.

Tumor Registry: None.

Professional Education: Medical student instruction in radiotherapy, radiobiology, and radioisotopes. Postgraduate training in radiobiology, radiation pathology, and radiation dosimetry.

Brazil: *Belo Horizonte*

Borges da Costa Hospital**
Avenida Alfredo Balena 190
Belo Horizonte
Minas Gerais–30,000 Brazil
Tel.: 226–7000

Director: Prof. Oswaldo Borges da Costa

Affiliation: Minas Gerais Federal University Medical Faculty.

Emphasis: Radiotherapy, curietherapy, surgery, and chemotherapy. Early detection and diagnostic services with emphasis on cancer of the uterine cervix.

Equipment: Conventional radiologic diagnostic and therapeutic equipment.

Cancer Personnel:

M.D. AND M.D./Ph.D.:   18   NURSES: 51
TECHNICAL PERSONNEL: 10
   TOTAL: 79

Cancer Patient Statistics:

BEDS: 111   NEW PATIENTS: 3345
AVERAGE STAY: 32

Library: 3000 volumes, 5 periodicals

Tumor Registry.

Professional Education: Postgraduate and graduate instruction in oncology.

Brazil: *Curitiba–Parana*

Erasto Gaertner Hospital
Rua Dr. Ovande do Amaral
Guabirotuba
Curitiba–Parana, Brazil
Tel.: 24–3682

Director: Antero sadi Pizzatto, M.D.

Admissions: Council of Department Heads

Affiliation: Liga Parananense de Combate ao Cancer.

Emphasis: Surgery, radiotherapy, chemotherapy, and immunotherapy. Control facilities for gynecologic cancer.

Equipment:

DIAGNOSTIC
Conventional X-ray equipment
Scintillation camera

THERAPEUTIC
Linear accelerator
Cobalt 60
Contact therapy

Cancer Personnel:

M.D. AND M.D./Ph.D.: 9 ft, 17 pt
TECHNICAL PERSONNEL: 5 ft
TOTAL: 32 full-time, 17 part-time

NURSES: 18 ft

Cancer Patient Statistics:

BEDS: 106
NO. IN-PATIENTS: 1803
AVERAGE STAY: 22

NO. OUT-PATIENTS: 7127
NEW PATIENTS: 1809

Library: 36 periodicals.

Tumor Registry.

Professional Education: Pediatric oncology and medical student instruction.

Brazil: *Porto Alegre*

Santa Rita Hospital*
Rue Sarmento Leite 183
90000 Porto Alegre, Brazil
Tel.: 25–74–22 (0512)

Directors: Edgar Diefenthaeler, M.D.; Meitor Cirnelima, M.D.

Affiliation: Associacao Sulriograndense de Combate ao Cancer Faculdade Catolica de Medicina.

Emphasis: Surgical, radiotherapeutic, and chemotherapeutic treatment with physical rehabilitation services. Special program in larynx rehabilitation. Research in myeloma and lymphoma.

Equipment:

DIAGNOSTIC
Conventional X-ray equipment
Endoscope
Iodine 131

THERAPEUTIC
8meV Megatron
Linear Accelerator
Telecobalt 60
Cesium 137
Dosimetry
Orthovoltage X-ray

Cancer Personnel:

M.D. AND M.D./Ph.D.:   5 ft, 25 pt   NURSES: 84 pt
TECHNICAL PERSONNEL: 4 pt
   TOTAL: 5 full-time, 113 part-time

Cancer Patient Statistics:

BEDS: 150   NO. OUT-PATIENTS: 1928
NO. IN-PATIENTS: 1224   NEW PATIENTS: 1096
AVERAGE STAY: 28

Library: 4000 volumes.

Tumor Registry.

Professional Education: Training for residents and general practitioners.

Brazil: *Recife*

Pernambuco Cancer Hospital*
Av. Cruz Cabuga 1597
Santo Amaro
Recife, Brazil
Tel.: 224 351

Director: Nelson B. Coutinho, M.D.

Affiliation: Sociedade Pernambucana de Combate ao Cancer.

Emphasis: Surgical, radiotherapeutic, chemotherapeutic, and immunotherapeutic treatment with rehabilitation facilities.

Equipment: Conventional diagnostic and therapeutic equipment.

Cancer Personnel:

M.D. AND M.D./Ph.D.:   8 ft, 33 pt   TECHNICAL PERSONNEL: 1 ft, 22 pt
Ph.D.:   5 pt   NURSES: 140 ft
   TOTAL: 149 full-time, 60 part-time

Cancer Patient Statistics:

BEDS: 160   NO. OUT-PATIENTS: 52,739
NO. IN-PATIENTS: 1739   NEW PATIENTS: 3493
AVERAGE STAY: 195

Cancer Library: None.

Tumor Registry: None

Professional Education: Graduate instruction in oncology.

Brazil: *Rio de Janeiro*

Brazilian National Cancer Institute
Praca Cruz Vermelha 23
20,000 Rio de Janeiro RJ Brazil
Tel.: (021) 222-7595

Director: Adayr Eiras de Araujo, M.D.

Affiliation: National Cancer Division, Ministry of Health.

Emphasis: Surgery, radiotherapy, chemotherapy, and immunotherapy programs.
Clinical research in immunotherapy, chemotherapy, and leukemia.

Equipment:

DIAGNOSTIC	THERAPEUTIC
Conventional X-ray equipment	20meV linear accelerator
Sonography	Cobalt
Tomography	Orthovoltage X-ray
Linear scanner	Superficial X-ray
Magna-scanner	Laminar flow unit
Gamma detection units	Blood cell separator

Cancer Personnel:

M.D. AND M.D./Ph.D.: 47 ft, 67 pt	TECHNICAL PERSONNEL: 30 ft
Ph.D.: 15 ft, 31 pt	NURSES: 145 ft, 60 pt
TOTAL: 237 full-time, 158 part-time	

Cancer Patient Statistics:

BEDS: 240	NO. OUT-PATIENTS: 96,179
NO. IN-PATIENTS: 2415	NEW PATIENTS: 1615
AVERAGE STAY: 28	

Library: 810 volumes, 70 periodicals.

Tumor Registry.

Professional Education: Continuing education courses and residency program.

Brazil: *Rio de Janeiro*

Mario Kroeff Hospital**
Rua Mage 326
Penha Circular CEP 20000
Rio de Janeiro, Brazil
Tel.: 2-80-45-55

Director: Agostino Do Passo

Affiliation: Brazilian Association of Cancer Assistance.

Emphasis: Surgery, chemotherapy, and radiotherapy. Clinical research in statistical studies of neoplastic processes.

Equipment: Conventional diagnostic and therapeutic equipment.

Cancer Personnel:

M.D. AND M.D./Ph.D.:   8 ft, 11 pt   NURSES: 37 ft, 8 pt
TECHNICAL PERSONNEL: 2 ft, 4 pt
   TOTAL: 47 full-time, 23 part-time

Cancer Patient Statistics:

BEDS: 148   NO. OUT-PATIENTS: 4943
NO. IN-PATIENTS: 890   NEW PATIENTS: 4180
AVERAGE STAY: 131

Library: 205 volumes, 5 periodicals.

Tumor Registry.

Professional Education: Postdoctoral training in radiology, nuclear medicine, surgery, chemotherapy, pathology, physics, and social work.

Brazil: *Sao Paulo*

Central Institute, A.C. Camargo Hospital, A. Prudente Foundation**
Rua Prof. Antonio Prudente, 211, P.B. 5271
01509 Sao Paulo, Brazil
Tel.: 278–8811

Director: Professor A.F. Gentil

Affiliation: Divisao Nacional de Cancer.

Emphasis: Treatment of less common tumors, leukemia, Hodgkin disease, and childhood tumors. Full range of treatment facilities with physical, occupational, and social rehabilitation services.

Equipment:

DIAGNOSTIC   THERAPEUTIC
Conventional X-ray equipment   Linear accelerator
                                     Contact therapy
                                     Orthovoltage X-ray
                                     Cesium
                                     Cobalt 60
                                     Isotopes

Cancer Personnel:

M.D. AND M.D./Ph.D.:   79
Ph.D.:   2
   TOTAL: 173

TECHNICAL PERSONNEL: 21
NURSES: 71

Cancer Patient Statistics:

BEDS: 324
NO. IN-PATIENTS: 5467
AVERAGE STAY: 16

NO. OUT-PATIENTS: 50,053
NEW PATIENTS: 4004

Library: 4957 volumes, 60 periodicals.

Tumor Registry.

Professional Education: Basic instruction in neoplastic process and specialization courses in surgery, medicine, and radium therapy.

Bulgaria: *Sofia*

Bulgarian Oncological Research Institute**
Plovdisko pole str. 6
1156 Sofia, Bulgaria
Tel.: 72 05 45

Director: Professor Gerassim Mitrov

Affiliation: Academy of Medicine.

Emphasis: Full range of surgery, chemotherapy, radiotherapy, and immuno-therapy with physical and rehabilitation services. Clinical research in lung, breast, stomach, colon, and rectal cancers.

Equipment:

DIAGNOSTIC
Conventional X-ray equipment

THERAPEUTIC
42meV Betatron
Telecobalt
Superficial X-ray
Isotopes

Cancer Personnel:

M.D. AND M.D./Ph.D.:   45
Ph.D.:   94
   TOTAL: 357

TECHNICAL PERSONNEL: 40
NURSES: 178

Cancer Patient Statistics:

BEDS: 265
NO. IN-PATIENTS: 2331
AVERAGE STAY: 41

NO. OUT-PATIENTS: 47,086
NEW PATIENTS: 2587

Library: 11,891 volumes, 137 periodicals.

Tumor Registry.

Professional Education: Postgraduate training in oncology, surgery, radiotherapy, and chemotherapy.

Canada: *Alberta*

Cross Cancer Institute
11560 University Ave.
Edmonton, Alberta, Canada T6G 1Z2
Tel.: (403) 432–8771

Director: R. Neil MacDonald, M.D.

Affiliation: University of Alberta.

Emphasis: Medical and radiation oncology. Initiation of a major radiobiology program; estrogen receptor laboratory and epidemiologic program.

Equipment:

DIAGNOSTIC
Estrogen receptor lab
Mammography/thermography
Colposcopy/tomographic-gamma
    camera
CT whole body scanner (1979)

THERAPEUTIC
6meV linear accelerators (2)
20meV linear accelerator
Cobalt 60
Superficial X-ray (2)

Cancer Personnel:

M.D. AND M.D./Ph.D.:   25
Ph.D.:   4
    TOTAL: 137

TECHNICAL PERSONNEL: 45
NURSES: 63

Cancer Patient Statistics:

BEDS: 76
NO. IN-PATIENTS: 2022
AVERAGE STAY: 9

NO. OUT-PATIENTS: 40,000
AVERAGE COST: $150.00
NEW PATIENTS: 2332

Library: 2682 volumes, 148 periodicals.

Tumor Registry.

Professional Education: Resident training in radiotherapy.

Canada: *British Columbia*

British Columbia Cancer Institute*
2656 Heather St.
Vancouver, British Columbia, V5Z 3J3, Canada
Tel.: 874–9321

Director: J.M.W. Gibson, M.D.

Affiliation: University of British Columbia.

Emphasis: Radiobiology with special reference to pi-meson therapy and the development of radiosensitivities. Clinical research in protocols for the treatment of lymphomata and participation in trials for the treatment of leukemia.

Equipment:

DIAGNOSTIC	THERAPEUTIC
Conventional X-ray equipment	Cobalt (4)
	Cesium
	280kV X-ray
	Superficial X-ray

Cancer Personnel:

M.D. AND M.D./Ph.D.:	9	TECHNICAL PERSONNEL:	10
Ph.D.:	9	NURSES:	44
TOTAL:	72		

Cancer Patient Statistics:

BEDS:	60	NO. OUT-PATIENTS:	23,502
NO. IN-PATIENTS:	2046	NEW PATIENTS:	2995
AVERAGE STAY:	14		

Cancer Library: None.

Tumor Registry: None.

Professional Education: Training of radiologists and undergraduate instruction. Resident training in gynecology, medicine, and surgery.

Canada: *British Columbia*

Manitoba Cancer Treatment and Research Foundation
700 Bannatyne Ave.
Winnipeg, Manitoba R3E 0V9, Canada
(204) 787–2241

Director: L.G. Israels, M.D.

Affiliation: University of Manitoba, Health Sciences Center; St. Boniface Hospital.

Emphasis: Cancer treatment and rehabilitation in pediatric and adult malignancies. Research on hematologic malignancies and solid tumors. Coordinating agency for Province cervical screening program and cancer statistics.

Equipment:

DIAGNOSTIC	THERAPEUTIC
CAT scanner	4meV Linac
Ultrasound	Cobalt 60
Nuclear medicine	Therac 40
Immunodiagnostic labs	

Cancer Personnel:

M.D. AND M.D./Ph.D.:   6 ft, 17 pt   TECHNICAL PERSONNEL: 49 ft, 1 pt
Ph.D.:   14 ft   NURSES: 31 ft
     TOTAL: 100 full-time, 18 part-time

Cancer Patient Statistics:

OUT-PATIENT FACILITY: 25,396   NEW PATIENTS: 1065

Library: 3475 volumes, 89 periodicals.

Tumor Registry.

Professional Education: Under- and postgraduate instruction in oncology for University of Manitoba. Continuing education for Province physicians.

Canada: *Ontario*

Ontario Cancer Foundation, London Clinic
Victoria Hospital, South St.
London, Ontario, Canada N6A 4G5
(519) 432–5241, ext. 391

Director: T.A. Watson, M.B., Ch.B.

Affiliation: University of Western Ontario.

Emphasis: Radiotherapy, chemotherapy, and nuclear medicine. Research in Hodgkin disease, radiation dosimetry, chemotherapy, and immunology.

Equipment:

DIAGNOSTIC	THERAPEUTIC
Conventional X-ray equipment	Theratron-80
Nuclear medicine	Betatron
	Therac 6
	Simulator
	Strontium plaque

Cancer Personnel:

M.D. AND M.D./Ph.D.: 10
Ph.D.: 7
   TOTAL: 41

TECHNICAL PERSONNEL: 17
NURSES: 7

Cancer Patient Statistics:

BEDS: 39
NO. IN-PATIENTS: 39+

NO. OUT-PATIENTS: 40,000
NEW PATIENTS: 2529

Library: 1200 volumes and periodicals.

Tumor Registry:

Professional Education: Training in therapeutic radiology. Graduate instruction in radiobiology, radiation physics, and nuclear medicine.

Canada: *Ontario*

The Ontario Cancer Institute
500 Sherbourne St.
Toronto, Ontario, Canada M4X 1K9
(416) 924-0671

Director: Raymond S. Bush, M.D.

Admissions: T. West

Affiliation: University of Toronto; Ontario Cancer Treatment and Research Foundation.

Emphasis: Radiation therapy, chemotherapy, and surgical consultation. Rehabilitation. Rehabilitation in head and neck protheses. Research in leukemia.

Equipment:

DIAGNOSTIC
Computer treatment planning
Thermography
Ultrasound and rectal probe
Body section CAT scanner
Gamma camera
Rectilinear scanner

THERAPEUTIC
35meV Varian linear accelerator
Cobalt
Irradiator
Full range of radiotherapy

Cancer Personnel:

M.D. AND M.D./Ph.D.: 49 ft, 2 pt
Ph.D.: 23 ft
   TOTAL: 373 full-time, 19 part-time

TECHNICAL PERSONNEL: 167 ft, 17 pt
NURSES: 134 ft

Cancer Patient Statistics:

BEDS: 172
NO. IN-PATIENTS: 5356
AVERAGE STAY: 10
NO. OUT-PATIENTS: 66,900

AVERAGE COST: $253.00
PAYMENT PLAN: all
NEW PATIENTS: 6127

Library: 6000 volumes, 1200 periodicals.

Tumor Registry: None.

Professional Education: Postgraduate training in medical biophysics. Under-graduate instruction in clinical, pathologic, and radiologic aspects of malignancies.

Canada: *Quebec*

Centre d'Oncologie, Hospital Notre-Dame
2065 Alexandre De Seve
Montreal, Quebec H27 2W5, Canada
(514) 876–7272

Director: Yvan Methot, M.D.

Affiliation: University of Montreal.

Emphasis: Radiation, medical, and surgical oncology. Use of colposcopy. Re-habilitation in ostomy and laryngectomy.

Equipment:

DIAGNOSTIC
CT scanner
Colposcopy
Conventional X-ray equipment

THERAPEUTIC
Cobalt
Afterloading
Cesium

Cancer Personnel:

M.D. AND M.D./Ph.D.: 22 ft, 5 pt
Ph.D.: 2 ft
  TOTAL: 49 full-time, 5 part-time

TECHNICAL PERSONNEL: 19 ft
NURSES: 6 ft

Cancer Patient Statistics:

BEDS: 150
NO. IN-PATIENTS: 323
AVERAGE STAY: 24

NO. OUT-PATIENTS: 12,154
NEW PATIENTS: 2193
AVERAGE COST: $254.00

Library: 500 volumes, 70 periodicals.

Tumor Registry.

Canada: *Saskatchewan*

Allan Blair Memorial Clinic
1555 Pasqua St.
Regina, Saskatchewan, S4T 4L8 Canada
(306) 527-9651

Director: Peter A.M. Walden, M.D.

Affiliation: Western Canada Cancer Agency; National Cancer Institute

Emphasis: Specialization in carcinoma of the endometrium, colorectal, and
ovarian carcinomas. Clinical research in carcinoma of the endometrium and
effect of combined radiation and chemotherapy.

Equipment: Conventional diagnostic and therapeutic equipment.

Cancer Personnel:

M.D. AND M.D./Ph.D.:	10	TECHNICAL PERSONNEL:	5
Ph.D.:	2	NURSES:	6
TOTAL:	23		

Cancer Patient Statistics:

NO. OUT-PATIENTS: 8661
NO. NEW PATIENTS: 2283

Library: 800 volumes, 68 periodicals.

Registry: Complete Province patient registry.

Professional Education: Programs for family practitioners, nurses, and technicians.

Canada: *Saskatchewan*

Saskatchewan Cancer Commission*
4003 Dewdney Ave.
Regina, Saskatchewan, S4T 4L8, Canada
(306) 523-8288

Director: D.H. Crofford

Affiliation: College of Medicine, University of Saskatchewan; Saskatchewan Dept.
of Public Health

Emphasis: Clinical research in Hodgkin disease and myeloma. Statistical research
in breast and G.I. tract cancer. Surgery, chemotherapy, and radiotherapy treatment.

Equipment:

DIAGNOSTIC
Conventional X-ray equipment
Gamma cameras
Scanners

THERAPEUTIC
Isocentric teletherapy
Betatron
Crystal detector
Superficial X-ray
Orthovoltage X-ray

Cancer Personnel:

M.D. AND M.D./Ph.D.: 20
Ph.D.: 6
   TOTAL: 47

TECHNICAL PERSONNEL: 8
NURSES: 13

Cancer Patient Statistics:

NO. IN-PATIENTS: 6717
AVERAGE STAY: 17

NO. OUT-PATIENTS: 33,167
NEW PATIENTS: 3146

Library: 3000 volumes, 80 periodicals.

Tumor Registry.

Professional Education: Resident training in therapeutic radiology. Undergraduate instruction in diagnostic and therapeutic radiology, nuclear medicine, and ionizing radiation.

Canada: *Saskatchewan*

Saskatoon Cancer Clinic*
University Hospital Clinic
Saskatoon, Saskatchewan, S7N 0W8, Canada
(306) 343–9565

Director: E.M. Brown, M.C.

Affiliation: Saskatchewan Cancer Commission.

Emphasis: Research into physics, radiotherapy, chemotherapy, immunotherapy, nuclear medicine, and epidemiology. Treatment by chemotherapy, radiotherapy, and surgery.

Equipment:

DIAGNOSTIC
Conventional X-ray equipment
Gamma cameras
Scanners

THERAPEUTIC
Isocentric teletherapy
Betatron
Crystal detector
Superficial X-ray
Orthovoltage X-ray

Cancer Personnel:

M.D. AND M.D./Ph.D.: 10   TECHNICAL PERSONNEL: 10
Ph.D.: 3   NURSES: 6
  TOTAL: 29

Cancer Patient Statistics:

NO. IN-PATIENTS: 2538   NO. OUT-PATIENTS: 12,892
AVERAGE STAY: 16   NEW PATIENTS: 1629

Cancer Library: None.

Tumor Registry.

Professional Education: Resident training in radiotherapy and nuclear medicine.

Chile: *Santiago*

Dr. C.P. Correa National Radium Institute**
Zanartu No. 1000, Casilla No. 6677, Correo No. 4
Santiago de Chile
Tel.: 37 6008

Director: Jose Rajevie Bravar, M.D.

Affiliation: Ministerio de Salud Publica; Servicio Nacional de Salud.

Emphasis: Surgery, radiotherapy/curietherapy, and chemotherapy. Clinical research on lymphocytes and mucopolysaccharides.

Equipment:

DIAGNOSTIC   THERAPEUTIC
Conventional X-ray equipment   Telecobalt (2)
Cesium sources   Orthovoltage X-ray
     Sealed radium
     Cesium sources

Cancer Personnel:

M.D. AND M.D./Ph.D.: 12 ft, 10 pt   NURSES: 68 ft
TECHNICAL PERSONNEL: 4 ft
  TOTAL: 84 full-time, 10 part-time

Cancer Patient Statistics:

BEDS: 92   NO. OUT-PATIENTS: 14,381
NO. IN-PATIENTS: 1120   NEW PATIENTS: 1485
AVERAGE STAY: 33

Library: 800 volumes, 10 periodicals.

Tumor Registry: None.

Professional Education: Postgraduate training and undergraduate instruction of physicians, nurses, and technicians with the University of Chile.

Columbia: *Bogota*

Instituto Nacional de Cancerologia
Calle La 9–85
Bogota, Columbia
Tel.: 466 019

Director: Julio Ospina, M.D.

Admissions: Cesar Mendoza, M.D.

Affiliation: Ministry of Public Health.

Emphasis: Radiotherapy, nuclear medicine, and surgery. Development of National Cancer Program with facilities for radiotherapy and chemotherapy. Research in nuclear medicine and treatment/rehabilitation for all malignancies.

Equipment:

DIAGNOSTIC	THERAPEUTIC
Conventional X-ray equipment	Cobalt (4)
Electron microscope	
Chromatography	

Cancer Personnel:

M.D. AND M.D./Ph.D.: 49 ft, 29 pt	TECHNICAL PERSONNEL: 45 ft
Ph.D.: 1 ft	NURSES: 84 ft
TOTAL: 179 full-time, 29 part-time	

Cancer Patient Statistics:

BEDS: 160	NO. OUT-PATIENTS: 22,857
NO. IN-PATIENTS: 2224	NEW PATIENTS: 2281
AVERAGE STAY: 15	

Library: 20,000 volumes.

Tumor Registry.

Professional Education: Postgraduate training in oncology.

Cuba: *Havana*

Cuban Institute of Oncology and Radiobiology*
29 & F Street
Havana 4, Cuba
Tel.: 32–7531

Director: Professor Zoilo Marinello

Affiliation: Ministry of Public Health.

Emphasis: Surgery, radiotherapy, and chemotherapy treatment; pediatric cancer care, rehabilitation and social services. Research in Hodgkin disease and early diagnosis.

Equipment:

DIAGNOSTIC	THERAPEUTIC
Conventional diagnostic X-ray equipment	Cobalt 60 (4)
	Nuclear medicine facilities

Cancer Personnel:

M.D. AND M.D./Ph.D.:	65	TECHNICAL PERSONNEL:	111
Ph.D.:	51	NURSES:	108
TOTAL:	335		

Cancer Patient Statistics:

BEDS:	405	NO. OUT-PATIENTS:	108,200
NO. IN-PATIENTS:	5075	NEW PATIENTS:	2400
AVERAGE STAY:	23		

Library: 2000 volumes, 200 periodicals

Tumor Registry.

Professional Education: Postgraduate training in oncology.

Czechoslovakia: *Bratislavia*

Slovakia Oncological Institute**
Heydukova ulica c. 10
88102 Bratislavia, Czechoslovakia
Tel.: 537 11, 575 41, 2, 3

Director: Peter Cepek, M.D., Ph.D.

Emphasis: Primary nonsurgical and radical surgical treatment of malignant diseases except skeleton and CNS. Research in immunology and early diagnosis.

Equipment:

DIAGNOSTIC
Conventional diagnostic X-ray
   equipment

THERAPEUTIC
Orthovoltage
Nuclear medicine facilities

Cancer Personnel:

M.D. AND M.D./Ph.D.: 50 ft, 1 pt
Ph.D.: 8 ft, 5 pt
   TOTAL: 242 full-time, 9 part-time

TECHNICAL PERSONNEL: 46 ft, 3 pt
NURSES: 138

Cancer Patient Statistics:

BEDS: 200
NO. IN-PATIENTS: 2594

AVERAGE STAY: 25
NO. OUT-PATIENTS: 31,957

Library: 8100 volumes, 2500 periodicals

Tumor Registry: None.

Professional Education: Postgraduate specialization in clinical oncology and in radiotherapy and gynecologic oncology.

Czechoslovakia: *Prague*

Institute of Radiotherapy
18000 Praha 8
Na Truhlarce 100, Czechoslovakia
Tel.: 84 39 45

Director: Vladimir Kubec, M.D.

Affiliation: Institute of National Health, Prague.

Emphasis: Nonsurgical cancer treatment, radiotherapy, and clinical oncology. Immunotherapy and chemotherapy. Basic research in chemical carcinogenesis, proteosynthesis, and brachytherapy.

Equipment:

DIAGNOSTIC
Conventional X-ray equipment
Electron microscope

THERAPEUTIC
Telecobalt (2)
Linear accelerator
Simulator
Afterloading

Cancer Personnel:

M.D. AND M.D./Ph.D.: 20 ft, 7 pt
Ph.D.: 6 ft
   TOTAL: 149 full-time, 7 part-time

TECHNICAL PERSONNEL: 50
NURSES: 73

Cancer Patient Statistics:

BEDS: 103
NO. IN-PATIENTS: 1424
AVERAGE STAY: 21

NO. OUT-PATIENTS: 47,553
NEW PATIENTS: 1286

Library: 7780 volumes.

Tumor Registry.

Professional Education: Postgraduate training in radiotherapy and oncology.

Denmark: *Aarhus*

Department of Radiotherapy and Oncology
Aarhus Municipal Hospital
8000 Aarhus C, Denmark
Tel.: 06–125–555

Director: Professor Sigvard Kaae, M.D.

Affiliation: University of Aarhus.

Emphasis: Radiotherapy and chemotherapy. Research in Hodgkin disease. Treatment of uterine and bladder cancers.

Equipment:

DIAGNOSTIC
Conventional X-ray equipment

THERAPEUTIC
Cobalt (2)
Linear accelerators (2)
Betatron

Cancer Personnel:

M.D. AND M.D./Ph.D.:   21
Ph.D.:   8
   TOTAL: 236

TECHNICAL PERSONNEL: 55
NURSES: 152

Cancer Patient Statistics:

BEDS: 160
NO. IN-PATIENTS: 4761
AVERAGE STAY: 10

NO. OUT-PATIENTS: 23,794
NEW PATIENTS: 1844

Library: 5000 volumes.

Tumor Registry: None.

Denmark: *Copenhagen*

Finsen Institute**
Strand Boulevarden 49
2100 Copenhagen, Denmark
Tel.: 01–260850

Director: J.H. Zeuthen

Emphasis: Radiotherapy, chemotherapy, and surgery treatment techniques. Research in multimodality therapies.

Equipment:

DIAGNOSTIC
Conventional diagnostic X-ray
    equipment
Electron microscope

THERAPEUTIC
Linear accelerators (3)
Cobalt (2)
Betatron

Cancer Personnel:

M.D. AND M.D./Ph.D.:   93 ft
Ph.D.:   32 ft
    TOTAL: 579 full-time, 8 part-time,
        39 volunteer

TECHNICAL PERSONNEL: 92 ft, 29
    volunteer
NURSES: 362 ft, 8 pt, 10 volunteer

Cancer Patient Statistics:

BEDS: 292
NO. IN-PATIENTS: 4831

AVERAGE STAY: 13
NO. OUT-PATIENTS: 267,536

Library: 10,000 volumes, 200 periodicals.

Tumor Registry.

Professional Education: Postgraduate training in oncology, radiotherapy, nuclear medicine.

Egypt: *Cairo*

Cairo University Cancer Institute*
Kasr El Aini St.
Cairo, Egypt
Tel.: 843661 842329

Director: Professor Ismail El-Sebai

Affiliation: Cairo University.

Emphasis: Surgery, radiotherapy and radiodiagnosis, and medical oncology.

Clinical research in bladder, head and neck, breast, colon, and rectal cancers, and in lymphoma.

Equipment: Conventional diagnostic and therapeutic X-ray equipment.

Cancer Personnel:

M.D. AND M.D./Ph.D.:   34   TECHNICAL PERSONNEL: 20
Ph.D.:   10   NURSES: 65
   TOTAL: 129

Cancer Patient Statistics:

BEDS: 300   NO. OUT-PATIENTS: 6440
NO. IN-PATIENTS: 2659   NEW PATIENTS: 2475
AVERAGE STAY: 33

Cancer Library: None.

Tumor Registry: None.

Professional Education: Postgraduate training and undergraduate education.

England: *London*

Charing Cross Hospital Medical Oncology and Radiotherapy
Oncology Departments*
Fulham Palace Road
London, England W68RF
Tel.: 01–748 2050

Directors: K. Bagshawe, M.D.; D. O'Connell, M.D.

Affiliation: University of London.

Emphasis: National treatment center for patients with trophoblastic tumors, gestational choriocarcinoma, malignant teratoma, leukemia, lymphoma, and solid tumors.

Equipment:

DIAGNOSTIC   THERAPEUTIC
Full range of diagnostic X-ray   Cobalt 60 (2)
   equipment   250kV X-ray
                                   Superficial X-ray
                                   Sealed and unsealed isotopes

Cancer Personnel:

M.D. AND M.D./Ph.D.:   17   TECHNICAL PERSONNEL: 20
Ph.D.:   45   NURSES: 50
   TOTAL: 132

Cancer Patient Statistics:

BEDS: 80
NO. IN-PATIENTS: 1600
AVERAGE STAY: 15

NO. OUT-PATIENTS: 10,000
NEW PATIENTS: 1500

Library: 350 volumes, 20 periodicals

Tumor Registry: None.

Professional Education: Instruction for biochemists and clinical pathologists.

England: *London*

Royal Marsden Hospital*
Fulham Road
London, England SW3
Tel.: 01 352 8171

Director: C.B. Cameron, M.D.

Affiliations: Institute of Cancer Research; South-West Thames Regional Cancer Service.

Emphasis: Diagnosis and treatment of leukemia, lymphomas, testicular tumors, childhood tumors, brain tumors, and cancer of the male and female genital tracts.

Equipment: Conventional diagnostic and therapeutic equipment.

Cancer Patient Statistics:

BEDS: 371
NO. IN-PATIENTS: 9000
AVERAGE STAY: 12

NO. OUT-PATIENTS: 80,000
NEW PATIENTS: 4000

Cancer Library: None.

Tumor Registry.

Professional Education: Postgraduate training in cancer nursing, radiotherapy, and nuclear medicine.

England: *Manchester*

Christie Hospital and Holt Radium Institute and Paterson Labs.*
Withington, Manchester, England M209BX
Tel.: 061 445–8123

Directors: D. Crowther, Ph.D.; E. Easson, M.D.; L. Lajtha, M.D.

Affiliation: University of Manchester.

Emphasis: Specialized cancer surgery relating to radiotherapy; head and neck, breast, urologic, gynecologic and reconstructive surgery. Clinical research in trials involving radiotherapy, surgery, and chemotherapy.

Equipment:

DIAGNOSTIC
Conventional X-ray equipment

THERAPEUTIC
Linear accelerators
Telecobalt
Superficial X-ray
Electron and neutron
Sealed and unsealed isotopes

Cancer Personnel:

M.D. AND M.D./Ph.D.:   42 ft, 21 pt
Ph.D.:   73 ft, 5 pt
   TOTAL: 471 full-time, 26 part-time

TECHNICAL PERSONNEL: 150 ft
NURSES: 206 ft

Cancer Patient Statistics:

BEDS: 360
NO. IN-PATIENTS: 6300
AVERAGE STAY: 13

NO. OUT-PATIENTS: 77,731
NEW PATIENTS: 5886

Library: 2000 volumes, 147 periodicals.

Tumor Registry.

Professional Education: Postgraduate training in radiotherapy, radiobiology, and experimental and social oncology.

England: *Newcastle-upon-Tyne*

Cancer Research Campaign Oncological Center
Newcastle General Hospital
Westgate Road
Newcastle-upon-Tyne, NE4 6BE, England
Tel.: 38811, ext. 655

Director: William M. Ross, M.D.

Admissions: William M. Ross, M.D.

Affiliation: Newcastle General Hospital.

Emphasis: Treatment and rehabilitation. Cancer research in national clinical trials.

Equipment:

DIAGNOSTIC
Conventional X-ray equipment

THERAPEUTIC
Full range of external beam, intra-cavitary, interstitial, and isotope equipment

Cancer Personnel:

M.D. AND M.D./PH.D.:   15
Ph.D.:   6
   TOTAL: 111

TECHNICAL PERSONNEL: 30
NURSES: 60

Cancer Patient Statistics:

BEDS: 90
NO. IN-PATIENTS: 1831
AVERAGE STAY: 13

NO. OUT-PATIENTS: 33,722
NEW PATIENTS: 5200

Library: 1000 volumes, 20 periodicals.

Tumor Registry.

Professional Education: Postgraduate training.

France: *Angers*

Paul Papin Cancer Center**
2 rue Moll
49036 Angers Cédéx, France
Tel.: 883746

Director: Jean Cheguillaume, M.D.

Affiliation: French Federation of Anticancer Centers; International Union Against Cancer.

Emphasis: Radiotherapy and surgery. Research in chemotherapy of breast cancer and complications of radiotherapy.

Equipment:

DIAGNOSTIC
Gamma camera
Total body scanner
Thermography
Sonography

THERAPEUTIC
Cobalt (2)
Linear accelerator
Cesium
Iridium

Cancer Personnel:

M.D. AND M.D./Ph.D.:   5 ft, 19 pt

TECHNICAL PERSONNEL: 20 ft

Ph.D.:   3 ft   NURSES: 67 ft, 3 pt
    TOTAL: 95 full-time, 22 part-time

Cancer Patient Statistics:

BEDS: 78   NO. OUT-PATIENTS: 14,004
NO. IN-PATIENTS: 2132   NEW PATIENTS: 940
AVERAGE STAY: 12

Library: 400 volumes, 112 periodicals.

Tumor Registry: None.

Professional Education: Postgraduate training and radiotherapy.

France: *Bordeaux*

Bergonié Foundation Regional Cancer Center**
180 rue de Saint-Genes
33076 Bordeaux Cédéx, France
Tel.: (56) 911325

Director: Professor Claude Lagarde, M.D.

Affiliation: University of Bordeaux.

Emphasis: Surgery, radiotherapy, and chemotherapy with emphasis on thyroid
and breast tumors. Research in experimental hematology and endocrinology.

Equipment:

DIAGNOSTIC   THERAPEUTIC
Mammography   Linear accelerator
Thermography   Telecobalt (2)
Xerography   Dosimetry
Conventional X-ray equipment   Superficial X-ray
                                                 Isotopes

Cancer Personnel:

M.D. AND M.D./Ph.D.:   19 ft, 15 pt   TECHNICAL PERSONNEL: 30 ft
Ph.D.:   7 ft, 3 pt   NURSES: 60 ft
    TOTAL: 116 full-time, 18 part-time

Cancer Patient Statistics:

BEDS: 206   NO. OUT-PATIENTS: 19,875
NO. IN-PATIENTS: 3194   NEW PATIENTS: 2022
AVERAGE STAY: 22

Library: 3000 volumes, 110 periodicals.

Tumor Registry: None.

Professional Education: Graduate training in oncology. Postdoctoral training for radiologists, surgeons, pathologists, and hematologists.

France: *Dijon*

George François Leclerc Anti-Cancer Center
1 Prof. Marion St.
21034 Dijon Cédéx, France
Tel.: (80) 66 81 36

Director: Professor Ferdinand Cabanne, M.D.

Affiliation: State Department of Health University; Dijon University

Emphasis: Specialization in radiotherapy and surgery. Research on comparative therapeutic trials and digestive tract cancers. Regional information data for tumors pathology. Regional registry for digestive tract cancers.

Equipment:

DIAGNOSTIC	THERAPEUTIC
Radiodiagnosis (4 rooms)	Cobalt (2)
Sonography	Isotope equipment
Thermography	32meV linear accelerators
Nuclear medicine	Curietherapy—afterloaders for gyne-
Scanner	cology with cesium (5)
Gamma camera	

Cancer Personnel:

M.D. AND M.D./Ph.D.:   22 ft, 16 pt   TECHNICAL PERSONNEL: 45 ft
Ph.D.:   2 pt   NURSES: 60 ft
   TOTAL: 127 full-time, 18 part-time

Cancer Patient Statistics:

BEDS: 186   NO. OUT-PATIENTS: 7339
NO. IN-PATIENTS: 1744   NEW PATIENTS: 1373
AVERAGE STAY: 29.21   AVERAGE COST: 597,00F/day

Library: 900 volumes, 100 periodicals.

Tumor Registry.

Professional Education: Medical school instruction and postgraduate training.

France: *Lille*

Oscar Lambret Center**
1 rue Frédéric Combemale, B.P. 3569
59020 Lille Cédéx, France
Tel.: 57 12 00

Director: Professor Alain Demaille

Affiliation: French Federation of Anticancer Centers.

Emphasis: Specialization in experimental cancer research. Treatment and rehabilitation of solid tumors, leukemias, and hematosarcomas. Research in prognosis factors and radiosensitivity of tumor cells.

Equipment:

DIAGNOSTIC	THERAPEUTIC
Conventional X-ray equipment	Orthovoltage X-ray
	Nuclear medicine

Cancer Personnel:

M.D. AND M.D./Ph.D.: 17 ft, 15 pt   TECHNICAL PERSONNEL: 90 ft
Ph.D.: 1 ft, 1 pt   NURSES: 155 ft
　　TOTAL: 263 full-time, 16 part-time

Cancer Patient Statistics:

BEDS: 304   NO. OUT-PATIENTS: 11,836
AVERAGE STAY: 26   NEW PATIENTS: 2306

Library: 3400 volumes, 112 periodicals.

Tumor Registry: None.

Professional Education: Radiotherapy and medical gynecology.

France: *Lyon*

Leon Berard Center**
28 rue Laennec
69373 Lyon Cédéx 2, France
Tel.: 16–78 74–08–36

Director: Professor Marcel Mayer

Affiliation: Lyon University, Faculty of Medicine.

Emphasis: Surgery, chemotherapy, radiotherapy, hormonotherapy, and immunotherapy. Clinical research in breast cancer and immunologic research on
melanoma.

Equipment:

DIAGNOSTIC
Conventional X-ray equipment

THERAPEUTIC
Cobalt 60
Betatron
Radium
Iridium

Cancer Personnel:

M.D. AND M.D./Ph.D.:   34 ft, 28 pt
Ph.D.:   8 ft
   TOTAL: 261 full-time, 28 part-time

TECHNICAL PERSONNEL: 55 ft
NURSES: 164 ft

Cancer Patient Statistics:

BEDS: 315
NO. IN-PATIENTS: 4660
AVERAGE STAY: 16

NO. OUT-PATIENTS: 42,284
NEW PATIENTS: 3617

Cancer Library: None

Tumor Registry: None.

Professional Education: Resident training.

France: *Marseilles*

J. Paoli—I. Calmettes Institute**
232, Bd de Sainte-Marguerite
13272 Marseilles Cédéx, France
Tel.: (91) 75 90 86

Director: Professor Xavier Serafino

Affiliation: French Federation of Anticancer Centers.

Emphasis: Special competence in the treatment of leukemia and Hodgkin disease and in the conservative treatment of breast cancer. Rehabilitation center with psychiatric services and maxillofacial prothesis unit. Full range of surgical, radio-therapeutic, chemotherapeutic, and immunotherapeutic treatment facilities.

Equipment:

DIAGNOSTIC
Conventional X-ray equipment

THERAPEUTIC
Betatron
Cobalt
Cesium
Superficial X-ray
Electron and neutron
Isotopes

Cancer Personnel:

M.D. AND M.D./Ph.D.: 22 ft, 59 pt   NURSES: 120 ft
TECHNICAL PERSONNEL: 55 ft, 5 pt
    TOTAL: 197 full-time, 64 part-time

Cancer Patient Statistics:

BEDS: 318   NO. OUT-PATIENTS: 6715
NO. IN-PATIENTS: 5343   NEW PATIENTS: 1628
AVERAGE STAY: 18

Library: 1444 volumes, 120 periodicals.

Tumor Registry.

Professional Education: Undergraduate instruction. Programs for specialization in anatomopathology, hematology, pneumology, and radiology.

France: *Montpellier*

Montpellier Regional Cancer Center*
Clinques Saint Eloi
34059 Montpellier Cédéx, France
Tel.: 63 28 73

Director: Professor Claude Romieu

Affiliation: University of Montpellier.

Emphasis: Surgery, radiotherapy, chemotherapy, and hormonotherapy. Clinical research in hypernutrition and hyperalimentation.

Equipment:

DIAGNOSTIC   THERAPEUTIC
Conventional X-ray equipment   Isotopes
Electron microscope   Linear accelerator

Cancer Personnel:

M.D. AND M.D./Ph.D.: 25   TECHNICAL PERSONNEL: 224
Ph.D.: 16
    TOTAL: 265

Cancer Patient Statistics:

NO. OUT-PATIENTS: 8054   NEW PATIENTS: 1424

Cancer Library. None.

Tumor Registry.

Professional Education: Postgraduate training and undergraduate instruction.

France: *Nantes*

Nantes Cancer Center**
Quai Moncousu
44035 Nantes Cédéx, France
Tel.: (40) 73 41 82

Director: Professor Joseph Tardiveau, M.D.

Affiliation: French Federation of Anticancer Centers.

Emphasis: Special competence in hematosarcomas, sarcomas, melanomas, breast,
uterine, testicular, and lung cancers. Clinical research in chemotherapeutic
techniques.

Equipment:

DIAGNOSTIC	THERAPEUTIC
Thermography	Orthovoltage X-ray
Xerography	Cobalt
Echotomography	Contact radiotherapy
Radioimmunology	Radium
	Iridium

Cancer Personnel:

M.D. AND M.D./Ph.D.: 10 ft, 9 pt,
   1 volunteer
     TOTAL: 64 full-time, 9 part-time,
     1 volunteer

TECHNICAL PERSONNEL: 5
NURSES: 44

Cancer Patient Statistics:

BEDS: 80
NO. IN-PATIENTS 1523
AVERAGE STAY: 16

NO. OUT-PATIENTS: 9225
NEW PATIENTS: 3530

Library: 2000 volumes, 50 periodicals.

Tumor Registry.

Professional Education: Medical student training in clinical oncology; postgraduate training in radiotherapy and radiodiagnosis.

France: *Nice*

Antoine-Lacassagne Center
36 Voie Romaine
06054 Nice, France
Tel.: 53 10 10

Director: Professor Claude M. Lalanne, M.D.

Admissions: Professor Claude M. Lalanne, M.D.

Affiliation: French Federation of Anticancer Centers.

Emphasis: Radiotherapy. Rehabilitation for larynx and breast cancer. Research in hormonotherapy, chemotherapy, and radiotherapy.

Equipment:

DIAGNOSTIC
Thermography
Echography
Nuclear medicine
Radioimmunology
Hematology

THERAPEUTIC
High-energy radiotherapy
Cobalt
32 meV linear accelerator

Cancer Personnel:

M.D. AND M.D./Ph.D.: 30 ft, 25 pt
Ph.D.: 12 ft
   TOTAL: 196 full-time, 25 part-time

TECHNICAL PERSONNEL: 54 ft
NURSES: 100 ft

Cancer Patient Statistics:

BEDS: 200
NO. IN-PATIENTS: 3276
AVERAGE STAY: 17

NO. OUT-PATIENTS: 33,508
NEW PATIENTS: 5405

Library: 400 volumes, 100 periodicals.

Tumor Registry.

Professional Education: Postgraduate training.

France: *Paris*

Foundation Curie Institut du Radium
26 rue d'Ulm
75231 Paris Cédéx 05, France
Tel.: 329 12 42

Director: Robert Calle, M.D.

Affiliation: French Federation of Anticancer Centers.

Emphasis: Surgery, radiotherapy, chemotherapy, and immunotherapy. Physical, occupational, and rehabilitation programs. Research on ionizing radiation and radioactive substances.

Equipment:

DIAGNOSTIC	THERAPEUTIC
Mammography	Betatron
Thermography	Linear accelerator
Nuclear medicine	Cobalt 60 (4)

Cancer Personnel:

M.D. AND M.D./Ph.D.:   23 ft, 20 pt   NURSES: 90 ft
    TOTAL: 113 full-time, 20 part-time

Cancer Patient Statistics:

BEDS: 183   NO. OUT-PATIENTS: 19,512
AVERAGE STAY: 13   NEW PATIENTS: 2476

Library: 4000 volumes, 100 periodicals.

Tumor Registry.

Professional Education: Postgraduate training in oncology, pathology surgery, cytology, radiotherapy, and radiodiagnosis. Graduate instruction in radiotherapy.

France: *Rouen*

Centre Regional de Lutte Contre le Cancer
Rue d'Amiens
76 038 Rouen Cédéx, France
Tel.: 16 (35) 98 20 27

Director: Professor Rene Laumonier

Admissions: Madame Auber

Affiliation: French Federation of Anticancer Centers.

Emphasis: Specializing in cancer of the breast and uterus. Surgery, radiotherapy, and chemotherapy. Research in Hodgkin disease.

Equipment:

DIAGNOSTIC
Gamma camera
Thermography
Seriography
Electron microscope

THERAPEUTIC
Betatron
Cobalt 60

Cancer Personnel:

M.D. AND M.D./Ph.D.: 25 ft, 11 pt
Ph.D.: 2 ft
   TOTAL: 152 full-time, 11 part-time

TECHNICAL PERSONNEL: 50
NURSES: 75

Cancer Patient Statistics:

BEDS: 170
NO. IN-PATIENTS: 1581
AVERAGE STAY: 105

NO. OUT-PATIENTS: 13,158
NEW PATIENTS: 1637

Library: 2000 volumes.

Tumor Registry.

Professional Education: Training in oncology, pathology, and hematology.

France: *Saint-Cloud*

Rene Huguenin Center
5 rue Gaston Latouche
92211 St-Cloud, France
Tel.: 602 70 50

Director: Jean Gest, M.D.

Emphasis: Specialization in breast cancer. Clinical research and treatment in breast and larynx cancer. Immunovirology.

Equipment:

DIAGNOSTIC
Mammography
Nuclear medicine

THERAPEUTIC
Linear accelerator

Cancer Personnel:

M.D. AND M.D./Ph.D.: 24 ft, 32 pt
Ph.D.: 2 ft, 2 pt
   TOTAL: 314 full-time, 39 part-time

TECHNICAL PERSONNEL: 133 ft, 5 pt
NURSES: 155

Cancer Patient Statistics:

BEDS: 261
AVERAGE STAY: 23

NO. OUT-PATIENTS: 27,361
NEW PATIENTS: 2634

Library: 2450 volumes, 220 periodicals.

Tumor Registry.

Professional Education: Instruction in radiotherapy and clinical oncology.

France: *Toulouse*

Claudius Regaud Center**
11 rue Piquemil
31300 Toulouse, France
Tel.: (61) 42 94 27

Director: Professor Pierre-François Combes, M.D.

Affiliation: Paul Sabatier University.

Emphasis: Radiotherapy and surgery. Clinical research in thermography detection and follow-up radiation treatment.

Equipment:

DIAGNOSTIC
Radiodiagnosis units
Scintography
Thermography

THERAPEUTIC
Cobalt 60 (2)
X-ray simulation
Dosimetry
Curietherapy

Cancer Personnel:

M.D. AND M.D./Ph.D.:   36 ft, 13 pt
Ph.D.:   6 ft, 1 pt
    TOTAL: 127 full-time, 15 part-time

TECHNICAL PERSONNEL: 33 ft
NURSES: 72 ft, 1 pt

Cancer Patient Statistics:

BEDS: 302
NO. IN-PATIENTS: 3172
AVERAGE STAY: 29

NO. OUT-PATIENTS: 24,542
NEW PATIENTS: 1557

Library: 500 volumes, 87 periodicals.

Tumor Registry.

Professional Education: Training for medical students, nurses, and technicians. Resident training in radiotherapy and nuclear medicine.

France: *Villejuif*

Gustave-Roussy Institute**
16 bis ave. Paul-Vaillant Couturier
94800 Villejuif, France
Tel.: 726–49–09

Director: Professor Pierre Denoix

Affiliation: French Federation of Anticancer Centers; International Union
Against Cancer.

Emphasis: Surgery, chemotherapy, and radiotherapy. Research in immunology,
endocrinology, and virology. Clinical research on radiosensitivity of human
tumor cells.

Equipment:

DIAGNOSTIC
Electron microscope
Conventional X-ray equipment

THERAPEUTIC
Telecobalt
Orthovoltage X-ray
Curietherapy

Cancer Personnel:

M.D. AND M.D./Ph.D.: 95 ft, 61 pt
Ph.D.: 98 ft, 74 pt
    TOTAL: 661 full-time, 149 part-time

TECHNICAL PERSONNEL: 110 ft
NURSES: 358 ft, 14 pt

Cancer Patient Statistics:

BEDS: 515
NO. IN-PATIENTS: 9348
AVERAGE STAY: 21

NO. OUT-PATIENTS: 106,684
NEW PATIENTS: 11,521

Library: 18,000 volumes, 500 periodicals.

Tumor Registry.

Professional Education: Training in oncology diagnosis and treatment.

France: *Vandoeuvre les Nancy*

Alexis Vautrin Center
R.N. 74-Brabois
54500 Vandoeuvre les Nancy, France
Tel.: (28) 55 81 66

Director: Professor Claude Chardot

Affiliation: French Federation of Anticancer Centers.

Emphasis: Surgery and radiotherapy. Research in breast tumors.

Equipment:

DIAGNOSTIC	THERAPEUTIC
Pathology/cytology lab	Linear accelerators
Angiography	Telecobalt
Sonography	Contact therapy
Conventional X-ray equipment	Simulator
	Curietherapy

Cancer Personnel:

M.D. AND M.D./Ph.D.:   19   OTHER PERSONNEL: 299
Ph.D.:   2
   TOTAL: 320

Cancer Patient Statistics:

BEDS: 200   NO. OUT-PATIENTS: 10,000
NO. IN-PATIENTS: 6000   NEW PATIENTS: 2400
AVERAGE STAY: 9

Library: 550 volumes.

Tumor Registry.

Professional Education: Postgraduate training and graduate instruction in oncology.

Germany (Democratic Republic): *Berlin-Buch*

Central Institute for Cancer Research**
   Lindenberger Weg 80
1115 Berlin-Buch, Germany
Tel.: 56 98 51

Director: S. Tanneberger, M.D.

Affiliation: Academy of Sciences of the German Democratic Republic.

Emphasis: Specialization in treatment of tumors of lung, gastrointestinal tract, and female breast. Chemotherapeutic, surgical, and radiotherapeutic treatment. Clinical research on early detection with nuclear medical, microbiologic, immunologic, and endocrinologic procedures.

Equipment:

DIAGNOSTIC	THERAPEUTIC
Conventional X-ray equipment	Orthovoltage X-ray

Cancer Patient Statistics:

BEDS: 217
NO. IN-PATIENTS: 2100

AVERAGE STAY: 28
NEW PATIENTS: 9000

Cancer Library: None.

Tumor Registry.

Germany (Federal Republic): *Essen*

West German Tumor Center
Hufelandstrasse 55
4300 Essen, Fed. Rep. of Germany
Tel.: 7991 2000

Director: Professor Carl G. Schmidt, M.D.

Affiliation: University of Essen.

Emphasis: Chemotherapy and radiotherapy. Research and treatment of hematologic disorders.

Equipment: Conventional diagnostic and therapeutic equipment.

Cancer Personnel:

M.D. AND M.D./Ph.D.: 16
Ph.D.: 6
  TOTAL: 122

TECHNICAL PERSONNEL: 60
NURSES: 40

Cancer Patient Statistics:

BEDS: 92
AVERAGE STAY: 12

NO. IN-PATIENTS: 14,000
NEW PATIENTS: 9800

Library: 20,000 volumes, 100 periodicals.

Tumor Registry: None.

Professional Education: Instruction and training in clinical oncology.

Greece: *Athens*

Hellenic Anticancer Institute**
171 Alexandras Ave.
Athens 603, Greece
Tel.: 642-1201

Director: A. Papaconstantinou

Emphasis: Full range of surgical, radiotherapeutic, chemotherapeutic, and immunotherapeutic treatment facilities. Clinical research on combined radiotherapy and chemotherapy treatment modalities.

Equipment:

DIAGNOSTIC	THERAPEUTIC
Conventional X-ray equipment	Betatron
Electron microscope	Telecobalt (3)
Magnascanner	Superficial X-ray (4)
Scintillation counters	Radium
	Isotopes

Cancer Personnel:

M.D. AND M.D./Ph.D.: 95 ft, 1 pt, 3 volunteer
Ph.D.: 17 ft, 2 pt, 1 volunteer
   TOTAL: 313 full-time, 3 part-time, 4 volunteer

TECHNICAL PERSONNEL: 61 ft
NURSES: 140 ft

Cancer Patient Statistics:

BEDS: 380
NO. IN-PATIENTS: 2355
AVERAGE STAY: 62

NO. OUT-PATIENTS: 31,331
NEW PATIENTS: 23,765

Library: 400 volumes, 108 periodicals.

Tumor Registry: None.

Professional Education: Postgraduate training in oncology, radiotherapy, radiodiagnosis, and surgery.

Greece: *Piraeus*

Metaxas Memorial Cancer Hospital*
51 Botassi St.
Piraeus 30, Greece

Director: V. Lisseos, M.D.

Affiliation: Hellenic Cancer Society.

Emphasis: Surgery, radiation, and chemotherapy. Prophylactic chemotherapy. Immunotherapy. Clinical research in the evaluation of new drugs and multimodality treatment protocols.

Equipment:

DIAGNOSTIC
Conventional X-ray equipment
Thermography

THERAPEUTIC
Orthovoltage X-ray

Cancer Personnel:

M.D. AND M.D./Ph.D.: 97
Ph.D.: 33
   TOTAL: 357

TECHNICAL PERSONNEL: 82
NURSES: 145

Cancer Patient Statistics:

BEDS: 365
NO. IN-PATIENTS: 4385
AVERAGE STAY: 24

NO. OUT-PATIENTS: 18,920
NEW PATIENTS: 3438

Cancer Library: None.

Tumor Registry: None.

Professional Education: Postgraduate training in oncology, gynecology, cytology, and radiation therapy.

Greece: *Thessalonika*

Theagenion Medical Institute*
2 Serron St.
Thessalonika, Greece
Tel.: 031 832 311

Director: Professor A. Christoforidis, M.D.

Emphasis: Radiotherapy, chemotherapy, and surgical treatment. Clinical research in the chemotherapy of malignant diseases.

Equipment:

DIAGNOSTIC
Conventional X-ray equipment
Electron microscope
Scanning spectrophotometer

THERAPEUTIC
Gamma ray
Betatron
Cobalt 60 (2)

Cancer Personnel:

M.D. AND M.D./Ph.D.: 40
Ph.D.: 8
   TOTAL: 148

TECHNICAL PERSONNEL: 50
NURSES: 50

Cancer Patient Statistics:

BEDS: 301   NEW PATIENTS: 2415
NO. OUT-PATIENTS: 14,857

Library: 1000 volumes, 80 periodicals.

Tumor Registry.

Professional Education: X-ray and radiotherapy training.

Hong Kong: *Kowloon*

M. & H.D. Institute of Radiology and Oncology
Queen Elizabeth Hospital
Kowloon, Hong Kong
Tel.: 3–840111, Ext. 405

Director: Hung-Chiu Ho, M.D., D.Sc.

Affiliation: Medical and Health Department of Hong Kong Government.

Emphasis: Radiation therapy, chemotherapy, and radiodiagnosis. Radiotherapy and radiodiagnosis technology. Mould Laboratory. Increasing epidemiologic study of nasopharyngeal and bronchial carcinomas, development of IgA anti-EB-VCA serum for early diagnosis of nasopharyngeal carcinoma, and improvement of radiotherapy techniques for treatment of nasopharyngeal carcinoma.

Equipment:

DIAGNOSTIC
CT head scanner
Ultrasound
Gamma camera

THERAPEUTIC
Linear accelerators (3)
35meV Betatron
9000 curie telecobalt

Cancer Personnel:

M.D. AND M.D./Ph.D.: 35   TECHNICAL PERSONNEL: 171
Ph.D.: 11   NURSES: 20 (out-patient only)
    TOTAL: 237

Cancer Patient Statistics:

BEDS: 350   NO. OUT-PATIENTS: 67,109
NO. IN-PATIENTS: 2636   NEW PATIENTS: 2729
AVERAGE STAY: 40   AVERAGE COST: HK$10–HK$80/day

Library: 620 volumes

Tumor Registry.

Professional Education: Training for radiologists and radiation therapist-oncologists.

Hungary: *Budapest*

Hungarian National Institute of Oncology*
Rath Gy. U. 7/9
1525 Budapest P.F. 21X11, Hungary
Tel.: 354–350

Emphasis: Surgical, radiologic, and chemotherapeutic treatment. Rehabilitation programs in surgery and gynecology.

Equipment:

DIAGNOSTIC	THERAPEUTIC
Conventional X-ray equipment	Orthovoltage X-ray
	Isotopes

Cancer Personnel:

M.D. AND M.D./Ph.D.: 45 ft, 12 pt	TECHNICAL PERSONNEL: 328 ft, 4 pt
Ph.D.: 20 ft, 6 pt	NURSES: 111 ft
TOTAL: 504 full-time, 22 part-time	

Cancer Library.

Tumor Registry.

Professional Education: Graduate and postgraduate instruction in oncoradiology and oncopathology.

India: *Ahmedabad*

Gujarat Cancer and Research Institute**
New Civil Hospital Campus
Asarwa, Ahmedabad 380016, India
Tel.: 66563

Director: T.B. Patel, M.B.B.S.

Affiliation: B.J. Medical College; Ahmedabad and Gujarat University

Emphasis: Surgery, radiotherapy, and chemotherapy. Rehabilitation with plastic and reconstructive surgery and prostheses. Conventional diagnostic and radiotherapeutic equipment.

Equipment:

DIAGNOSTIC	THERAPEUTIC
Conventional X-ray equipment	Radiotherapy equipment

Cancer Personnel:

M.D. AND M.D./Ph.D.:   68 ft, 4 pt   NURSES: 118 ft
TECHNICAL PERSONNEL: 22 ft
  TOTAL: 208 full-time, 4 part-time

Cancer Patient Statistics:

BEDS: 200   NO. OUT-PATIENTS: 66,417
NO. IN-PATIENTS: 3457   NEW PATIENTS: 4262
AVERAGE STAY: 16

Library: 916 volumes, 715 periodicals.

Tumor Registry.

Professional Education: Undergraduate and postgraduate medical education in surgery, radiology, radiotherapy, medicine, and anesthesia.

India: *Bombay*

Tata Memorial Center
Dr. Ernest Borges Marg
Parel, Bombay, India
Tel.: 448 341

Director: D.J. Jussawalla, M.D.

Affiliation: University of Bombay.

Emphasis: Surgery, radiotherapy, and chemotherapy. Rehabilitation programs. Epidemiologic research.

Equipment:

DIAGNOSTIC   THERAPEUTIC
700 Ma X-ray   Cobalt 60
Isotope scanners   Cesium 130
Electron microscope   Linear accelerator

Cancer Personnel:

M.D. AND M.D./Ph.D.:   78   TECHNICAL PERSONNEL: 873
Ph.D.:   117   NURSES: 120
  TOTAL: 1188

Cancer Patient Statistics:

BEDS: 210   NO. OUT-PATIENTS: 700/day
NO. IN-PATIENTS: 5344   NEW PATIENTS: 16,000
AVERAGE STAY: 15

Library: 8700 volumes, 140 periodicals

Tumor Registry.

India: *Hyderabad*

Mehdi Nawaz Jung Cancer Hospital and Radium Institute
Red Hills
Hyderabad 500004 (Andhra Pradesh) India
Tel.: 38421

Director: V.V. Subba Rao, M.D.

Affiliation: Osmania University.

Emphasis: Surgery, radiotherapy, chemotherapy, and nuclear medicine. Research in radiotherapy and on chemotherapy trials for ovarian cancer.

Equipment:

DIAGNOSTIC	THERAPEUTIC
Conventional X-ray equipment	Cathetron
Isotope scanner	Afterloading
Spectrometer	Cobalt 60 (2)
Teletherapy simulator	Kilovoltage X-ray (2)

Cancer Personnel:

M.D. AND M.D./Ph.D.: 13	NURSES: 22
TECHNICAL PERSONNEL: 25	
TOTAL: 60	

Cancer Patient Statistics:

BEDS: 160	NO. OUT-PATIENTS: 96,000
NO. IN-PATIENTS: 2900	NEW PATIENTS: 6000
AVERAGE STAY: 30	

Library: 1000 volumes

Tumor Registry.

Professional Education: Postgraduate training in radiotherapy, clinical oncology, and nuclear medicine.

India: *Madras*

Cancer Institute (W.I.A.)
Adyar, Madras 600 020, India
Tel.: 412 714

Director: S. Krishnamurthi, M.D.

Affiliation: Universities of Madras, Kerala, and Nagpur.

Emphasis: Radiotherapy, radiation medicine and medical oncology. Rehabilitation with maxillofacial reconstruction. The Institute is the major radiotherapy and chemotherapy center for the country.

Equipment:

DIAGNOSTIC	THERAPEUTIC
Mammography	Afterloading
Selective angiography	Cobalt 60
Ultrasonography	Linear accelerator
Rectilinear scanner	Cesa gammatron
Endoscope	

Cancer Personnel:

M.D. AND M.D./Ph.D.:   26 ft, 7 pt   TECHNICAL PERSONNEL: 94 ft
Ph.D.:   10 ft   NURSES: 38 ft
        TOTAL: 168 full-time, 7 part-time

Cancer Patient Statistics:

BEDS: 250   NO. OUT-PATIENTS: 10,094
NO. IN-PATIENTS: 1972   NEW PATIENTS: 3602
AVERAGE STAY: 42

Library: 2162 volumes.

Tumor Registry.

Professional Education.   Postgraduate training in oncology and immunology.

Iran: *Tehran*

Taj Pahlavi Cancer Institute
P.O. Box 14/1154
Tehran, Iran
Tel.: 920 005

Director: Professor Atarod Mojtabai, M.D.

Affiliation: Tehran University.

Emphasis: Surgery, radiotherapy, and chemotherapy. Research in early cancer detection, intestinal lymphoma, and Hodgkin disease.

Equipment:

DIAGNOSTIC
Conventional X-ray equipment
Electron microscope

THERAPEUTIC
Cobalt (4)
Simulator
Superficial X-ray

Cancer Personnel:

M.D. AND M.D./Ph.D.: 22 ft, 20 pt
Ph.D.: 2 ft
   TOTAL: 119 full-time, 20 part-time

TECHNICAL PERSONNEL: 40 ft
NURSES: 55 ft

Cancer Patient Statistics:

BEDS: 150
NO. IN-PATIENTS: 900
AVERAGE STAY: 21

NO. OUT-PATIENTS: 10,000
NEW PATIENTS: 2000

Library: None.

Tumor Registry.

Professional Education: Postgraduate training in pathology, cytopathology, radiotherapy, and surgery.

Iraq: *Baghdad*

Institute of Radiology and Nuclear Medicine*
Alwiyah Baghdad, Iraq
Tel.: 96056

Director: Ali Al-Hindawi, Ph.D.

Affiliation: Ministry of Health.

Emphasis: Radiotherapy and chemotherapy for the entire range of cancer sites.

Equipment:

DIAGNOSTIC
Conventional X-ray equipment
Gamma camera
Scanner
Renogram

THERAPEUTIC
6meV linear accelerators
Cobalt 60 (2)
Orthovoltage X-ray (3)
Superficial X-ray

Cancer Personnel:

M.D. AND M.D./Ph.D.: 10
Ph.D.: 17
   TOTAL: 51

TECHNICAL PERSONNEL: 3
NURSES: 21

Cancer Patient Statistics:

BEDS: 100   AVERAGE STAY: 9
NO. IN-PATIENTS: 3081   NEW PATIENTS: 1741

Library: 450 volumes, 9 periodicals

Tumor Registry.

Professional Education: Training of radiographers and training in radiotherapy and nuclear medicine.

Ireland: *Dublin*

St. Anne's City Hospital for Diseases of the Skin and Cancer
Northbrook Rd.
Dublin 6, Ireland
Tel.: 01–976–778

Director: Patrick A. Browne, M.D.

Admissions: Sister Marie Semple

Affiliation: St. Luke's Hospital; Royal College of Surgeons.

Emphasis: Limited special surgery. Malignant diseases amenable to treatment by radiotherapy and/or chemotherapy. Full range of surgical and radiotherapeutic facilities.

Equipment:

DIAGNOSTIC	THERAPEUTIC
Radioisotope scanner	Cobalt 60
Beta counting unit	Kilovoltage X-ray

Cancer Personnel:

M.D. AND M.D./Ph.D.: 1 ft, 18 pt   TECHNICAL PERSONNEL: 3 ft
Ph.D.: 3 ft   NURSES: 26 ft
    TOTAL: 33 full-time, 18 part-time

Cancer Patient Statistics:

BEDS: 60   NO. OUT-PATIENTS: 10,773
NO. IN-PATIENTS: 1370   NEW PATIENTS: 1538
AVERAGE STAY: 12

Library: None.

Tumor Registry.

Professional Education: Graduate instruction for Royal College of Surgeons and dental students.

Ireland: *Dublin*

St. Luke's Hospital Radiotherapy and Clinical Oncology Center
Highfield Rd.
Rathgar, Dublin 6, Ireland
Tel.: 974 552

Director: Professor M.J. O'Halloran

Admissions: Medical Director

Affiliation: Trinity College, University College; Medical Teaching Hospitals.

Emphasis: Radiotherapy, chemotherapy, immunotherapy and hormonotherapy. Research in head and neck carcinoma trial, breast trial; studies with ascorbic acid and malignancy. Protocol for trial on rectal carcinoma.

Equipment:

DIAGNOSTIC	THERAPEUTIC
Image intensifier	Cobalt 60 (2)
Monitor-pituitary implants	8meV Dynaray and electron
Nuclear medicine	100 kV X-ray
	300 kV X-ray (2)
	Radium
	Linear accelerator

Cancer Personnel:

M.D. AND M.D./Ph.D.: 7	TECHNICAL PERSONNEL: 35
Ph.D.: 7	NURSES: 66
TOTAL: 115	

Cancer Patient Statistics:

BEDS: 154	NO. OUT-PATIENTS: 32,107
NO. IN-PATIENTS: 154	NEW PATIENTS: 3394
AVERAGE STAY: 14	

Library: 34 journals and texts.

Hospital Registry.

Professional Education: Postgraduate training in radiology.

Israel: *Haifa*

The Northern Israel Oncology Center
Rambam Medical Center
Aba Khoushy School of Medicine
Technion, Haifa, Israel
Tel.: (04) 52 82 71

Director: Eliezer Robinson, M.D.

Affiliation: Aba Khoushy School of Medicine.

Emphasis: Radiotherapy, chemotherapy, and immunotherapy. Research in experimental model systems and development of computer systems in patient management.

Equipment:

DIAGNOSTIC	THERAPEUTIC
Gamma cameras (2)	Cobalt unit
Whole body scanner	Linear accelerator
SNF counting instrument	Orthovoltage X-ray

Cancer Personnel:

M.D. AND M.D./Ph.D.:   17 ft,
2 volunteer
Ph.D.:   4 ft
    TOTAL: 105 full-time, 2 volunteer

TECHNICAL PERSONNEL: 52 ft
NURSES: 32 ft

Cancer Patient Statistics:

BEDS: 75
AVERAGE STAY: 20

NO. OUT-PATIENTS: 120/day
NEW PATIENTS: 1500

Library: 500 volumes.

Tumor Registry.

Professional Education: Student and physician workshops and seminars.

Italy: *Cagliari*

Cagliari Oncological Hospital*
Via Jenner
Cagliari, Italy
Tel.: 070–280966

Directors: Loddo Sante, M.D.; Carlo Demontis, M.D.

Emphasis: A full range of surgical, chemotherapeutic, radiotherapeutic and, within limits, immunotherapeutic treatment facilities with physical and social rehabilitation.

Equipment:

DIAGNOSTIC
Rull range of radiologic equipment

THERAPEUTIC
Rull range of radiotherapeutic equipment
Nuclear medicine

Cancer Personnel:

M.D. AND M.D./Ph.D.:   75
Ph.D.:   9
  TOTAL: 289

TECHNICAL PERSONNEL: 39
NURSES: 166

Cancer Patient Statistics:

BEDS: 288
NO. IN-PATIENTS: 2048
AVERAGE STAY: 30

NO. OUT-PATIENTS: 6500
NEW PATIENTS: 1809

Library: 1000 volumes, 30 periodicals.

Tumor Registry.

Italy: *Milan*

National Cancer Institute of Milan
Via Venezian 1
20133 Milano, Italy
Tel.: 02/2390

Director: Umberto Veronesi, M.D.

Admissions: Sergio Di Pietro, M.D.

Affiliation: Headquarters, WHO Melanoma Group.

Emphasis: Specialization in breast cancer, malignant melanoma, and lymphomas. Radiotherapy. Research in adjuvant chemotherapy on breast cancer, conservative treatment of early breast cancer, surgery and immunotherapy of melanoma.

Equipment:

DIAGNOSTIC
Conventional X-ray equipment
Electron microscope

THERAPEUTIC
Cobalt (2)
Betatron
Linear accelerator

Cancer Personnel:

M.D. AND M.D./Ph.D.: 109　　TECHNICAL PERSONNEL: 67
Ph.D.: 30　　　　　　　　　　NURSES: 404
　　TOTAL: 610

Cancer Patient Statistics:

BEDS: 510　　　　　　　　　NO. OUT-PATIENTS: 98,387
NO. IN-PATIENTS: 6773　　　NEW PATIENTS: 19,391
AVERAGE STAY: 26

Library: 2600 volumes.

Tumor Registry.

Professional Education: Postgraduate training in clinical oncology.

Italy: *Naples*

Senatore Pascale Foundation
Via Mariano Semmola Cappella dei Cangiani
Napoli, Italy
Tel.: 255100 463340

Director: Professor Giovanni D'errico, M.D.

Affiliation: Scientific Institute and Prevention Center.

Emphasis: Radiotherapy, chemotherapy, and immunology. Research in biochemistry, immunology, and oncologic pathology.

Equipment:

DIAGNOSTIC　　　　　　　　THERAPEUTIC
Conventional X-ray equipment　　17meV Betatron
Electron microscope　　　　　Telecobalt (2)
　　　　　　　　　　　　　　Superficial X-ray (2)
　　　　　　　　　　　　　　Isotopes

Cancer Personnel:

M.D. AND M.D./Ph.D.: 29 ft, 43 pt,　TECHNICAL PERSONNEL: 52 ft
　50 volunteer　　　　　　　　　NURSES: 152 ft
Ph.D.: 27 ft, 6 pt, 21 volunteer
　　TOTAL: 260 full-time, 49 part-
　　　time, 71 volunteer

Cancer Patient Statistics:

BEDS: 395　　　　　　　　　NO. OUT-PATIENTS: 21,450
AVERAGE STAY: 20

Library: 1200 volumes, 150 periodicals.

Tumor Registry: None.

Professional Education: Training of radiologic technicians.

Italy: *Torino*

Turin Oncological Institute**
31 via Cavour
10123 Torino, Italy
Tel.: 882666

Director: L. Caldarola, M.D.

Affiliation: University of Turin, Faculty of Medicine and Surgery.

Emphasis: Treatment and rehabilitation including surgery, antiblastic therapy, hormonotherapy, radiotherapy, and physiotherapy.

Equipment: Conventional radiotherapy equipment.

Cancer Personnel:

M.D. AND M.D./Ph.D.: 2 ft, 27 pt, 4 volunteer	TECHNICAL PERSONNEL: 5
Ph.D.: 3 ft	NURSES: 8
TOTAL: 18 full-time, 27 part-time, 4 volunteer	

Cancer Patient Statistics:

BEDS: 230	AVERAGE STAY: 24
NO. IN-PATIENTS: 2427	NO. OUT-PATIENTS: 43,277

Cancer Library.

Tumor Registry: None

Professional Education: Postgraduate training in clinical oncology.

Japan: *Nagoya*

Aichi Cancer Center
81–1159 Kanokoden Tashiro-Cho
Chikusa-KU, Nagoya, Japan
Tel.: 052–762–6111

Director: Hajime Imanaga, M.D.

Admissions: Hajime Imanaga, M.D.

Affiliation: Japan Cancer Center Association.

Emphasis: Chemotherapy, radiotherapy, and immunotherapy. Treatment of all cancers. Experimental pathology.

Equipment:

DIAGNOSTIC
Tomography
Angiography
X-TV unit
Polytome

THERAPEUTIC
Betatron
Linear accelerator
Treatment simulator

Cancer Personnel:

M.D. AND M.D./Ph.D.:   98
Ph.D.:   8
   TOTAL: 596

TECHNICAL PERSONNEL: 240
NURSES: 250

Cancer Patient Statistics:

BEDS: 335
NO. IN-PATIENTS: 2226
AVERAGE STAY: 57

NO. OUT-PATIENTS: 106,349
NEW PATIENTS: 1098

Library: 17,943 volumes.

Tumor Registry.

Japan: *Tokyo*

Japanese Foundation for Cancer Research**
Kami-Ikebukuro 1–371
Toshima-ku, Tokyo 170, Japan
Tel.: (03) 918–0111

Director: Haruo Sugano, M.D.

Emphasis: Detection and treatment of early cancers, especially alimentary tract, cervical, and lung cancers. Chemotherapeutic treatment of leukemia and lymphoma. Clinical research of early gastric cancer.

Equipment:

DIAGNOSTIC
Conventional X-ray equipment
Mammography
Echomammography
Fluorography

THERAPEUTIC
Cobalt 60
Radiotherapy

Cancer Personnel:

M.D. AND M.D./Ph.D.:   66 ft, 6 pt
Ph.D.:   29 ft, 3 pt
   TOTAL: 479 full-time, 27 part-time

TECHNICAL PERSONNEL: 121 ft, 5 pt
NURSES: 263 ft, 13 pt

Cancer Patient Statistics:

BEDS: 320
NO. IN-PATIENTS: 2701
AVERAGE STAY: 36

NO. OUT-PATIENTS: 226,577
NEW PATIENTS: 43,794

Library: 1600 volumes and periodicals.

Tumor Registry.

Professional Education: Training for physicians in mass-screening of stomach cancers, courses for cytologic technicians and diagnostic X-ray technicians.

Japan: *Tokyo*

National Cancer Center**
5-1-1, Tsukiji
Chuo-ku, 104 Tokyo, Japan
Tel.: (03) 542-2511

Director: Nakahara Waro, Ph.D., M.D.

Affiliation: Ministry of Health and Welfare.

Emphasis: Surgery, chemotherapy, and radiotherapy. Treatment of brain tumors, malignant eye tumors, surgical treatment of lung cancer with combined irradiation and chemotherapy.

Equipment: Conventional X-ray and radiotherapeutic equipment.

Cancer Personnel:

M.D. AND M.D./Ph.D.:   102 ft, 28 pt
Ph.D.:   121 ft
   TOTAL: 491 full-time, 45 part-time

TECHNICAL PERSONNEL: 45 ft, 5 pt
NURSES: 223 ft, 12 pt

Cancer Patient Statistics:

BEDS: 445
NO. IN-PATIENTS: 2169
AVERAGE STAY: 56

NO. OUT-PATIENTS: 11,176
NEW PATIENTS: 2090

Library: 28,723 volumes, 541 periodicals.

Professional Education: Postgraduate training for physicians in clinical oncology.

Korea: *Seoul*

Cancer Research Hospital and Korea Atomic Energy Research Institute*
2 Chung-Dong
Sudaemun-Ku, Seoul 120, Korea (Rep.)
Tel.: 72–7887

Director: Jang Kyu Lee, M.D., Ph.D.

Emphasis: Full range of surgical, radiotherapeutic, and chemotherapeutic facilities. Clinical research on patients following mastectomy and radiotherapy.

Equipment:

DIAGNOSTIC	THERAPEUTIC
Conventional X-ray equipment	Cobalt teletherapy (3)
	Superficial X-ray
	Radium
	Isotopes

Cancer Personnel:

M.D. AND M.D./Ph.D.: 16	TECHNICAL PERSONNEL: 21
Ph.D.: 1	NURSES: 35
TOTAL: 73	

Cancer Patient Statistics:

BEDS: 100	NO. IN-PATIENTS: 80,629
NO. IN-PATIENTS: 510	NEW PATIENTS: 2269
AVERAGE STAY: 25	

Library: 1500 volumes, 45 periodicals.

Tumor Registry: None.

Professional Education: Instruction in nuclear medicine, radiotherapy, and chemotherapy for physicians.

Mexico: *Mexico City*

C.M.N. Oncological Hospital**
Av. Cuauhtemoc 330
Mexico 7, D.F. Mexico
Tel.: 771–05–25

Director: Mauricio Garcia-Sainz, M.D.

Emphasis: Comprehensive cancer diagnosis and treatment with surgery, radiotherapy, and chemotherapy. Clinical research in biochemistry and immunology.

Equipment:

DIAGNOSTIC
Conventional X-ray equipment

THERAPEUTIC
Cobalt 60 (3)
Linear accelerator
Cathetron

Cancer Personnel:

M.D. AND M.D./Ph.D.: 74
Ph.D.: 2
   TOTAL: 412

TECHNICAL PERSONNEL: 92
NURSES: 244

Cancer Patient Statistics:

BEDS: 186
NO. IN-PATIENTS: 5101
AVERAGE STAY: 9

NO. OUT-PATIENTS: 122,058
NEW PATIENTS: 5581

Library: 599 volumes, 79 periodicals.

Tumor Registry: None.

Professional Education: Postgraduate training in medical and surgical oncology and radiotherapy.

Mexico: *Mexico City*

National Cancer Institute*
Av. Ninos Heroes 151
Mexico City 7, Mexico
Tel.: 578-6051

Director: Jose Noriega, M.D.

Affiliations: International Union Against Cancer; Secretaria de Salubridad y Asistencia

Emphasis: Immunology. Cytology and pathology laboratory. Tissue-culture laboratory.

Cancer Personnel:

M.D. AND M.D./Ph.D.: 10 ft, 26 pt
Ph.D.: 2 ft
   TOTAL: 78 full-time, 26 part-time

TECHNICAL PERSONNEL: 27 ft
NURSES: 39

Cancer Patient Statistics:

BEDS: 61
NO. IN-PATIENTS: 1341

AVERAGE STAY: 12
NEW PATIENTS: 4106

Cancer Library: None.

Tumor Registry.

Professional Education: Resident training in radiological, surgical, and internal medical oncology.

Netherlands: *Amsterdam*

Netherlands Cancer Institute
Antoni van Leeuwenhoek Hospital
Plesmanlaan, 121 Amsterdam
Tel.: 0 20–512–9111

Director: I.S. Sindram

Admissions: B. Warendorp

Emphasis: Treatment and rehabilitation for breast and throat cancers. Clinical research on tumor immunology and experimental chemotherapy and radiotherapy. Basic research in fundamental biochemistry.

Equipment:

DIAGNOSTIC	THERAPEUTIC
Conventional X-ray equipment	Conventional X-ray equipment
Electron microscope	Neutron generator

Cancer Personnel:

M.D. AND M.D./Ph.D.: 33 ft, 22 pt	TECHNICAL PERSONNEL: 344 ft
Ph.D.: 51 ft	NURSES: 118

TOTAL: 546 full-time, 22 part-time

Cancer Patient Statistics:

BEDS: 180	NO. OUT-PATIENTS: 51,316
NO. IN-PATIENTS: 2815	NEW PATIENTS: 3003
AVERAGE STAY: 21	

Library: 23,000 volumes.

Tumor Registry.

Professional Education: Programs in radiotherapy and internal and surgical oncology.

Netherlands: *Rotterdam*

Dr. Daniel Den Hoed Clinic/Rotterdam Radiotherapy Institute
Groene Hilledijk 301, P.B. 5201
Rotterdam, Netherlands
Tel.: 010–857–700

Director: D.M. van der Veldt, M.D.

Admissions: Professor B.H.P. van der Werf-Messing, M.D.

Affiliation: Erasmus University.

Emphasis: Radiotherapy, chemotherapy, endocrinological techniques, and surgery. Clinical research on radiation techniques and experimental radiotherapy. Nuclear medicine research on radiopharmacology.

Equipment:

DIAGNOSTIC	THERAPEUTIC
Conventional X-ray equipment	2 Linacs
CT scanner	Betatron
	Cobalt
	Cathetron

Cancer Personnel:

M.D. AND M.D./Ph.D.: 35	TECHNICAL PERSONNEL: 144
Ph.D.: 13	NURSES: 91
TOTAL: 183	

Cancer Patient Statistics:

BEDS: 150	NO. OUT-PATIENTS: 52,000
NO. IN-PATIENTS: 3150	NEW PATIENTS: 3032
AVERAGE STAY: 15	

Library: 3000 volumes.

Tumor Registry.

Professional Education.   Postgraduate training in radiotherapy, oncology, and nuclear medicine. Nurses training in oncology. Graduate and undergraduate instruction in radiotherapy, surgery, and tumor pathology.

Norway: *Oslo*

Det Norske Radium Hospital
Montebelo, Oslo 3, Norway
Tel.: 55 40 80

Director: Kolborn Pollen

Affiliation: Norsk Hydros Institute for Cancer Research.

Emphasis: Radiotherapeutic-oriented radiobiological research. Treatment in radiotherapy, chemotherapy, and hormonotherapy.

Equipment:

DIAGNOSTIC	THERAPEUTIC
Transmission microscope	Cobalt 60
Scanning electron microscope	Linear accelerators
Conventional X-ray equipment	Betatron

Cancer Personnel:

M.D. AND M.D./Ph.D.:   96 ft, 3 pt
Ph.D.:   20
 TOTAL: 485 full-time, 157 part-time, 120 volunteer

TECHNICAL PERSONNEL: 159 ft, 4 pt
NURSES: 210 ft, 150 pt, 120 volunteer

Cancer Patient Statistics:

BEDS: 336
NO. IN-PATIENTS: 7443
AVERAGE STAY: 15

NO. OUT-PATIENTS: 32,280
NEW PATIENTS: 3002

Library: 1600 volumes, 250 periodicals.

Tumor Registry.

Professional Education: Undergraduate instruction in oncology. Postgraduate training for oncologists and physicists. Radiotherapy and diagnosis for radiographers and nurses.

Norway: *Oslo*

Norwegian National Hospital**
Pilestredet 32, Oslo 1, Norway
Tel.: 20 10 50

Director: Tryggve Hauan

Affiliation: University of Oslo.

Emphasis: Surgical, chemotherapeutic, and radiotherapeutic treatment facilities. Clinical research on the effect of radiation and studies of end-results of treatment of Wilms' tumor.

Equipment: Conventional diagnostic and therapeutic X-ray equipment.

Cancer Personnel:

M.D. AND M.D./Ph.D.:   23
Ph.D.:   1
 TOTAL: 124

TECHNICAL PERSONNEL: 20
NURSES: 80

Cancer Patient Statistics:

BEDS: 81
NO. IN-PATIENTS: 2292
AVERAGE STAY: 12

NO. OUT-PATIENTS: 4000
NEW PATIENTS: 1000

Library: 4000 volumes, 30 periodicals.

Tumor Registry: None.

Professional Education: Postgraduate training in most specialties.

Peru: *Lima*

Peruvian National Neoplastic Disease Institute**
Avenida Alfonso Ugarte 825
Lima, Peru
Tel.: 28–96–60, 23–6979

Director: Eduardo Caceres, M.D.

Emphasis: Cancer of the uterine cervix, breast, and stomach. Rehabilitation with prostheses, speech therapy, and psychologic services.

Equipment:

DIAGNOSTIC
Conventional X-ray equipment
Mammography
Nuclear medicine

THERAPEUTIC
Cobalt (3)
Linear accelerator
250kV therapy equipment
Superficial X-ray
Radium

Cancer Personnel:

M.D. AND M.D./Ph.D.: 30 ft, 51 pt
Ph.D.: 6 ft, 1 pt
   TOTAL: 218 full-time, 52 part-time

TECHNICAL PERSONNEL: 37
NURSES: 145

Cancer Patient Statistics:

BEDS: 143
NO. IN-PATIENTS: 43,944
AVERAGE STAY: 14.5 days

NO. OUT-PATIENTS: 86,788 (visits)
NEW PATIENTS: 5743/yr

Library: 1216 volumes, 181 periodicals.

Tumor Registry.

Professional Education: Resident training in clinical sciences. School of Cyto-technology.

Poland: *Gliwice*

Institute of Oncology, Gliwice Branch
44-101 Gliwice, Poland
ul. Armii Czerwonej 15
Tel.: 31-10-61

Director: Jeremi Swiecki, M.D.

Affiliation: Warsaw Institute of Oncology.

Emphasis: Radiotherapy, oncological surgery, and oncological gynecology.

Equipment:

DIAGNOSTIC	THERAPEUTIC
Tomography	Curietherapy
Mammography	Roentgen and Co–60 therapy
Anatomopathologic researches	Isotope–therapy–J-131
Cytology	
Lymphography	
Isotope–diagnostic–J-131	

Cancer Personnel:

M.D. AND M.D./Ph.D.: 62	TECHNICAL PERSONNEL: 312
Ph.D.: 37	NURSES: 80
TOTAL: 491	

Cancer Patient Statistics:

BEDS: 305	NO. OUT-PATIENTS: 15,055
NO. IN-PATIENTS: 3463	NEW PATIENTS: 4638
AVERAGE STAY: 31	

Library: 4158 volumes, 160 periodicals.

Tumor Registry.

Professional Education: Postgraduate training in pathology, oncology, surgery, and radiotherapy.

Poland: *Krakow*

Krakow Institute of Oncology*
Garncarska 11
31-115 Krakow, Poland
Tel.: 266-80

Director: Professor Hann Kolodziejska-Wertheim, M.D.

Affiliation: Warsaw Institute of Oncology.

Emphasis: Specialization in chemotherapy of breast cancer, lymphomas, and gastrointestinal tract cancers. Radiotherapy, surgery, and chemotherapy. Clinical research in cellular immunologic reactions in breast cancer.

Equipment:

DIAGNOSTIC	THERAPEUTIC
Conventional X-ray equipment	Cobalt 60
	Betatron
	Radium 226
	Cesium 137

Cancer Personnel:

M.D. AND M.D./Ph.D.:   33 ft, 5 pt   TECHNICAL PERSONNEL: 43 ft, 5 pt
Ph.D.:   12 ft, 1 pt   NURSES: 39 ft
    TOTAL: 127 full-time, 11 part-time

Cancer Patient Statistics:

BEDS: 122   NO. OUT-PATIENTS: 26,455
NO. IN-PATIENTS: 1708   NEW PATIENTS: 4000
AVERAGE STAY: 21

Library: 4837 volumes, 120 periodicals.

Tumor Registry.

Professional Education: Postgraduate training in radiotherapy, cancer surgery and pathology.

Poland: *Warsaw*

Maria Sklodowska-Curie Memorial Institute of Oncology
00–973 Warsaw, 15 Waweleska St.
Warsaw, Poland
Tel.: 22–12–76

Director: Tadeusz Kosarowski, M.D.

Admissions: Ryszard Sosinski

Affiliation: Ministry of Health and Social Welfare.

Emphasis: Treatment in breast, colorectal, stomach, uterine, ovarian, and head and neck cancers. Research in "ledakrin" as a chemotherapeutic agent. Rehabilitation in breast cancers.

Equipment:

DIAGNOSTIC
Xeromammography
Thermography
Nuclear medicine
Electron microscope

THERAPEUTIC
Betatron
Linear accelerators (2)
Cobalt (5)
Afterloading
Isotopes

Cancer Personnel:

M.D. AND M.D./Ph.D.: 230
Ph.D.: 27
  TOTAL: 817

TECHNICAL PERSONNEL: 359
NURSES: 201

Cancer Patient Statistics:

BEDS: 647
NO. IN-PATIENTS: 8251
AVERAGE STAY: 24

NO. OUT-PATIENTS: 86,211
NEW PATIENTS: 15,349

Library: 12,000 volumes.

Tumor Registry.

Professional Education: Postgraduate training in oncologic surgery, radiotherapy, gynecology, and chemotherapy.

Portugal: *Lisbon*

Portuguese Institute of Oncology—Francisco Gentil*
rua Prof. Lima Basto
Lisbon 4, Portugal
Tel.: 76 3140/9

Director: Professor Jose Conde, M.D.

Affiliation: Ministry of Education and Culture.

Emphasis: Surgery, chemotherapy, and radiotherapy treatment. Rehabilitation and prostheses. Experimental pathology and genetics.

Equipment:

DIAGNOSTIC
Conventional X-ray equipment

THERAPEUTIC
Linear accelerator
Cobalt 60 (2)
Cesium
X-ray equipment
Radium

Cancer Personnel:

M.D. AND M.D./Ph.D.:   177 ft, 10 pt
Ph.D.:   55 ft
   TOTAL: 855 full-time, 10 part-time

TECHNICAL PERSONNEL: 153 ft
NURSES: 470 ft

Cancer Patient Statistics:

BEDS: 454
NO. IN-PATIENTS: 5723
AVERAGE STAY: 23

NO. OUT-PATIENTS: 138,606
NEW PATIENTS: 3712

Cancer Library: None.

Tumor Registry: None.

Professional Education: Residency training in oncology. Training for cytologists.

Puerto Rico: *Rio Piedras*

I. Gonzales Martinez Oncologic Hospital
Puerto Rico Medical Center
Box 1811, Hato Rey
Rio Piedras, Puerto Rico
(809) 765–7070

Director: Ramon E. Llubet, M.D.

Affiliation: University of Puerto Rico Medical Campus.

Emphasis: Treatment with surgery, chemotherapy, radiotherapy, and nuclear medicine. Research in gynecology, surgery, urology, medicine, and radiotherapy.

Equipment:

DIAGNOSTIC
Conventional radiology equipment

THERAPEUTIC
Conventional radiotherapy equipment
Nuclear medicine

Cancer Personnel:

M.D. AND M.D./Ph.D.:   11 ft, 25 pt,
  75 volunteer
Ph.D.:   1 ft, 3 pt, 2 volunteer
   TOTAL: 117 full-time, 28 part-time, 77 volunteers

TECHNICAL PERSONNEL: 22 ft
NURSES: 83 ft

Cancer Patient Statistics:

BEDS: 140
NO. IN-PATIENTS: 110/day
AVERAGE STAY: 20 days

NO. OUT-PATIENTS: 18,226
NEW PATIENTS: 1522

Library: 1000 volumes.

Tumor Registry.

Puerto Rico: *Santurce*

Puerto Rico Cancer Control Program**
Dept. of Health
Santurce 00926, Puerto Rico
(809) 766-2514

Director: Isidro Martinez, M.D.

Affiliation: Department of Health.

Emphasis: Surgery, radiotherapy, and chemotherapy with facial and breast prostheses and rehabilitation. Clinical research on cancer of colon and rectum; research on cancer immunology.

Equipment: Conventional diagnostic and therapeutic equipment.

Cancer Personnel:

M.D. AND M.D./Ph.D.:   2 ft, 12 pt
Ph.D.:   4 ft
   TOTAL: 40 full-time, 12 part-time

TECHNICAL PERSONNEL: 17 ft
NURSES: 17

Cancer Patient Statistics:

BEDS: 195
NO. IN-PATIENTS: 5533
AVERAGE STAY: 19

NO. OUT-PATIENTS: 23,822
NEW PATIENTS: 5846

Library: 1916 volumes and periodicals.

Tumor Registry: None.

Romania: *Bucharest*

Institute of Oncology
Bd. 1 Mai No. 11, Sector 8
7000 Bucharest
Tel.: 50.20.70 or 50.33.98

Director: Dr. Octav Costachel, Professor

Affiliation: Ministry of Health.

Emphasis: Cancer immunology; radiotherapy, chemotherapy, immunotherapy and surgery.

Equipment:

DIAGNOSTIC
X-ray
Digital thermograph
Scanner thermograph
Radioisotope scanner

THERAPEUTIC
Cobalt
Cesium
Radium and cobalt needles
X-ray

Cancer Personnel:

M.D. AND M.D./Ph.D.: 155
TECHNICAL PERSONNEL: 89
   TOTAL: 427

NURSES: 183

Cancer Patient Statistics:

BEDS: 340
NO. IN-PATIENTS: 2720
AVERAGE STAY: 30

NO. OUT-PATIENTS: 44,176 (visits)
NEW PATIENTS: 1880

Library: 41,417 volumes.

Tumor Registry.

Romania: *Cluj-Napoca*

Cluj-Napoca Oncological Institute
3400 Cluj-Napoca Str.
Republicii 34–36, Romania
Tel.: 23920

Director: Ion Kiricuta, M.D.

Affiliation: Ministry of Health.

Emphasis: Specialization in treatment of female genitalia and rectal cancers. Rehabilitative plastic surgery for radionecrosis. Basic and clinical research in nonspecific immunotherapy of cancer.

Equipment:

DIAGNOSTIC
Conventional X-ray equipment

THERAPEUTIC
Cesium
Telecobalt
Radium
Orthovoltage X-ray
Superficial X-ray

Cancer Personnel:

M.D. AND M.D./Ph.D.: 48 ft, 5 pt
Ph.D.: 28 ft, 1 pt
   TOTAL: 436 full-time, 6 part-time

TECHNICAL PERSONNEL: 182 ft
NURSES: 178 ft

Cancer Patient Statistics:

BEDS: 402
NO. IN-PATIENTS: 5059
AVERAGE STAY: 23

NO. OUT-PATIENTS: 28,369
NEW PATIENTS: 1944

Library: 4795 volumes, 311 periodicals.

Tumor Registry.

Professional Education: Postgraduate and graduate instruction in association with the Institute of Medicine and Pharmacy.

Romania: *Itasi*

Jassy Radiological Clinic
33, Bd. Independentei
6600–Itasi 5, Romania
Tel.: 13720, 11301

Director: Professor Gheorghe Chisleag, M.D., D.Sc.

Affiliations: Ministry of Education and Teaching; University of Jassy, Faculty of Medicine; Ministry of Health.

Emphasis: Radiotherapy, chemotherapy, and rehabilitation. Clinical research on the earlier detection of tumors and computerized programs for the treatment of pelvic cancer. All patient costs are subsidized by the Ministry of Health and the Ministry of Education and Teaching.

Equipment:

DIAGNOSTIC
Conventional X-ray equipment

THERAPEUTIC
Telecobalt
250kV X-ray
Superficial X-ray
Sealed cobalt 60 sources

Cancer Personnel:

M.D. AND M.D./Ph.D.: 12
Ph.D.: 2
TOTAL: 49

TECHNICAL PERSONNEL: 11
NURSES: 24

Cancer Patient Statistics:

BEDS: 105
NO. IN-PATIENTS: 1815
AVERAGE STAY: 26

NO. OUT-PATIENTS: 18,215
NEW PATIENTS: 1102

Library: 1050 volumes, 15 periodicals.

Tumor Registry.

Professional Education: Training in the specialties of radiodiagnosis and radiotherapy.

Scotland: *Edinburgh*

Radiotherapy Institute, Western General Hospital
Crewe Road
Edinburgh EH4 2XU Scotland
Tel.: 031 332 2525

Director: Professor William Duncan

Affiliations: University of Edinburgh; Medical Research Council

Emphasis: Specialization in fast-neutron therapy, hyperthermia, breast and
urologic cancer, and malignant lymphoma.

Equipment:

DIAGNOSTIC	THERAPEUTIC
Conventional X-ray equipment	Cyclotron
Ultrasonography	Linear accelerators
EMI head scanner	300kV X-ray
Nuclear medicine cameras	Superficial X-ray
Whole body scanner	Isocentric neutron unit

Cancer Personnel:

M.D. AND M.D./Ph.D.: 20 ft, 2 pt	TECHNICAL PERSONNEL: 28 ft
Ph.D.: 10 ft	NURSES: 16 ft, 10 pt
TOTAL: 74 full-time, 12 part-time	

Cancer Patient Statistics:

BEDS: 112	NO. OUT-PATIENTS: 17,000
NO. IN-PATIENTS: 112	NEW PATIENTS: 2500
AVERAGE STAY: 12	

Library: None.

Tumor Registry.

Professional Education: Postgraduate training in radiation therapy and oncology.
Undergraduate instruction for medical and dental students; nursing education.

Scotland: *Glasgow*

West of Scotland Cancer Intelligence Unit
Greater Glasgow Health Board, Ruchill Hospital
520 Bilsland Drive, Glasgow G20 9NB, Scotland, U.K.
Tel.: 041 946-7120

Director: C.R. Gillis, M.D.

Affiliations: International Agency for Research on Cancer; International Association of Cancer Registries.

Emphasis: Epidemiology of cancers of alimentary tract. Natural history of ovarian cancer. Epidemiology and treatment of lung cancer. Evaluation of cancer treatment. This is not a treatment facility.

Cancer Personnel:

    M.D. AND M.D./Ph.D.:   1   TECHNICAL PERSONNEL: 14
    Ph.D.:   3
      TOTAL: 18

Library: 200 volumes.

Tumor Registries.

Professional Education: Training and seminars in the evaluation of cancer treatment.

South Africa: *Bloemfontein*

O.F.S. Institute of Isotopes and Radiation
National Hospital
Bloemfontein, 9300 South Africa
Tel.: 7-0411, ext. 646

Director: Professor J.D. Anderson

Admissions: Professor J.D. Anderson

Affiliations: University of O.F.S.—Faculty of Medicine; Royal College of Radiologists, London; Royal Society of Medicine, London; S.A. College of Medicine.

Emphasis: Consultative clinics in lymphomas, leukemia, breast cancer, urology, gynecology, and dermatology. Basic research in radiobiology.

Equipment:

    DIAGNOSTIC   THERAPEUTIC
    Nuclear medicine   Superficial X-ray

DIAGNOSTIC	THERAPEUTIC
Gamma cameras	250kV X-ray (2)
Whole body counter	Linear accelerators (3)
B-gamma counter	
Simulators	
Tomography	

Cancer Personnel:

M.D. AND M.D./Ph.D.: 7	TECHNICAL PERSONNEL: 30
Ph.D.: 8	NURSES: 22
TOTAL: 67	

Cancer Patient Statistics:

BEDS: 150	NO. OUT-PATIENTS: 12,271
NO. IN-PATIENTS: 150	NEW PATIENTS: 1813
AVERAGE STAY: 30	

Library: 250 volumes.

Tumor Registry: None.

Professional Education: Radiotherapy training.

South Africa: *Cape Town*

Groote Schuur Hospital
Radiotherapy Department
Observatory, Cape 7925, South Africa
Tel.: 47 3311, ext. 2450

Director: Professor G.R.H. Sealy

Affiliation: University of Cape Town.

Emphasis: Radiotherapy and chemotherapy. Research in improved methods of treatment modalities.

Equipment:

DIAGNOSTIC	THERAPEUTIC
Conventional X-ray equipment	Cobalt (4)
	Hyperbaric chamber
	Linear accelerator
	Isotopes

Cancer Personnel:

M.D. AND M.D./Ph.D.: 14 ft, 4 pt	TECHNICAL PERSONNEL: 50 ft
Ph.D.: 4 ft	NURSES: 15 ft
TOTAL: 83 full-time, 4 part-time	

Cancer Patient Statistics:

BEDS: 80
NO. IN-PATIENTS: 150/month
AVERAGE STAY: 14

NO. OUT-PATIENTS: 54,000
NEW PATIENTS: 2700

Library: University of Cape Town Medical Library.

Tumor Registry: None.

Professional Education: Postgraduate training in radiotherapy and oncology.

South Africa: *Johannesburg*

Dept. of Radiation Therapy, Johannesburg General Hospital
P.B. X39
Johannesburg, 200 South Africa
Tel.: 724–1121

Director: Professor N.G. de Moor

Affiliation: University of the Witwatersrand.

Emphasis: Cancer of the breast and cervix, pediatric tumors, head and neck cancer, Hodgkin and non-Hodgkin lymphoma, osteogenic sarcoma, and thyroid cancer and disease.

Equipment:

DIAGNOSTIC	THERAPEUTIC
Scanning unit	18meV Linac
Gamma camera	Cobalt (2)
Whole body counter	HVX, MVX
CT scanner	Radium
Estrogen receptors	Isotopes

Cancer Personnel:

M.D. AND M.D./Ph.D.: 3
TECHNICAL PERSONNEL: 20
  TOTAL: 26

NURSES: 3

Cancer Patient Statistics:

BEDS: 550
NO. IN-PATIENTS: 230
AVERAGE STAY: 60

NO. OUT-PATIENTS: 50,000
NEW PATIENTS: 2200

Library: 1000 volumes, 300 periodicals.

Tumor Registry: None.

Professional Education: Degree program in radiation therapy.

Sweden: *Goteborg*

Institute for Radiotherapy
Sahlgrenska, Sjukhuset, S–413 45, Goteborg, Sweden
Tel.: 031–601 000

Director: Gustav Notter, M.D.

Emphasis: Radiotherapy and cytostatic therapy for all types of cancer. Research
in normal and malignant tissues.

Equipment:

DIAGNOSTIC	THERAPEUTIC
Simulator	Linear accelerator
Gamma cameras	Cobalt 60
Rectilinear scanner	Afterloading
Thyreoide uptake measurement	200kV X-ray
	Iridium 192 implants

Cancer Personnel:

M.D. AND M.D./Ph.D.:   16   NURSES: 41
TECHNICAL PERSONNEL: 11
    TOTAL: 71

Cancer Patient Statistics:

BEDS: 120   NO. OUT-PATIENTS: 16,000
NO. IN-PATIENTS: 6250   NEW PATIENTS: 1500
AVERAGE STAY: 6

Library: 500 volumes, 10 periodicals.

Tumor Registry: None.

Professional Education: Postgraduate training in radiotherapy and clinical
oncology.

Sweden: *Lund*

Lund University Radiotherapy Department*
Lasarettet i Lund
S–221 85 Lund, Sweden
Tel.: 046 117 100

Director: Professor Martin Lindgren, M.D.

Affiliation: University of Lund.

Emphasis: Treatment of solid tumors with surgical and radiologic techniques. Clinical research in pancreatic and ovarian cancer.

Equipment:

DIAGNOSTIC
Conventional X-ray equipment

THERAPEUTIC
Conventional X-ray equipment
Supervoltage X-ray (6)
Simulator

Cancer Personnel:

M.D. AND M.D./Ph.D.: 16 ft
Ph.D.: 3 ft
    TOTAL: 83 full-time, 4 part-time

TECHNICAL PERSONNEL: 45 ft, 2 pt
NURSES: 24 ft, 2 pt

Cancer Patient Statistics:

BEDS: 98
NO. IN-PATIENTS: 2500
AVERAGE STAY: 15

NO. OUT-PATIENTS: 19,000
NEW PATIENTS: 2200

Cancer Library.

Tumor Registry.

Professional Education: Main center for oncology education in area.

Sweden: *Stockholm*

Radiumhemmet, Karolinska Institute
10401 Stockholm, Sweden
Tel.: 08/340 500

Director: Professor Jerzy Einhorn

Affiliation: WHO Collaborating Center for Research and Treatment of Urinary Bladder Cancer.

Emphasis: WHO Center (only one, worldwide) specializing in urinary bladder and prostatic cancer. All nonsurgical tumor treatment.

Equipment: Full range of diagnostic and therapeutic equipment.

Cancer Personnel:

M.D. AND M.D./Ph.D.: 28

Cancer Patient Statistics:

BEDS: 135

NO. OUT-PATIENTS: 120,000

Library: 4000 volumes, 49 periodicals.

Tumor Registry.

Professional Education: Postgraduate training and graduate instruction in radio-therapy and oncology.

Switzerland: *Basel*

University of Basel, Kantonsspital, Medical Center
Department of Oncology
Hebelstrasse
1 Ch-4056 Basel, Switzerland
Tel.: 061/25 25 25

Director: Professor J.P. Obrecht, M.D.

Emphasis: Surgical, chemotherapeutic, radiotherapeutic, and immunothera-peutic treatment. Occupational and social rehabilitation services.

Equipment: Conventional diagnostic and therapeutic equipment.

Cancer Personnel:

M.D. AND M.D./Ph.D.:   6 ft,
  2 volunteer
TECHNICAL PERSONNEL: 4 ft, 5 pt
  TOTAL: 11 full-time, 7 part-time,
    2 volunteer

NURSES: 1 ft, 2 pt

Cancer Patient Statistics:

NO. IN-PATIENTS: 2000
AVERAGE STAY: 14

NO. OUT-PATIENTS: 4355
NEW PATIENTS: 119

Cancer Library: None.

Tumor Registry.

Professional Education: Postgraduate training for residents, interns, and staff.

Tunisia: *Tunis*

Institute Salah Azaiz
Boulevard du 9 Avril
Bab Saadoun, Tunis, Tunisia
Tel.: 260–622

Director: Nejib Mourali, M.D.

Affiliation: Tunisian Ministry of Public Health.

Emphasis: Treatment and research in immunology, surgery, and radiotherapy.

Equipment:

DIAGNOSTIC	THERAPEUTIC
Isotope exploration	Cobalt 60 (2)
Mammography	Cesium
Lymphography	
Thermography	

Cancer Personnel:

M.D. AND M.D./Ph.D.: 19 ft, 6 pt	TECHNICAL PERSONNEL: 32 ft
Ph.D.: 3 ft	NURSES: 95 ft

TOTAL: 149 full-time, 6 part-time

Cancer Patient Statistics:

BEDS: 190	NO. OUT-PATIENTS: 18,000
NO. IN-PATIENTS: 2627	NEW PATIENTS: 1393
AVERAGE STAY: 23	

Library: 500 volumes

Tumor Registry.

Professional Education: Graduate instruction in oncology.

Turkey: *Ankara*

Ankara Oncology Hospital and Institute
Etimesgut-Ankara, Turkey
Tel.: 110182

Director: Lutfi Koselioglu, M.D.

Admissions: Erol Atalay

Affiliation: Ministry of Health and Welfare.

Emphasis: Specializing in adult and pediatric cancer; breast, head and neck, skin, and gynecologic cancer. Clinical research in bone metastases and radium therapy.

Equipment:

DIAGNOSTIC	THERAPEUTIC
Scanning unit	Cobalt
Beta camera	Cesium

DIAGNOSTIC	THERAPEUTIC
Gamma camera	Deep therapy
Radiodiagnostic	Dermopan
	Pleasiotherapy

Cancer Personnel:

M.D. AND M.D./Ph.D.: 29		TECHNICAL PERSONNEL: 33
Ph.D.: 5		NURSES: 55
TOTAL: 122		

Cancer Patient Statistics:

BEDS: 330	NO. OUT-PATIENTS: 12,822
NO. IN-PATIENTS: 3462	NEW PATIENTS: 2900
AVERAGE STAY: 28	

Library: 1200 volumes.

In-hospital Registry.

Professional Education: Postgraduate training in medical oncology, surgery, and radiotherapy.

Venezuela: *Caracas*

Padre Machado Oncological Hospital**
Calle El Degredo
Los Castanos El Cementerio Caracas DF, Venezuela
Tel.: 617749 618211

Directors: A. Calvo; I. Gonzalez

Affiliation: Sociedad Anticancerosa de Venezuela.

Emphasis: Surgical, radiotherapeutic, and chemotherapeutic facilities with psychiatric and rehabilitation services. Research on the screening and early detection of gastric, lung, breast, and gynecologic cancers.

Equipment:

DIAGNOSTIC	THERAPEUTIC
Conventional X-ray equipment	Telecobalt (2)
	Superficial X-ray
	Radium
	Cesium

Cancer Personnel:

M.D. AND M.D./Ph.D.:   20 ft, 30 pt,
  24 volunteer
Ph.D.:   2 ft
  TOTAL: 163 full-time, 30 part-time,
    24 volunteer

TECHNICAL PERSONNEL: 23 ft
NURSES: 118 ft

Cancer Patient Statistics:

BEDS: 150
NO. IN-PATIENTS: 1401
AVERAGE STAY: 27

NO. OUT-PATIENTS: 41,081
NEW PATIENTS: 1067

Library: 3200 volumes, 140 periodicals.

Tumor Registry.

Professional Education: Postgraduate training in oncology, surgery, radiotherapy, medical oncology, and gastroenterology.

Wales (U.K.): *Cardiff*

South Wales Radiotherapy and Oncology Service**
Velindre Hospital
Whitchurch, Cardiff, Wales
Tel.: 63325

Director: T. Deeley, M.B. Ch.B.

Affiliation: South Glamorgan Area Health Authority.

Emphasis: Radiotherapy and chemotherapy. Clinical research of controlled trials in the investigation of hyperbaric oxygen, radiotherapy, and chemotherapy combinations and the treatment of ovarian tumors.

Equipment:

DIAGNOSTIC
Conventional X-ray equipment

THERAPEUTIC
Linear accelerators
Telecobalt
Afterloading cathetron
Whole body strontium
Hyperbaric facility
Orthovoltage X-ray
Superficial X-ray
Radium

Cancer Personnel:

M.D. AND M.D./Ph.D.:   17
  TOTAL: 77

NURSES: 60

Cancer Patient Statistics:

BEDS: 100
NO. IN-PATIENTS: 1500
AVERAGE STAY: 24

NO. OUT-PATIENTS: 35,000
NEW PATIENTS: 2500

Cancer Library: None.

Tumor Registry: None.

Professional Education: Graduate and postgraduate training and instruction in radiology.

Yugoslavia: *Belgrade*

Ksenofon Sahovic Institute**
Pasterova 14
11000 Belgrade, Yugoslavia
Tel.: 685–059

Director: Mladomir Pantelic, M.D.

Affiliation: University of Belgrade, Medical Faculty.

Emphasis: Treatment of leukemia, Hodgkin disease, and advanced cases of breast cancer. Surgery, chemotherapeutic, and immunotherapeutic treatment facilities.

Equipment: Conventional diagnostic and therapeutic equipment.

Cancer Personnel:

M.D. AND M.D./Ph.D.: 29
Ph.D.: 2
  TOTAL: 91

NURSES: 60

Cancer Patient Statistics:

BEDS: 201
NO. IN-PATIENTS: 2551
AVERAGE STAY: 29

NO. OUT-PATIENTS: 31,684
NEW PATIENTS: 1551

Library: 1500 volumes, 15 periodicals.

Tumor Registry: None.

Professional Education: Postgraduate training in oncology and surgery.

B

Organizations Devoted to Rehabilitation of Cancer Patients and Their Families

LEUKEMIA SOCIETY OF AMERICA, INC.

Leukemia Society of America, Inc.
Executive Director: Meade P. Brown
211 East 43 Street
New York, New York 10017

Alabama Chapter
Executive Director: Jerry L. Freeman
President: Ronald J. Creel
244 Goodwin Crest Drive
Suite 104
Birmingham, Alabama 35209
(205) 942-9032

Arizona Chapter
Executive Director: Mrs. MaryLou Passmor
President: Leonard J. Mark
3318 North 2nd Street
Phoenix, Arizona 85012
(602) 264-7116

SF Area Chapter
Director: Orval D. Williams
Associate Director: Mrs. Betty Edmonds
President: Mrs. Delores J. Swig
323 Geary Street
San Francisco, California 94102
(415) 781-4270

Greater Los Angeles Chapter
Executive Director: Miss Joyce I.
  Hobday
President: Roy M. Brewer
606 Wilshire Blvd.—Suite 406
Santa Monica, California 90401
(213) 451-5961

San Diego County Chapter
Executive Director: Ben D. Griffith
President: Robert Deane
4379 30th Street—Suite 7
San Diego, California 92104
(714) 280-1461

Tri-County Chapter
Executive Director: Mrs. Winn MacEwan
President: William J. Anthony
9778 Katella Avenue—Suite 203
Anaheim, California 92804
(714) 539-9511

COLORADO

Colorado Chapter
Executive Director: Mrs. Charlotte
  Owens
President: Lewis Westbrook
601 Broadway—Room 217
Denver, Colorado 80203
(303) 572-3000

CONNECTICUT

Central Connecticut Chapter
Executive Director: John J. Namnoum
President: Michael D. Saffer
175 Grand Avenue
P.O. Box 49
Fair Haven Station
New Haven, Connecticut 06513
(203) 777-6397

Fairfield County Chapter
Executive Director: Jean A. Perusse
President: David Oliphant
1051 Post Road
P.O. Box 1203
Darien, Connecticut 06820
(203) 655-8297

Northern Connecticut Chapter
Executive Director: John J. Namnoum
President: Earl L. Kemmler
44 State Street
Hartford, Connecticut 06103
(203) 524-5953

DELAWARE

Delaware Chapter
Executive Director: Joseph Basile
President: Paul L. Newhart
Goldsborough Building
1102 West Street—Room 605
Wilmington, Delaware 19801
(302) 654-5262

DISTRICT OF COLUMBIA

Greater Washington Chapter
Executive Director: Mrs. Gisele
  Rountzounis
President: Robert B. Gibbons
1625 Eye Street, N.W.
Washington, D.C. 20006
(202) 223-2656

FLORIDA

Central Florida Chapter
Executive Director: Royce G. Olson
President: Thomas D. Purdy
3191 Maguire Blvd.—Suite 214
Orlando, Florida 32803
(305) 898-0733

Northern Florida Chapter
Executive Director: Herbert L. Marsh
President: C. Foster Wright, D.V.M.
101 Century 21 Drive—Suite 104
Jacksonville, Florida 32216
(904) 725-3677

Palm Beach Area Chapter
Executive Director: Miss Rosemary
  Stevens
President: Everett H. Aspinwall, Jr.
119 Datura Street
West Palm Beach, Florida 33401
(305) 659-0746

Southern Florida Chapter
Executive Director: Mrs. Dorothy
  Grant
President: Robert H. Newman
1701 Congress Building
111 N.E. Second Avenue
Miami, Florida 33132
(305) 522-0121 *(Broward)
(305) 373-2624 (Dade)

Sun Coast Chapter
Executive Director: Mrs. Amy
  Newbury
President: George C. Tsourakis
3125 Fifth Avenue North
Suite 315
St. Petersburg, Florida 33713
(813) 822-3752

GEORGIA

Georgia Chapter
Executive Director: Robert M.
  Clark, Jr.
1430 West Peachtree St., N.W.
Atlanta, Georgia 30309
(404) 892-8008

ILLINOIS

Greater Chicago Chapter
Executive Director: Mrs. Dorothy
  Stark
President: Peter A. Loutos
5 East Washington Street
Room 1522
Chicago, Illinois 60602
(312) 726-0003

KANSAS

Kansas Chapter
Executive Director: Mrs. Ann
  Stephenson
President: Phil Gerdes
1405 South Hydraulic
Wichita, Kansas 67211
(316) 262-2417

*Use for long-distance call.

KENTUCKY

Kentucky Chapter
Executive Director: Mrs. Joyce F.
  Horan
President: Donald J. Zeman
3715 Bardstown Road
Room 408
Louisville, Kentucky 40218
(502) 451-8140

LOUISIANA

Louisiana Chapter
President: Donald Ward
302-3 Masonic Temple Bldg.
333 St. Charles Avenue
New Orleans, Louisiana 70130
(504) 525-0437

MARYLAND

Maryland Chapter
Executive Director: Miss Phyllis E.
  Keyser
President: James S. Watson
One Spinners Court
Randallstown, Maryland 21133
(301) 655-2244

MASSACHUSETTS

Central Massachusetts Chapter
Executive Director: James A.
  Fitzgerald, Jr.
President: Gerald Teran
340 Main Street—Suite 953
Worcester, Massachusetts 01608
(617) 756-3501

Greater Boston Chapter
Executive Director: Joseph A. Galvin
President: Richard P. Curran
739 Boylston Street
Boston, Massachusetts 02116
(617) 262-5970

Western Massachusetts Chapter
Executive Director: Miss Anne O'Leary
President: Leon M. Cote
115 State Street
Springfield, Massachusetts 01103
(413) 788-0586

MISSOURI

Metropolitan Kansas City Chapter
Executive Director: Tim Wood
President: Robert V. Lewellen
Barickman Building
427 West 12th Street—Room 301
Kansas City, Missouri 64105
(816) 842-0053

Metropolitan St. Louis Chapter
Executive Director: Rollin E. Fisher
President: William M. Ward, Jr.
1612 Big Bend Boulevard
St. Louis, Missouri 63117
(314) 644-3633

NEW JERSEY

Central New Jersey Chapter
Executive Director: James Monaco
President: Michael P. Friedman, M.D.
1496 Morris Avenue
Union, N.J. 07083
(201) 687-3450

Northern New Jersey Chapter
Executive Director: Mrs. Lorraine
   Seidel
President: Phil Pampinella
1855 Springfield Ave.—2nd Floor
Maplewood, New Jersey 07040
(201) 761-5858

Southern New Jersey Chapter
Executive Director: Edward W. Godin
President: Kyle W. Will
1001 Kings Highway North
Suite 105
Cherry Hill, New Jersey 08034
(609) 667-7400

NEW YORK

Central New York Chapter
Executive Director: Malcolm Alama
President: Joseph Corona
3001 James Street
Syracuse, New York 13206
(315) 437-5516

Long Island Chapter
Executive Director: Miss Josephine C.
   Cassidy
President: Theodore Butler
40 Jerusalem Ave.
Hicksville, New York 11801
(516) 938-3900

Monroe County Chapter
Executive Director: Miss Neilia Brooks
President: William Moore
1835 St. Paul Street
Rochester, New York 14621
(716) 342-4200

New York City Chapter
Executive Director: Frank V. Whitley
President: Frederick T. Dombo, Jr.
405 Lexington Avenue
Room 4220
New York, New York 10017
(212) 682-3015

Upstate New York Chapter
Executive Director: Mrs. Madeleine
   McClure
President: Raymond J. Kinley
313 Washington Avenue
Albany, New York 12206
(518) 462-5414

Westchester/Hudson Valley Chapter
Executive Director: William E. Doyle
President: Ted Kamp
Harwood Building—5th Floor
Scarsdale, New York 10583
(914) 725-4422

Western New York Chapter
Executive Director: Thomas Van
   Volkenburg
President: Earl C. LaRocca
3606 Main Street
Eggertsville, New York 14226
(716) 833-5400

OHIO

Central Ohio Chapter
Executive Director: Mrs. Margery
    Perkins
President: Mrs. H. Richard P.
    Neihof
22 East Gay Street
Columbus, Ohio 43215
(614) 221–3129

Greater Dayton Area Chapter
Executive Director: Miss Mary Lou
    Hemmerich
President: Mrs. Bertha Winfield
2637 Oakley Avenue
Kettering, Ohio 45419
(513) 299–3817

Northern Ohio Chapter
Executive Director: Mrs. Sarah
    Rasmussen
President: John T. Corrigan
215 Euclid Avenue
Cleveland, Ohio 44114
(216) 621–6727

OKLAHOMA

Oklahoma Chapter
Executive Director: Ronald M.
    Cardwell
President: M.C. Duncan
The May-Ex Building
Suite 100A
3022 N.W. Expressway
Oklahoma City, Oklahoma 73112
(405) 947–3359

PENNSYLVANIA

Central Pennsylvania Chapter
Executive Director: Mrs. Esther Beatty
President: Chester F. Fisher
4815 (R) Jonestown Road
Harrisburg, Pennsylvania 17109
(717) 652–6520

Eastern Pennsylvania Chapter
Executive Director: John C. Rigas
President: Mrs. Charles A. Burton
969½ Bristol Pike
Andalusia, Pennsylvania 19020
(215) 638–4480

Western Pennsylvania Chapter
Executive Director: Mrs. Thelma Storck
President: Frank H. McKean
907 Empire Building
507 Liberty Avenue
Pittsburgh, Pennsylvania 15222
(412) 261–2118

RHODE ISLAND

Rhode Island Chapter
Executive Director: Mrs. Catherine
    Giorgi
President: Edward G. Nowak, Jr.
145 Wayland Avenue
Providence, Rhode Island 02906
(401) 331–2908

TEXAS

Greater Dallas/Ft. Worth Chapter
Executive Director: W. Jerry Thomas
President: Mrs. A.D. Martin, Sr.
Davis Building—Suite 1900D
1309 Main Street
Dallas, Texas 75202
(214) 748–6975

South/Central Texas Chapter
President: Frank O. Gebhardt
106 Broadway
San Antonio, Texas 78205
(512) 225–4404

Texas Gulf Coast Chapter
Executive Director: Mrs. Mary Wilmeth
President: Doyle Stuckey
3311 Richmond Avenue—Suite 335
Houston, Texas 77006
(713) 529–8709

VIRGINIA

Virginia Chapter
Executive Director: Eugene Flanegan
President: Samuel J. Trapani
2101 Executive Drive
Tower Box 21
Hampton, Virginia 23666
(804) 838–5384

WISCONSIN

Wisconsin Chapter
Executive Director: Rudolph F.
    Feuerschutz, Jr.
President: James W. Nicla
411 East Nason
Milwaukee, Wisconsin
(414) 271–4880

THE UNITED OSTOMY ASSOCIATION, INC.

United States of America

ALABAMA

Anniston Area Chapter
Mrs. Margaret Weissinger
1515 McCall Dr.
Anniston, Alabama 36201
(205) 236–1870

Birmingham Chapter
Bruce C. Day
6008 Wendy Circle
Birmingham, Alabama 35213
(205) 595–5163

Gadsden Chapter
Mrs. Joyce Nelson
Gadsden State Jr. College
Gadsden, Alabama 35903
(205) 546–0484, ext. 20

Mobile Ostomy Association
Mrs. Margaret P. Hanes
2707 Eldorado Dr.
Mobile, Alabama 36605
(205) 473–1476

Ostomy Association of Montgomery
Allen Sellers
3388–A McGehee Rd.
Montgomery, Alabama 36111

Ostomy Association of North Alabama
President: Doug Spivey
11319 Dellcrest Dr., S.E.
Huntsville, Alabama 35803
(205) 881–8786

Selma, Alabama, Chapter
Mr. W.J. Patterson
318 City View Ave.
Selma, Alabama 36701
(205) 874–4155

ARIZONA

Colostomy Club of Greater Phoenix
President: Mr. Andy Tomlinson
4825 N. 72nd Way
Scottsdale, Arizona 85251
(602) 946–6314

Mission Ostomy Chapter of Tucson
P.O. Box 4822
Tucson, Arizona 85717

Ostomy Association of Yuma
800 E. 26th Pl.
Yuma, Arizona 85364
(602) 344–4544

Phoenix Ileostomy Chapter, Inc.
President: Bob Drake
2513 E. Cambridge
Phoenix, Arizona 85008
(602) 956-6875

ARKANSAS

Central Arkansas Ostomy Association
   at Little Rock
President: Ed Brister
6227 Asher Ave.
Little Rock, Arkansas 72204
(501) 565-3934

Fort Smith Chapter
President: Miss Judy Stephens
5 Homestead Terrace
Fort Smith, Arkansas 72904
(501) 783-5973

Pine Bluff, Arkansas, Chapter
President: Ms. Martha Jo Berry
2813 Colonial
Pine Bluff, Arkansas 71601
(501) 536-5136

CALIFORNIA

Cascade Chapter
President: Mrs. Vivian V. Jones
1645 El Cerrito Dr.
Red Bluff, California 96080
(916) 527-7090

Central Valley Ostomy Association
Georgie Lee Davis
2321 Viola Ave.
Modesto, California 95351

Fresno Chapter
President: Shirley Laird
5836 E. Ramona
Fresno, California 93727

Golden Gate Chapter
P.O. Box 6545
Oakland, California 94614
(415) 893-4334

Ileostomy Association of Los
   Angeles, Inc.
1710 N. La Brea Ave., Suite 101
Los Angeles, California 90046
(213) 876-8110

Ileostomy—Colostomy Group of
   San Diego County
President: George A. Lowin
P.O. Box 81324
San Diego, California 92138

Kern Ostomy Association
Edith Schultz
2414 Cotton St.
Bakersfield, California 93304

Monterey County California Chapter
Jack Hall
3757 Raymond Way
Carmel, California 93921
(408) 624-4700

Napa Valley Chapter
President: Del Lorenzo
1890 Adrian St.
Napa, California 94558

Orange County Chapter
President: Merrill N. Couchman
2548 Santiago Ave.
Santa Ana, California 92706
(714) 543-1765

Ostomy Association of Greater
   Chico
President: Bill Alberson
1181 East Ave.
Chico, California 95926
(916) 343-7879

Ostomy Association of the Inland
   Empire
P.O. Box 2903, Arrowhead Station
San Bernardino, California
(714) 986-7455

Ostomy Association of San Gabriel/
   Pomona Valley
President: Neil A. Geariety
P.O. Box 2074
La Puente, California 91746
(213) 331-8266

Redwood Ostomy Association
c/o American Cancer Society
19 Fifth St.
Eureka, California 95501
(707) 433–2510

Sacramento Ostomy Association
President: John Meyer
4026 Las Pasas Way
Sacramento, California 95825
(916) 487–5594

San Mateo County California Chapter
President: Edythe Miller
P.O. Box 544
Redwood City, California 94063
(415) 345–6214 (business)
(415) 364–5152 (residence)

Santa Barbara Ostomy Association
Oliver Yang
998 Cienequitas Rd.
Santa Barbara, California 93110
(805) 687–1184

Santa Clara Valley Chapter
P.O. Box 305
Santa Clara, California 95052
(408) 243–1081 (residence)
(408) 275–7631 (business)

Santa Cruz County Chapter
President: Mrs. Eleanor Wettlaufer
P.O. Box 236
Aptos, California 95003
(408) 688–2712

Sonoma County Chapter
President: Ethel Kinney
P.O. Box 73
El Vearno, California 95433
(707) 996–3351

Yuba–Sutter Area Chapter
President: Ms. Annette Megas
2789 Roosevelt Rd.
Yuba City, California 95991
(916) 674–5918

COLORADO

Larimer County, Colorado, Chapter
President: Mrs. Helen E. Spencer
2525 E. Mulberry #93
Fort Collins, Colorado 80521
(303) 484–1815

Metropolitan Denver Chapter
President: Donald Busi
11303 Melody Dr., Apt. 207
Northglenn, Colorado 80234
(303) 451–5022

Northern Colorado Ostomy Association
President: Mr. Francis Carpenter
1612 15th Ave.
Greeley, Colorado 80631
(303) 352–8078

Pikes Peak Ostomy Association
Rev. Bonaventure Bandi
2227 N. Tejon
Colorado Springs, Colorado 80907

Valley Ostomy Association
Miss Rosalie Herrera
P.O. Box 1531
Grand Junction, Colorado 81501
(303) 243–4632

CONNECTICUT

Bristol Area Ostomy Association
Helena Kuttner
26 Beach Ave.
Terryville, Connecticut 06786
(203) 589–4983

Fairfield County Chapter
President: Mrs. Patricia J. Childs
115 Hurlbutt St.
Wilton, Connecticut 06897
(203) 762–8836

Greater Bridgeport Area Ostomy
    Association
Mr. Sal Astengo
577 Wood Ave.
Bridgeport, Connecticut 06604
(203) 335–0595

Greater Danbury Chapter
President: Marilyn F. Dores
179 So. King St.
Danbury, Connecticut 06810
(203) 748-7970

Hartford Ostomy Association
Mrs. Bette Hagist
P.O. Box 351
Bloomfield, Connecticut 06002
(203) 523-7581

Lower Naugatuck Valley Ostomates
  Association
Treasurer: Mrs. Grace Wolfe
29 Glen Circle
Seymour, Connecticut 06483
(203) 888-9694

Manchester Area Ostomy Association
President: Mrs. Anne McNeil
5 Lawton Rd.
Manchester, Connecticut 06040

Meriden—Middlesex Chapter
c/o American Cancer Society
Meriden Rd., Rt. 66
Middletown, Connecticut 06457
(203) 347-2523

New Haven Ostomy Association
Mrs. Helen Turbert
169 Gilbert St.
West Haven, Connecticut 06516
(203) 933-2346

New London County Ostomy
  Association
Secretary: Gilbert J. Sandri
288 Indigo St.
Mystic, Connecticut 06355
(203) 536-0758

Quinebaug Valley Chapter
Mrs. Ruth H. Stevenson
Box 68
Woodstock, Connecticut 06281
(203) 928-4659

Waterbury, Connecticut, Chapter
President: Joseph Zotter
47 Hutchinson St.
Waterbury, Connecticut 06810
(203) 755-5466

DELAWARE

Delmarva Ostomy Association
President: Mrs. Doris T. Fletcher
Box 93A, Rt. #2
Delmar, Delaware 19940
(302) 846-9571

Wilmington, Delaware, Chapter
President: Robert V. Canning
5111 Governor Printz Blvd.
Wilmington, Delaware 19809
(302) 764-0401

DISTRICT OF COLUMBIA

Metropolitan Washington Chapter
President: Mrs. Alice B. McLaughlin
c/o Washington Hospital Center
Room 1B-42, 110 Irving St. N.W.
Washington, D.C. 20010
(202) 541-6019

FLORIDA

Broward Ostomy Association
President: Mrs. Bertha Kronheimer
P.O. Box 6083
Hollywood, Florida 33021
(305) 565-0324

Coral Gables Ostomy Association
President: Arthur L. Brown
9261 S.W. 56th Terrace
Miami, Florida 33165

Greater Orlando, Florida, Chapter
President: Mr. Bryce W. Eanes
1020 Ibsen Ave.
Orlando, Florida 23809
(305) 855-4347

H.O.P.E. of North Florida Ostomy
  Association (Jacksonville area)
President: Richard Peck
Sunnymead Dr.
Jacksonville, Florida 32211
(904) 725-4954

Lake County, Florida, Chapter
President: Vonna Hill
Rt. 1, Box 562
Mt. Dora, Florida 32757
(904) 383-6686

Miami Ileostomy and Colostomy
Association
President: Harold Kolbert
1135 103rd St.
Bay Harbor Island
Miami, Florida 33154

Ocala, Florida, Chapter
President: Ida C. Kanarr
5739 N.E. 14th Ave.
Ocala, Florida 32670

Ostomy Association of Central
Florida
President: Thomas Burslem
618 Conestoga Circle
Orlando, Florida 32808
(305) 293-1221

Ostomy Association of Sara-Tee
President: Fleda Tubbs
1929 5th Ave. Dr.
Bradenton, Florida 33505
(813) 748-3227

Ostomy Association of Southwest
Florida (Naples–Ft. Myers Area)
Kenneth M. Jennings
641 Travers Ave.
Fort Myers, Florida 33901

Palm Beach County Ostomy
Association
President: Mrs. Mildred Laframboise
40 Robalo Ct.
North Palm Beach, Florida 33408
(305) 622-2089

Pensacola Ostomy Association
President: Wanda Huebschman
P.O. Box 5344
Pensacola, Florida 32505

Polk County Ostomy Society
President: Douglas MacDonald
1439 Lemon St.
Clearwater, Florida 33516
(813) 447-5178

St. Petersburg Chapter
President: David Kuperman
6190 30th Ave. N.
St. Petersburg, Florida 33710
(813) 347-7470

Space Coast Ostomy Association
Robert D. McClaran
430 Franklyn Ave.
Idialantic, Florida 32903

Tallahassee Area Chapter
Vice-President: Vivian Scarborough
3121 Sharer Rd.
Tallahassee, Florida 32303
(904) 385-6723

The Tampa Bay Ostomy Society
President: Anna Salla
4103 Norma Ave.
Tampa, Florida 33611
(813) 839-3974

Venice Area Ostomy Association
President: Malcom B. Weaver
859 Mobile Gardens
Englewood, Florida 33533
(813) 474-1059

GEORGIA

Albany, Georgia, Chapter
Ivy J. Fender
2522 Briarwood Dr.
Albany, Georgia 31707
(912) 436-8280

Athens—Northeast Georgia Ostomy
Association
President: John Hannay
139 No. Homewood Dr.
Athens, Georgia 30601

Augusta Area Chapter
President: Mrs. Andrea Daniel
707 Aumond Rd.
Augusta, Georgia 30904
(404) 736-5381

Cartersville Area Chapter
President: Dr. L.P. Davis
P.O. Box 764
Cartersville, Georgia 30120

Coastal Georgia Ostomy Association
President: Hymon Friedman
45B Lamara Apt.
Savannah, Georgia 31404
(912) 925-4192

Columbus—Fort Benning Ostomy
   Society
James R. Self
2840 Sue Mack Dr.
Columbus, Georgia 31904
(404) 561-8078

Golden Isles Ostomy Association
President: Robert Bean
421 Newcastle St.
Brunswick, Georgia 31520

Greater Atlanta Ostomy Association
President: Mrs. Beth Carr
1159 Larkfield Dr. N.E.
Atlanta, Georgia 30328
(404) 394-7289

Middle Georgia Ostomy Association
Mrs. Deane Ellis
514 Ashby Way
Warner Robins, Georgia 31093
(912) 923-1464

Northwest Georgia Ostomy Association
President: Dave Lawton
7 Forest Lane
Rome, Georgia 30161

South Georgia Ostomy Association
John Lounsbrough
Box 114
Naylor, Georgia 31641

HAWAII

Hawaii Island Ostomy Association
President: Ernest A. Smith
156 Makalani St.
Hilo, Hawaii 96720

Honolulu Ostomy Association
President: Evelyn Trapido
3615 Alani Dr.
Honolulu, Hawaii 96822

Maui Ostomy Association
Mr. Edwin Kokobun
2138 Kolo Lane
Wailuku, Hawaii 96793

IDAHO

Boise Area, Idaho Chapter
President: Mrs. Connie Taylor
924 14th Avenue South
Nampa, Idaho 83651
(208) 466-3219

ILLINOIS

Aurora, Illinois, Chapter
Mr. Robert Riney
1725 Lyndale
Aurora, Illinois 60504
(312) 897-2524

Capital Ostomy Association, Inc.
President: Michael W. Gillespie
R.R. 2, Winch Ln., Box 138
Springfield, Illinois 62707
(217) 546-0774

Champaign—Urbana Chapter
President: Ann Shanholtzer
1415 Honeysuckle Lane
Champaign, Illinois 61820

Charleston/Mattoon Area Chapter
President: Ms. Bernita Burk
P.O. Box 813, 308 So. 16th
Mattoon, Illinois 61938
(217) 235-4106

Colostomy Association of Chicago, Inc.
President: Harriet Klemptner
6136 N. Washtenaw
Chicago, Illinois 60659
(312) 262-3999

Danville, Illinois, Chapter
President: Inez Montgomery
Box 144
Indianola, Illinois 61850
(217) 284-3237

Elginland Ostomy Association
President: Mrs. Marjorie M. Muzik
624 Braeburn Rd.
Dundee, Illinois 60118
(312) 426-7808

Greater Joliet Area Ostomy Association
Secretary: Marie Kosteic
1025 Frederick St.
Joliet, Illinois 60435
(815) 723-7491

Ileoptomists, Inc.
Mrs. Shirley Ross
333 Sherman Ave.
Evanston, Illinois 60202
(312) 869-4439

Illiana Chapter
Mrs. Marilyn P. Hay
113 Westwood Dr.
Park Forest, Illinois 60466
(312) 748-3879

Illinois Valley Ostomy Association
P.O. Box 592
Streator, Illinois 61364

Kankakee Ostomy Association, Inc.
President: William Grimm
1875 Meadowview
Kankakee, Illinois 60901
(815) 939-2608

Lake County Ostomy Association
Mrs. Charles Presley
2035 No. Jackson St.
Waukegan, Illinois 60085
(312) 623-0427

North Suburban Chicago Chapter
President: Ms. Bonnie Bachmann
303 Anthony Road
Buffalo Grove, Illinois 60090
(312) 537-9065

Peoria Area Chapter
President: Sharon Mollenhauer
c/o Proctor Community Hospital
5409 No. Knoxville Ave.
Peoria, Illinois 61614
(309) 691-4702

Quad City Chapter
President: W. Robert Bergren
P.O. Box 576
Moline, Illinois 61265
(309) 786-4253

Rock County, Wisconsin, Chapter
President: Mrs. Margaret Larsen
441 Whittemore Dr.
South Beloit, Illinois 61080

Rockford Ostomy Association
President: Bill Swanson
P.O. Box 1641
Rockford, Illinois 61110
(815) 399-4508

Short Circuit Club of Decatur and
  Area, Inc.
President: Mr. Dale Colee
4488 Hale Dr.
Decatur, Illinois 62526
(217) 428-6657

Southern Illinois Ostomy Association
  (Mt. Vernon Area)
President: Paul R. Watson
533 No. Shelby
Salem, Illinois 62881
(618) 548-2969

Vermillion Ostomy Association of
  Pontiac
President: Mrs. Alfretta Bond
1419 N. Aurora
Pontiac, Illinois 61764
(815) 844-7301

Wheaton, Illinois, Chapter
President: Mrs. Ardeth Zamsky
528 N. Ardmore Apt. 1-E
Villa Park, Illinois 60181
(312) 279-2100

INDIANA

Evansville Chapter
Mrs. Bettye Hassel
R.R. #7, Box 215
Evansville, Indiana 47712
(812) 963-3200

Fort Wayne Chapter
c/o Kathleen Wood
1021 W. Wayne St.
Fort Wayne, Indiana 46804
(219) 743-5303

Indianapolis Chapter
President: W. Dean Lacy
4228 No. Catherwood
Indianapolis, Indiana 46226
(317) 546-0481

Kokomo, Indiana, Chapter
Francis Richard Elliott, Jr.
P.O. Box 146 (346 N. Union St.)
Russiaville, Indiana 46979
(317) 883-7466

Lafayette Ostomy Society
President: Cecil Atkinson
222 E. Railroad St.
Remington, Indiana 47977

La Porte County Ostomy Group
Secretary: Raymond Jagodka
202 Roosevelt St.
La Porte, Indiana 46350
(219) 324-2648

Muncie, Indiana, Chapter
Mr. Rick Carnagua
515 Colony Dr.
Yorktown, Indiana 47396

Ostomy Club of St. Joseph County
Staff Rep.: Miss Elaine Lubbers
521 W. Colfax
South Bend, Indiana 46601
(219) 234-3136

Richmond Area Ostomy Association
President: Tom Fields
810 E. Delaware
Cambridge City, Indiana 47374

Terre Haute Chapter
President: John Niklasch
12 Salem Pl.
Terre Haute, Indiana 47803
(812) 877-2895

Wabash Valley Chapter
Vincent Foster
1323 Church St.
Vincennes, Indiana 47591
(812) 882-5706

IOWA

Ames, Iowa, Chapter
Treasurer: Karen Hoiberg
c/o Mary Greely, Memorial Hospital
117 11th St.
Ames, Iowa 50010
(515) 239-2011

Des Moines Chapter
c/o Iowa Lutheran Hospital
Penn at University
Des Moines, Iowa 50316
(515) 283-5125

Dubuque, Iowa, Chapter
President: Ruth M. Turnis
701½ Wilson Avenue
Dubuque, Iowa 52001
(319) 588-4176

Fort Dodge Ostomy Society
720 South 17th Street
Fort Dodge, Iowa 50501

Iowa City Area Ostomates
Miss Gladys Scott
Rt. 2, Box 75
Iowa City, Iowa 52240

North Iowa Area Chapter
President: Mrs. Louise Mock
615 5th Ave. N.E.
Clarion, Iowa 50525
(515) 532-3669

Oskaloosa, Iowa, Area Chapter
President: Homer Stufflebeam
606 W. Jefferson
Bloomfield, Iowa 52538
(515) 644-2368

Siouxland Ostomy Association
President: Lawrence Pearson
2326 So. Palmetto St.
Sioux City, Iowa 51106
(712) 276-3816

Waterloo, Iowa, Area Chapter
President: Ms. Eileen Shirk
1633 Howard Ave.
Waterloo, Iowa 50702
(319) 291-6993

KANSAS

Fort Scott, Kansas, Chapter
Mr. Lloyd J. Feagins
1615 Charles St.
Fort Scott, Kansas 66701
(316) 223-1243

Salina, Kansas, Chapter
Ms. Donna Short
316 E. Bond
Salina, Kansas 67401
(913) 825-6877

Topeka Chapter
President: Herbert Ring
6760 Aylesbury
Topeka, Kansas 66814

Wichita Ostomy Association
President: Miss Beth Boy
523 Chestnut
Holstead, Kansas 67056

KENTUCKY

Bluegrass Chapter
President: Ruben Roberts
104 Manitoba Lane
Lexington, Kentucky 40503
(606) 272-7567

Kentuckiana Chapter
President: Christine Bensing
3921 Cane Run Rd.
Louisville, Kentucky 40211
(502) 774-5370

LOUISIANA

Acadiana Ostomy Association
Mrs. Gloria Aucoin
107 N. Mall
Lafayette, Louisiana 70503
(318) 235-7673

Baton Rouge Area Ostomy Association
P.O. Box 64938
Baton Rouge, Louisiana 70896
(504) 344-7463 (American Cancer
    Society Office)

Greater New Orleans Ostomy
    Association
President: Edward Boettner
P.O. Box 53156
New Orleans, Louisiana 70153
(504) 945-1768

Shreveport Louisiana Chapter
Mrs. Mae Trahan
2313 Tillman
Bossier City, Louisiana 71010
(318) 742-8557

MAINE

Androscoggin Ostomy Association
Mr. Gerald N. Bouffard
42 Bushey Circle
Lewiston, Maine 04240
(207) 782-3663

Aroostook Ostomy Association
President: Ernestine McKay
34 Dyer St.
Presque Isle, Maine 04769

Augusta Ostomy Association
President: Robert Butler
Welch's Point
E. Winthrop, Maine 04343

Bath, Maine, Chapter
Ms. Cheryl St. Pierre
Box 2066, Old Bath Rd.
Brunswick, Maine 04011

Central Maine Area Ostomy Association
Mrs. Bettina Barker
26 Island Ave.
Fairfield, Maine 04937
(207) 453-6586

Greater Portland Area Chapter
President: Francis W. Reilly
7 Rogers Rd.
Yarmouth, Maine 04096
(207) 846-5160

Ostomy Association of Eastern
    Maine
President: Paul E. Martin
33 6th St.
Bangor, Maine 04401

Ostomy Association of Rumford
President: Mrs. Mary L. Drown
R.F.D.
Dixfield, Maine 04224
(207) 562-7724

Anne Arundel County, Maryland,
   Ostomy Association, Inc.
President: Mrs. Peggy M. Williamson
14th St., Andrews Crossover
Severna Park, Maryland 21146
(301) 987-1641

Baltimore Ostomy Association
President: Ben Ettin
6972 Milbrook Park Dr.
Baltimore, Maryland 21215
(301) 484-6276

Cumberland, Maryland, Chapter
President: Catherine Yocum
P.O. Box 532
Cumberland, Maryland 21502
(301) 786-4158

Easton—Cambridge Chapter
President: Mrs. Doris Turkington
R.D. #1
Denton, Maryland 21629
(301) 479-1575

Frederick County, Maryland, Chapter
President: Mrs. Cecilia Costlow
607 Schley Ave.
Frederick, Maryland 21701
(301) 662-3167

Metropolitan Maryland Ostomy
   Association
President: Horace Saunders
9803 E. Light Dr.
Silver Spring, Maryland 20903
(301) 434-2647

Metropolitan Maryland Youth Ostomy
   Group
Advisor: Horace Saunders
344 University Blvd., West
Silver Spring, Maryland 20901

Southern Maryland Counties Chapter
c/o American Cancer Society
West Hyattsville, Maryland 20782
(301) 864-0370

Washington County Ostomy Association
President: Mrs. Doris Worthington
1829 Gilbert Ave.
Hagertown, Maryland 21740
(301) 733-5425

MASSACHUSETTS

Berkshire County Chapter
Ms. Sybil-Ann Sherman
26 Front St.
Williamstown, Massachusetts 02167
(413) 445-4595

Franklin County, Massachusetts, Chapter
President: Mrs. Carol A. Jones
39 Shattuck St.
Greenfield, Massachusetts 01301
(413) 773-8619

Merrimack Valley Ostomy Association
Mr. Chester Bradley
9 Gage St.
Methuen, Massachusetts 01844

Northern Worchester County Chapter
President: Mrs. Marilyn Dolan
99 Woodside Ave.
Leominster, Massachusetts 01453
(617) 537-1307

Ostomy Association of Boston, Inc.
247 Commonwealth Ave.
Boston, Massachusetts 02116
(617) 267-3665

Ostomy Association of Cape
   Cod, Inc.
Col. John J. Dalton (Retired)
Box 371
Crowell Rd.
Chatham, Massachusetts 02633

Ostomy Association of Greater
   Springfield, Inc.
P.O. Box 172
Springfield, Massachusetts 01118
(413) 783-5387

MICHIGAN

Ann Arbor, Michigan, Chapter
President: Mrs. Dorothy Hellems
212 Third St.
Ann Arbor, Michigan 48103
(313) 663-1970

Battle Creek Chapter
Mrs. Mary E. Ross
841 Beadle Lake
Battle Creek, Michigan 49017
(616) 964-4386

Coldwater Area Ostomy Society
President: Royce Olmstead
194 W. State St.
Coldwater, Michigan 49036
(517) 278-2435

Flint Area Chapter
Mr. Keith L. Ketzier
62058 Kenwood Dr.
Flint, Michigan 48504

Greater Detroit Chapter
18055 James Couzens Highway
Detroit, Michigan 48235
(313) 341-9715

Jackson Ostomy Association
President: Ouida Beck
939 Chittock St.
Jackson, Michigan 49203
(517) 782-3194

Kalamazoo Ostomy Association
President: Cathie Nouggle
3330 Lincolnshire
Kalamazoo, Michigan 49001

Muskegon Area Ostomy Association
President: Marselien Meloche
2616 Bellevue Rd.
Muskegon, Michigan 49441
(616) 759-0066 or 828-4296

Oakland County, Michigan, Chapter
Mrs. Raymond Glander
726 Labadie Ct.
Rochester, Michigan 48063
(313) 651-1108

Ostomy Association of Greater
Lansing
President: Walter Parker
714 S. Cochran
Charlotte, Michigan 48813

Ottawa County, Michigan, Chapter
President: Mr. Paul Babcock
414 Duncan Ct.
Grand Haven, Michigan 49417
(616) 842-3234

Straits Area Ostomy Association
Mrs. Dan Houser, Jr.
Box 2664, Wildwood Harbor Rd.
Boyne City, Michigan 49712
(616) 582-6848

Tri–City Ostomy Association
Mrs. Edith Anders
801 Linwood Dr.
Midland, Michigan 48640
(517) 835-8890

MINNESOTA

Mankato Area Chapter
President: Max Embacher
Rte. #4, Box 171
Mankato, Minnesota 56001
(507) 625-5349

Minneapolis, Minnesota, Chapter
Secretary: Mrs. Marianne Phelps
5649 Vera Cruz Avenue N.
Crystal, Minnesota 55429
(612) 537-7991

North St. Louis County, Minnesota,
Chapter
Mrs. Betty Peterson
1031 3rd St. South
Virginia, Minnesota 55792
(218) 749-2294

Redstone Area Ostomy Group
Miss Charlotte Hess
5½ So. Minnesota St.
New Ulm, Minnesota 56073
(507) 354-3653

Rochester Area Ostomy Group
Mr. Art Hanft
3732 3rd Pl. N.W.
Rochester, Minnesota 55901

St. Paul Ostomy Association
P.O. Box 30487
St. Paul, Minnesota 55175

Wilmar Area Ostomy Society
Mrs. Evelyn Aistrup
711 E. 5
Wilmar, Minnesota 56201

MISSISSIPPI

Gulf Coast Ostomy Association
President: Donald H. Myers
Edgewater Garden, Apt. 8–E
Biloxi, Mississippi 39531
(601) 388–4229

Ostomy Association of Jackson
President: Mrs. Nadine Leverette
P.O. Box 16604
Jackson, Mississippi 39206
(601) 956–2428

MISSOURI

Cape Girardeau, Missouri, Area Chapter
c/o American Cancer Society
1427 Thomas Dr.
Cape Girardeau, Missouri 63701
(314) 334–8187

Columbia, Missouri, Chapter
President: Mrs. Betty J. Pavitt
1110 Primrose Lane
Jefferson City, Missouri 65101
(314) 635–3561

Joplin Ostomy Association
President: Sam Engle
902 Cherry
Lamar, Missouri 64759

Kansas City Chapter
President: Adeline Werner
4446 Harrison
Kansas City, Missouri 64110
(816) 753–2806

Ostomy Association of St. Louis
President: Elnore Sturm
960 Briarton Dr.
St. Louis, Missouri 63126

St. Joseph, Missouri, Area Chapter
Mr. Virgil E. Jackson
Rt. 3, Box 113
Maysville, Missouri 64469
(816) 449–5787

Springfield Area Ostomy Association
President: Mrs. Ruth Turner
Box 267
Marionville, Missouri 65705
(417) 463–2483

MONTANA

Billings Area Ostomy Association
Mr. Fred Brown
1804 Colton Blvd.
Billings, Montana 59102

Butte, Montana, Area Chapter
President: Ms. Jean Svedahl
RFDA 192A Opportunity
Anaconda, Montana 59711
(406) 797–3474

Great Falls Ostomy Association
Box 6021
Great Falls, Montana 59601

NEBRASKA

Central Nebraska Chapter
President: Mrs. Mary Wortman
Rt. #3, Box 80
Wood River, Nebraska 68883
(308) 583–2401

Lincoln Ostomy Association
c/o American Cancer Society
Lancaster County Unit
4740 "A" St., Room 2
Lincoln, Nebraska 68510

Omaha, Nebraska, Chapter
c/o American Cancer Society
Nebraska Division, Inc.
6910 Pacific St.
Omaha, Nebraska 68106
(402) 551–2422

Western Nebraska Ostomy Association
at Chadron
President: Mrs. Susan Howell
634 Main
Chadron, Nebraska 69337
(308) 432–3910

NEVADA

Reno Ostomy Chapter
President: Miles Setty
P.O. Box "B"
Sparks, Nevada 89431
(702) 825–0767

Southern Nevada Ostomy Association
President: Troy McDonald
808 Capenter
Las Vegas, Nevada 89107
(702) 870–0428

NEW HAMPSHIRE

Granite State Ostomy Association
Mr. Ronald Knee
P.O. Box 96
Concord, New Hampshire 03301
(603) 224–1807

Greater Manchester Ostomy Association
Mr. Russell Aiken
49 Alfred St.
Manchester, New Hampshire 03104

Northeast Vermont Ostomy Association
President: Robert Elliot
Box 361
Lancaster, New Hampshire 03584
(603) 788–3575

Northern New Hampshire Chapter
President: Irving Whitney
76 Broadway
Concord, New Hampshire 03301

Ostomy Association of Southern New
Hampshire
President: Stanley Morton
35 Tyler St.
Nashua, New Hampshire 03060

NEW JERSEY

Audubon Area Chapter
President: Irene B. Sheppard
1 Wyoming Ave.
Audubon, New Jersey 08106
(609) 547–8541

Belleville–Montclair, New Jersey,
Chapter
President: Larry DeMayo
24 Mountain Way
Cedar Grove, New Jersey 00709

Bergen County Ostomy Association
Secretary: Sandy Frazier
80 North Walnut St.
Ridgewood, New Jersey 07450
(201) 444–1167

Hudson County Ostomy Association
Mr. Alfred Sharlow
531 Day Ave.
Ridgefield, New Jersey 07657

Ileostomy Association of Northern
New Jersey (Englewood Area)
Secretary: Mrs. Dorothy LaVigne
84 Cedar Lane
Teaneck, New Jersey 07666
(201) 692–0143

Jersey Shore Ostomy Association
Ms. Regina Pickover
33 Pal Dr.
Asbury Park, New Jersey 07712

Mercer County Ostomy Association
President: James R. Jones
269 Main St.
Groveville, New Jersey 08620

Millville Area Chapter
Rev. Russell C. Gromest
910 E. Main St.
Millville, New Jersey 08332
(609) 825–5919

Morris County Ostomy Association
Mr. John H. Monahan
51 White Birch Lane
Parsippany, New Jersey 07054
(201) 887–5877

Ostomy Association of Central
New Jersey (New Brunswick Area)
President: John Segar
22 Linsley Pl.
Metuchen, New Jersey 08840

Ostomy Association of New Jersey, Inc.
(Essex County)
President: Eileen Lutsky
50 N. Cottage Pl.
Westfield, New Jersey 07090
(201) 233-1683

Ostomy Association of Ocean County
100 Terrace Ave.
Toms River, New Jersey 08753
(201) 349-5280

Ostomy Association of Somerset
County
President: Robert Hay
703 Dunellen
Dunellen, New Jersey 08812

Ostomy Association of Union County
President: Mordechai S. Sobel
231 Birchwood Rd.
Linden, New Jersey 07036
(201) 486-0041

Salem County New Jersey Chapter
President: Clarence MacNeal, Jr.
18 Fenwick Dr.
Carney's Point, New Jersey 08069
(609) 299-0906

NEW MEXICO

Las Cruces Area Chapter
Secretary: Mrs. Ruby F. Larson
Rt. 3, Box 626B
Las Cruces, New Mexico 88001
(505) 382-5915

Ostomy Association of Albuquerque
President: R.L. Fourcher
P.O. Box 80024
Albuquerque, New Mexico 87108
(505) 294-1736

NEW YORK

Albany Area Ostomy Association
President: Mrs. Linda K. Boyd
7 Barclay St.
Albany, New York 12209
(518) 449-8722 (c/o American
Cancer Society)

Auburn, New York, Chapter
Mrs. Kay Cole, R.N.
7 Parsons St.
Auburn, New York 13021
(315) 252-5726

Brooklyn Ileostomy Association, Inc.
President: Harold Rosenblaum
1212 Newkirk Ave.
Brooklyn, New York 11230
(212) 859-0390

Chautauqua County, New York,
Chapter
Ms. Sue Crytzer
c/o WCA Hospital
207 Foote Ave.
Jamestown, New York 14701
(716) 487-0141

Colostomy Club of Brooklyn, Inc.
President: Joseph Margolis
3685 Bedford Ave.
Brooklyn, New York 11229

Colostomy Society of New York, Inc.
Mr. David Widman
P.O. Box 517
General Post Office
New York, New York 10001
(212) 221-1246

Corning Ostomy Chapter
Ms. Rose Plitt
RD #3
Addison, New York 14830
(607) 458-5414

Fingerlakes Ostomy Association
(Geneva, N.Y., Area)
Mr. Donald W. Dobbin
35 Columbia St.
Geneva, New York 14456

Fulton County, New York, Chapter
c/o American Cancer Society
25 Bleecker St.
Gloversville, New York 12078
(518) 725-3518

Genesee Valley Ostomy Association
c/o Monroe County Cancer and
     Leukemia Association
1441 East Ave.
Rochester, New York 14610

Greater Orange Area Chapter
c/o American Cancer Society
11-15 King St.
Middletown, New York 10940
(914) 343-5612 or 733-1021

Greater Utica Chapter
President: Mrs. Jean Stern, R.N.
109 Laurel Pl.
Utica, New York 13502

Ileostomy Association of New
     York, Inc.
QT New York
1540 Broadway, Suite 30
New York, New York 10036
(212) 824-2057

Jefferson County, New York, Chapter
President: Wayne H. Boniface
436 Paddock St.
Watertown, New York 13601
(315) 788-6893

Long Island Colostomy Association
President: Charles Bergman
3 Sunset Dr.
Huntington, New York 11743

Long Island Ileostomy Association, Inc.
Mr. Ted Horn
1027 Stafford Rd.
Valley Stream, New York 11580
(516) 872-9277

Mid-Hudson Chapter
Mr. Thomas C. Haen
Dutch Garden, Apt. 55F
Poughkeepsie, New York 12601
(914) 452-6599

Niagara Frontier Ostomy Association
c/o Mrs. Mae Mesner
74 Homesgarth Ave.
Cheektawaga, New York 14225

Oneida City Area Chapter
President: Miss Mildred A. Ridley
116 E. Sands St.
Oneida, New York 13421
(315) 363-2675

Orleans County Chapter
Mrs. Mary S. Lamont
3035 Densmore Rd.
Albion, New York 14411
(716) 589-6056

Ostomy Association of Oneonta
President: Mr. D.M. Charles
Underwood Dr.
Otego, New York 13825

Ostomy Club of Delaware County
President: Paul Miller
Mt. Pleasant
Walton, New York 13856

Ostomy Club of Rockland County
President: Lewis Rosenburg
57 Lillian Pl.
Pomona, New York 10972
(914) 354-7186

Oswego County, New York, Chapter
President: Mrs. Ruth Kelly
4440 E. River Rd.
RD #4
Oswego, New York 13126

Rensselaer County Ostomy Society
President: Kenneth L. Foster
339 Third St.
Troy, New York 12180
(518) 274-2700

Schenectady Ostomy Association
Mr. J. Stanley Lansing
3 Drott Dr.
Scotia, New York 12301

Southern Tier Ostomy Management
Association
Miss Jean M. Laux, R.N., E.T.
c/o Our Lady of Lourdes Hospital
169 Riverside Dr.
Binghamton, New York 13905
(607) 798-5111 or 798-5157

Staten Island, New York, Chapter
President: Ms. Marguerite McAndrews
117 Haven Ave.
Staten Island, New York 10306
(212) 351-2603

Suffolk Ostomy Association
President: Kermit Lesler
206 Liberty Ave.
Babylon, New York 11702
(516) 669-8176

Syracuse Ostomy Association
Mrs. Ruth Breese
304 Garden City Dr.
Mattydale, New York 13211
(315) 454-0650

Twin Tier Ostomy Association
President: Charles F. Roe
122 Eastview Dr.
Horseheads, New York 14845
(607) 373-8357 (business)
(607) 739-4337 (residence)

Westchester County, New York,
Chapter
President: Ethel Wagman
P.O. Box 93
Mt. Vernon, New York 10552
(914) 699-4689

NORTH CAROLINA

Asheville Ostomy Association
President: Norma Miller, R.N.
35 Swanger Rd.
Asheville, North Carolina 28805

Charlotte Chapter
President: Mrs. Letha Black
223 Montana Circle
Concord, North Carolina 28025
(704) 786-6666

Gaston Area Ostomy Association
Secretary: Mrs. J.B. Shuford
314 Linden Circle
Gastonia, North Carolina 28052

Piedmont Ostomy Association
President: George B. Campbell
P.O. Box 8511
Greensboro, North Carolina 27410
(919) 855-1430

Raleigh Area Chapter
Mr. Joseph M. Rowe
Medical Services Pharmacy
4818 Six Forks Rd.
Raleigh, North Carolina 27609
(919) 787-7181

Winston—Salem Area Ostomy
Association
President: Miss Hazel Jarratt
909 Warren Ave.
Winston—Salem, North Carolina 27107
(919) 723-3321

NORTH DAKOTA

Bismarck—Mandan Area Chapter
President: Edwin B. Harrison, Jr.
P.O. Box 504
Mandan, North Dakota 58554
(701) 223-1623

Fargo-Moorhead Chapter
President: Beverly Fox
P.O. Box 2622
Fargo, North Dakota 58102

Grand Forks Area Chapter
President: Mrs. Nicholas Kohanowski
3532 10th Ave. North
Grand Forks, North Dakota 58201
(701) 772-6589

Minot Area Chapter
President: Mr. Edmond P. Dreyer
1130 N.W. 1st St.
Minot, North Dakota 58701
(701) 839-2063

OHIO

Akron Chapter
President: Carlos Jackson
3235 Greenwich Rd.
Norton, Ohio 44230

Alliance, Ohio, Chapter
President: Jerry L. Antram
4875 Union Ave. N.E.
Homeworth, Ohio 44634
(216) 823-1743

Central Ohio Chapter
Dr. Ned A. Parrett
2815 Woodstock Rd.
Columbus, Ohio 43221
(614) 457-5480

Chillicothe Area Ostomy Association
of United Ostomy Association
Vice-President: John H. Miller
468 E. Water St.
Chillicothe, Ohio 45601

Cincinnati Ileostomy—Colostomy
Association
President: Donna McCabe
6936 Hearne Rd.
Cincinnati, Ohio 45211
(513) 574-6968

Cleveland Ostomy Association, Inc.
President: John Velardo
1100 Dorsh Rd.
South Euclid, Ohio 44121
(216) 381-5716

Dayton Ostomy Chapter
Esther Reimueller
329 Imogene Rd.
Dayton, Ohio 45405
(513) 277-0347

Lorain County Ostomy Association
President: Raymond Lee Kruger
913 Salem Ave.
Elyria, Ohio 44035

Marion, Ohio, Area Chapter
President: Mrs. Dawn E. Watters
1016 Chateau Dr.
Marion, Ohio 43302

Mt. Vernon, Ohio, Chapter
President: Mrs. June Ferguson
11 N. Park St.
Mt. Vernon, Ohio 43050

Portsmouth, Ohio, Chapter
President: Everett E. McElyea
224 Calvert Ln.
West Portsmouth, Ohio 45662
(614) 858-4659

Sandusky Ostomy Association
President: William J. Baratt
241 42nd St.
Sandusky, Ohio 44870
(419) 625-8643

Springfield, Ohio, Chapter
President: Dorothy Everhart
1229 Glenmore Dr.
Springfield, Ohio 45503
(513) 399-7067

Stark County Chapter
President: John Moulos
1521 Tremont S.W.
Massillion, Ohio 44646
(216) 832-8150

Toledo Area Ostomy Association
President: Phillip Brewster
Rt. #1, Box 213R
Swanton, Ohio 43558

Youngstown Chapter
c/o Youngstown Hospital Association
North Side Unit, Gypsy Lane and
Goletta
Youngstown, Ohio 44501
(216) 755-8811

OKLAHOMA

Bartlesville Ostomy Association
Coordinator: Jane Phillips
Episcopal Memorial Medical Center
Continuing Education Center
410 E. Frank Phillips Blvd.
Bartlesville, Oklahoma 74003
(918) 534-1210

Canadian Valley Ostomy Association
President: Mrs. Neva Chelf
Rt. 2, Box 14
Wewoka, Oklahoma 74884
(405) 257-2708

Enid Chapter
President: Neil Sisson
1117 N. 12th
Enid, Oklahoma 73701
(405) 234-6533

Norman, Oklahoma, Chapter
Secretary: John A. Shaw
P.O. Box 216
Norman, Oklahoma 73169
(405) 329-4799

Ostomy Association of Oklahoma
   City, Inc.
Mrs. Clara Speers
2336 N.W. 38th St.
Oklahoma City, Oklahoma 73112

Ponca City Ostomy Association
President: Mrs. Nancy Skach
1024 So. Pine
Stillwater, Oklahoma 74074

Tulsa Ostomy Association
D.O. Givens
5934 S. Birmingham Pl.
Tulsa, Oklahoma 74105

OREGON

Coos Bay Area Chapter
Richard Grossman
2235 Commercial
North Bend, Oregon 97459
(503) 756-7070

Lane County Ostomy Association
President: J. Gordon Smith
290 Woodlane Dr.
Springfield, Oregon 97477

Oregon Ostomy Association
10237 N. Leonard
Portland, Oregon 97203
(503) 286-8998

Willamette Valley Ostomy Association
P.O. Box 3062
Salem, Oregon 97302
(503) 581-5521

PENNSYLVANIA

Abington Area Ostomy Association
President: Mrs. Mary Keys
204 Newington Dr.
Hatboro, Pennsylvania 19040
(215) 675-4278

Antnracite Ostomy Association
President: Linda Frew
124 W. Arch St.
Frackville, Pennsylvania 17931

Beaver Pennsylvania Area Chapter
President: Norma H. Stroeter
1315 3rd St.
Beaver, Pennsylvania 15009
(412) 774-5384

Berwick Area Chapter
President: Ms. Betty G. Peters
532 E. Sixth St.
Berwick, Pennsylvania 18603
(717) 752-4454

Bucks County Ostomy Association
President: Thomas B. Noble
St. Peters Village
St. Peters, Pennsylvania 19470
(215) 469-9290

Butler County Chapter
President: Mrs. Evelyn Wigton
175 Muddy Creek Rd.
Butler, Pennsylvania 16001
(412) 282-4195

Central Montgomery County,
   Norristown Chapter
President: Edward Fleming
1820 Pine St.
Norristown, Pennsylvania 19401
(215) 275-1137

Central Pennsylvania Ostomy Society
President: Walter E. Wenrich
R.D. #3, Box 138
Altoona, Pennsylvania 16601
(814) 942-7092

Children's Tristateostomy Association
President: Mrs. Libby Sukarochana
716 Thompson Run Road
Pittsburgh, Pennsylvania 15237

C.I.R.A., Inc.
Mr. Max Turner
4609 C Street
Philadelphia, Pennsylvania 19120
(215) 324-1553

Delaware County Ostomy Association
President: Mrs. Becky Huntsman
P.O. Box 54
Elwyn, Pennsylvania 19063
(215) 352-6238

Erie Ostomy Association
President: Gladys Gustavson
P.O. Box 8082
Erie, Pennsylvania 16505
(814) 838-3670

Franklin–Oil City, Pa., Chapter
President: Mrs. Dottie E. Eckel
Dempseytown Rd., R.D. #3, Box 395
Franklin, Pennsylvania 16323
(814) 437-6132

Greensburg–Keystone Chapter
P.O. Box 901
Greensburg, Pennsylvania 15601
(412) 468-4853

Harrisburg Ostomy Association
Riland Scheidler
188 Pine St.
Millersburg, Pennsylvania 17061

Johnstown, Pa., Chapter
President: Mabel M. Yoder
Joseph Johns Towers #1002
Johnstown, Pennsylvania 15901
(814) 536-4581

Lackawanna County Ostomy Association
President: Alex Rinaldi
715 Terrace St.
Dunmore, Pennsylvania 18512
(717) 342-6445

Lancaster Ostomy Association
President: Miss Christina Kock
c/o American Cancer Society
625 Manor St.
Lancaster, Pennsylvania 17603

Lehigh Valley Ostomy Association
President: Donald Scurry
333 East North St.
Bethlehem, Pennsylvania 18018

Luzerne County, Pa., Chapter
President: Walter W. Kay
39 Bedford
Forty-Fort, Pennsylvania 18704
(717) 287-3040

Mercer County, Pa., Chapter
Secretary: Mrs. Wanda R. Yurkon
E. Lake Dr.
R.D. #2
Transfer, Pennsylvania 16154
(412) 962-5451; 347-5217

Ostomy Association of Berks County
President: William H. Conboy
P.O. Box 1355
Reading, Pennsylvania 19601

Pittsburgh Chapter
President: James A. Cowan
830 Wainwright Dr.
Pittsburgh, Pennsylvania 15228
(412) 561-4607

Pottstown Area, Pa., Chapter
President: Thomas B. Noble
St. Peters, Pennsylvania 19470
(215) 469-9290

Williamsport Ostomy Association
President: Elizabeth Lyon
255 Broad St.
Montoursville, Pennsylvania 17754
(717) 368-8575

RHODE ISLAND

Rhode Island Ostomy Club
President: William McPeak
64 Eagle Rd.
Cranston, Rhode Island 20920
(401) 943-1238

SOUTH CAROLINA

Charleston Ostomy Association
President: Albert V. Ewan
1214 MacQueen Ave.
Charleston, South Carolina 29407
(803) 766-2256

Greenville, S.C., Chapter
President: Thomas C. Griffith
1511 Easley Bridge Rd.
Greenville, South Carolina 29611

Spartanburg Chapter
Mr. Elmer Bradey
102 Skyuka Circle
Landrum, South Carolina 29356
(803) 457–2332

SOUTH DAKOTA

Black Hills Ostomy Association
President: Mrs. Ann Neil
1701 Ninth St.
Rapid City, South Dakota 57701

Sioux Falls Area Chapter
President: Henry A. Dingman
5104 W. 40th St.
Sioux Falls, South Dakota 57106
(605) 334–6555

TENNESSEE

Chattanooga Ostomy Association
President: Mrs. Sandra Barksdale
7111 Leslie Dell Lane
Chattanooga, Tennessee 37421

Knoxville Ostomy Association
Secretary: Mrs. Terry Tudor
109 Chatham Lane
Oak Ridge, Tennessee 37830
(615) 483–9841

Memphis Area Ostomy Group
President: Sidney Schiffman
1306 Lynnfield Rd., Apt. 1
Memphis, Tennessee 38138

Tri-City Ostomy Association
President: Mrs. Ralph Linfoot
Rt. #3, Box 122
Limestone, Tennessee 37681
(615) 257–2399

TEXAS

Abilene and Big Country, Texas,
    Chapter
President: Tom Abram
2433 No. 3rd, Apt. 131
Abilene, Texas 79603
(915) 673–4863

Austin, Texas, Chapter
President: Carol Laubach
5718 Wellington Dr.
Austin, Texas 78723

Beaumont Chapter
Ms. Tanya Morgan
1215 East Dr.
Beaumont, Texas 77706

Corpus Christi, Texas, Chapter
President: Roy J. Hanson
Emerson Drive
Corpus Christi, Texas 78415
(512) 853–3112

Dallas Area Chapter
President: Ben Bold
2747 Oakland St.
Garland, Texas 75041
(214) 278–0505

Fort Worth Area Chapter
President: Jack Jackson
2135 South Collins
Arlington, Texas 76010

Golden Spread Ostomy Association
R. Earl O'Keefe
P.O. Box 871
Amarillo, Texas 79167
(806) 374–0361

Houston Ostomy Association
P.O. Box 25164
Houston, Texas 77005
(806) 461–5949

Longview Area Chapter
President: Mrs. Shirley Rohrbach
205 Bobby Street
Longview, Texas 75601
(214) 757–5318

Lubbock Ostomy Association
Earl Holley
3007 56th Street
Lubbock, Texas 79413
(806) 799–1606

Ostomy Association of El Paso
Vice-President: Mrs. Jere Schalla
5332 Annette
El Paso, Texas 79924
(915) 751–0542

San Antonio, Texas, Chapter
Josephine Carman
126 Tophill Rd.
San Antonio, Texas 78209
(512) 826–4420

Sherman Area Chapter
Mrs. Louis Scott
Box 717
Sherman, Texas 75090
(214) 892–6506

Tyler, Texas, Chapter
Secretary: Esther Hudson
1206 Garden Valley Rd.
Tyler, Texas 75701
(214) 592–4103

Waco Ostomy Association
President: William J. Apodaca
Box 359
Mart, Texas 76664

West Texas Ostomy Association
Secretary: Phylis Crews
Box 3970
San Angelo, Texas 76901

Wichita Falls Ostomy Association
President: Francis Crook
P.O. Box 4362
Wichita, Texas 76308
(817) 322–5829

UTAH

Ogden Ostomy Association
c/o American Cancer Society
707 24th St.
Ogden, Utah 84010
(801) 295–5378

Ostomy Association of Utah
President: Nancy Rodgers
548 South 200 East
Bountiful, Utah 84010

VERMONT

Northeast Vermont Ostomy Association
President: Robert Elliot
Box 361
Lancaster, New Hampshire 03584
(603) 788–3575

Ostomy Association of Rutland
President: Mrs. Pauline Dickinson
P.O. Box 218
Center Rutland, Vermont 05736
(802) 773–3505

Ostomy Association of Vermont
President: John Chadwick
52 East Terr.
So. Burlington, Vermont 05401

VIRGINIA

Bluefield Area Chapter
Mrs. Lillie Taylor
Rte. 1, Box 83
Pounding Mill, Virginia 24637

Danville Area Chapter
President: Mrs. Brenda Shelton
Rte. #3, Box 34
Danville, Virginia 24541
(804) 797–9597

Fredericksburg, Virginia, Chapter
Mrs. Patty Farmer
P.O. Box 164
Milford, Virginia 22514
(804) 633–5227

Peninsula Ostomy Association
President: George L. D'Amelio
35 Kenwood Dr.
Hampton, Virginia 23666

Richmond Ostomy Association
President: Jack F. Irwin
1314 Claremont
Richmond, Virginia 23227
(804) 353–7550

Tidewater Ostomy Association
1129 East Little Creek Rd.
Norfolk, Virginia 23518

WASHINGTON

Aberdeen–Grays Harbor Chapter
President: Donald Schuldt
P.O. Box 497
Cosmopolis, Washington 98537
(206) 532–7797

Greater Seattle Chapter
President: Betty Case
4028 S.W. Trenton
Seattle, Washington 98136
(206) 935–5391

Kirkland Eastside Chapter
Secretary: Jacqueline C. Jackson
3803 East Ames Lake Dr.
Redmond, Washington 98052
(206) 333–4223

Mount Vernon, Washington, Chapter
President: Cecil Weyrich
2023 North Ave.
Anacortes, Washington 98221
(206) 293–6281

Ostomates of Eastern Washington
President: Mrs. Dwight B. Aden, Sr.
No. 3226 Milton
Spokane, Washington 99205
(509) 325–5298

Ostomy Association of Yakima
Linda Parten
Rte. 6, Box 351
Yakima, Washington 98902

Tacoma, Washington, Chapter
Mrs. Roberta E. Brewer
9636 Maple Avenue, SW
Tacoma, Washington 98499
(206) 588–3913

WEST VIRGINIA

Bluefield Area Chapter
Mrs. Lillie Taylor
Rte. 1, Box 83
Pounding Mill, Virginia 24637

Charleston Area Ostomy Association
President: Sophie A. Reski
4308 Lancaster Avenue, SE
Charleston, West Virginia 25304
(304) 925–0857

Huntington, West Virginia, Area
Chapter
President: Thomas Bauserman
616 South Terrace
Huntington, West Virginia 25705
(304) 522–3042

West Virginia Ostomy Association
President: Mr. Dwight C. Davis
P.O. Box 1916
Clarksburg, West Virginia 26301
(204) 624–4103

Wheeling Area Chapter
President: Rev. Ronald C. Riggs
2 Romney Rd.
Wheeling, West Virginia 26003

WISCONSIN

Chippewa Valley Ostomy Association
Robert L. Frye
1446 Hoover Ave.
Eau Clair, Wisconsin 54701

Kenosha—Racine Area
President: Beverly Luskin
630 78th St.
Kenosha, Wisconsin 53140
(414) 652–8108

La Crosse, Wisconsin, Chapter
Mrs. Martha Schultz
R. #1, Boma Rd.
Bridel Coulee
La Crosse, Wisconsin 54601
(608) 788–0258

Madison, Wisconsin, Chapter
Douglas Sorge
5917 Riva Rd.
Madison, Wisconsin 53711
(208) 271–0914

Milwaukee Ileostomy and Colostomy
    Association
c/o American Cancer Society
6401 West Capitol Dr.
Milwaukee, Wisconsin 53216
(414) 461–1100

North Central Wisconsin Ostomy
    Association
President: Daniel P. Hazen
726 Chicago Ave.
Wausau, Wisconsin 54401

Rock County, Wisconsin, Chapter
President: Mrs. Margaret Larsen
441 Whittemore Dr.
South Beloit, Illinois 61080

WYOMING

Central Wyoming Ostomy Association
President: Ron Emerson
3064 Alma
Casper, Wyoming 82601

Southeast Wyoming Ostomy Association
President: Elmer Dyekman
3432 Luckie Rd.
Cheyenne, Wyoming 82001
(307) 634–3668

CANADA

ALBERTA

Calgary Ostomy Society
Mr. George Glowacki
#91, 210 86th Avenue SE
Calgary, Alberta T2H 1N6
(403) 253–6272

Edmonton Chapter
Mrs. Sheelah A. Zapf
6314 152A Avenue
Edmonton, Alberta
(403) 476–8313

Medicine Hat, Alberta, Chapter
President: Miss E.E. Smith
730 Third St. SE
Medicine Hat, Alberta
(403) 526–3337

BRITISH COLUMBIA

Island Ostomy Association
Vic Gottfred
357 Linden Ave.
Victoria, British Columbia VBV 4G1

Okanagan Mainline Ostomy Association
President: J.W. Newis
Box 651
Kelowna, British Columbia V1Y 7P2
(604) 762–4422

Vancouver Chapter
President: David W. Oram
P.O. Box 86473
North Vancouver, British Columbia
   V7L 1B1
(604) 988–1589

MANITOBA

The Winnipeg Ostomy Association
President: Mr. A. Foreman
1106–2080 Pembina Highway
Winnipeg, Manitoba R3T 2G9
(204) 269–6784

NEW BRUNSWICK

Fredericton, New Brunswick and
   District Chapter
Mrs. Joan Trainor
112 Park St.
Fredericton, New Brunswick E3A-2J5

Saint John Ostomy Association
President: Corliss A. Percy
226 Douglas Avenue
Saint John, New Brunswick

NOVA SCOTIA

Metropolitan Halifax Chapter
Mrs. Bette Yetman
5 Bowser Ave.
Dartmouth, Nova Scotia B2W 1L8
(902) 434–8154

ONTARIO

Belleville, Trenton, Quinte Ostomy
   Association
President: Mr. V. Wannamaker
20 Gearin St.
Trenton, Ontario K8V 3X1
(613) 392–8971

Brantford and District Ostomy
   Association
President: James A. Hamilton
16 Sheffield Ave.
Brantford, Ontario
N3S 6V8
(519) 752–0215

Cornwall and District Ostomy
   Association
President: Ellen F. Robinson
29 Cumberland St.
Cornwall, Ontario K6J 4G8
(613) 933–5895

Eastern Ontario Ostomy Association
P.O. Box 5706
Ottawa, Ontario K2C 3M1
(613) 733-0499

Hamilton and District Colostomy
and Ileostomy Association
President: Mrs. Olive Taylor
2130 King St., East, Apt. 409
Hamilton, Ontario L8K 4W7
(416) 547-4629

Ileostomy Association of Toronto
President: Mollie Gafney
P.O. Box 732, Terminal A
Toronto, Ontario
(416) 922-1134

London and District Ostomy
Association
President: Mrs. S. Tebbutt
207 Raymond Ave.
London, Ontario N6A 2N2

Niagara Ostomy Association
c/o Canadian Cancer Society
112 Queenston St.
Delphin House
St. Catharines, Ontario
(416) 684-6455

Oshawa and District Ostomy
Association
President: Mrs. Susan Mills
R.R. #2
Bowmanville, Ontario L1C 3K3
(416) 725-8631

South Waterloo and Guelph Area
Chapter
President: James Holley
27 Vanier Dr., Apt. 905
Guelph, Ontario

Thunder Bay Ostomy Association
President: Bob Seymour
Box 2151
Thunder Bay, Ontario

Toronto Colostomy Association
President: Ron Maitland
P.O. Box 5624, Terminal A
Toronto, Ontario M5W 1N8
(416) 481-6171

QUEBEC

Association Des Stomises De
L'Estrie, Inc. (English Section)
S. Pierrette Cote
1136 Craig
Sherbrooke, Quebec J1H 4H3

Ileostomy—Colostomy Association of
Montreal
President: Mrs. Shirley Heft
375 Dufferin Rd.
Hampstead, Quebec H3X 2Y8
(514) 481-8995

SASKATCHEWAN

Regina Ostomy Chapter
President: Ken Matchett
281 Coldwell Rd.
Regina, Saskatchewan S4R 4L4
(306) 543-6655

Saskatoon Ostomy Association
President: Dr. J.W. Stephenson
520 9th St., E.
Saskatoon, Saskatchewan

THE INTERNATIONAL ASSOCIATIONS OF LARYNGECTOMEES

United States of America

ALABAMA

Birmingham
Decatur

Gadsden
Montgomery
Tuscaloosa

ARIZONA

Mesa
Phoenix
Tucson

ARKANSAS

Fort Smith
Little Rock

CALIFORNIA

Fresno
Long Beach
Los Angeles
Redding
Riverside
Sacramento
San Diego
San Francisco
San Jose
Santa Ana
Santa Maria
Vallejo

COLORADO

Denver
Pueblo

CONNECTICUT

Bridgeport
Darien
New Britain
New Haven
New London

DELAWARE

Wilmington

DISTRICT OF COLUMBIA

Washington

FLORIDA

Clearwater
Daytona Beach
Ft. Lauderdale
Fort Myers
Jacksonville
Palm Beach
Pensacola
St. Petersburg
Sarasota

GEORGIA

Atlanta
Columbus

IDAHO

Boise

ILLINOIS

Aurora
Belleville
Central
Chicago
Evanston
Rockford
Rock Island

INDIANA

Evansville
Fort Wayne
Indianapolis
Lafayette
Muncie
South Bend
Terre Haute

IOWA

Sioux City

KANSAS

Independence
Wichita

KENTUCKY

Lexington
Louisville
Owensboro

LOUISIANA

New Orleans
Alexandria

MAINE

Portland
Waterville

MARYLAND

Baltimore
Cumberland
Hagerstown
Silver Spring

MASSACHUSETTS

Boston
Taunton

MICHIGAN

Detroit
Grand Rapids
Kalamazoo
Marquette
Mt. Pleasant

MINNESOTA

Duluth
Minneapolis
St. Paul

MISSISSIPPI

Jackson

MISSOURI

Columbia
Joplin
Kansas City
St. Joseph
St. Louis
Sedalia

NEBRASKA

Omaha

NEVADA

Las Vegas

NEW HAMPSHIRE

Manchester

NEW JERSEY

Bergenfield
Collingswood
East Orange
Elizabeth
Jersey City
Menlo Park
Paterson
Pleasantville
Red Bank
Toms River

NEW MEXICO

Albuquerque
Roswell

NEW YORK

Albany
Amsterdam
Bay Shore
Binghamton
Buffalo
Catskill
Corning-Elmira
East Meadow
Glens Falls
Jamestown
Newburgh
New York
Parishville
Rhinebeck
Rochester
Saratoga Springs
Schenectady
Syracuse

Troy
Utica
Watertown
White Plains

NORTH CAROLINA

Charlotte
Raleigh
Winston-Salem

OHIO

Akron
Bowling Green
Canton
Cincinnati
Cleveland
Columbus
Dayton
Kent
Lorain
Marietta
Martins Ferry
Toledo
Youngstown
Zanesville

OKLAHOMA

Enid
Oklahoma City
Tulsa

OREGON

Portland

PENNSYLVANIA

Allentown
Altoona
Danville
Erie
Harrisburg
Kingston
Lancaster
New Castle
Norristown
Philadelphia

Pittsburgh
Reading
Upper Darby
Williamsport

RHODE ISLAND

Providence

SOUTH CAROLINA

Anderson
Charleston
Spartanburg

SOUTH DAKOTA

Vermillion

TENNESSEE

Bristol
Chattanooga
Jackson
Memphis
Nashville

TEXAS

Amarillo
Beaumont
Dallas
Fort Worth
Houston
Lubbock
Odessa
San Antonio
Wichita Falls

UTAH

Salt Lake City

VIRGINIA

Charlottesville
Lynchburg
Merrifield
Newport News
Norfolk

Richmond
Roanoke

WASHINGTON

Pasco
Seattle
Spokane
Tacoma

WEST VIRGINIA

Charleston
Huntington

WISCONSIN

Green Bay
Madison
Milwaukee
Oshkosh
Stevens Point
Waukesha

International

AUSTRALIA

Melbourne
Sydney

BELGIUM

Brussels

CANADA

Calgary, Alberta
Montreal, Quebec
St. Catherines, Ontario
Toronto, Ontario
Vancouver, British Columbia
Victoria, British Columbia
Winnipeg

CHINA, REPUBLIC OF

Taipei, Taiwan

ENGLAND

London

INDIA

Bombay

ISRAEL

Tel-Aviv

JAMAICA

Kingston

JAPAN

Kurasiki City
Tokyo

NEW ZEALAND

Auckland
Wellington

SCOTLAND

Glasgow

SOUTH AFRICA

Cape Town
Durban, Natal

VENEZUELA

Caracas

Associate Members

Mrs. Bette Burch
P.O. Box 2726
St. Thomas, Virgin Islands 00801

Mr. Gus Dittman
Route 3 - Box 351
Fort Atkinson, Wisconsin 53538

Mrs. Karen D. Jorgensen
Redvers, Saskatchewan
Canada SOC 2HO

Mr. Harry Meyers
710 Stanford Avenue
Newark, New Jersey 07106

Mr. Obert R. Williams
R.R. 1
Vienna, South Dakota 57271

Mr. Athanase Yoskas
Jean Moreas Str. 12-14
Athens 401, Greece

United States of America

ALABAMA

BIRMINGHAM

Cora Brand, President
Lost Chord Club of Birmingham
1401 10th St. S.E.
Cullman, Alabama 35055

DECATUR

M.B. Bowling, President
New Voice Club of North Alabama
Route 1
Decatur, Alabama 35601

GADSDEN

Wyatt Wilkinson, President
Lost Chord Club of Northeast Alabama
610 Glenport Ave., E.
Gadsden, Alabama 35903

MONTGOMERY

Rev. W.O. Phillips, President
Montgomery Laryngectomee Association
2044 Tullis Dr.
Montgomery, Alabama 36111

TUSCALOOSA

Tom M. Clements, President
West Alabama Lost Chord Club
37 Darret Grove
Tuscaloosa, Alabama 35401

ARIZONA

MESA

Jacqueline Johnston, President
Lost Chord Club of Arizona
6059 E. Dodge Street
Mesa, Arizona 85205

PHOENIX

Frank J. Cascio, President
New Voice Club of Arizona
133 W. Ruth
Phoenix, Arizona 85021

TUCSON

Dorothy Anthony, President
Dale Walker New Voice Club
1533 W. Gretchen Dr.
Tucson, Arizona 85705

ARKANSAS

FORT SMITH

O.W. Benoit, President
Arkansas Razorback Lost Chord Club II
4723 Arlington Ave.
Fort Smith, Arkansas 72901

LITTLE ROCK

Bob Shoemaker, President
Razorback Lost Chord Club
103 Conway Blvd.
Conway, Arkansas 72032

CALIFORNIA

FRESNO

Mrs. Tennessee Nelson, President
Lost Chord Club of Central California
4321 N. Cedar Ave.
Fresno, California 93726

LONG BEACH

Bob Kroll, President
Western Pals Lost Chord Club
1958 Rolling Vista Dr.
Lomita, California 90717

LOS ANGELES

R.C. Lindgren, President
Lost Chord Club of Southern Calif., Inc.
975 San Pasqual St.
Pasadena, California 91106

Valdemar Mikkolsen, President
Los Angeles Co.—USC Medical Center
    Lost Chord Club
5326 Cahuenga Blvd., 5
North Hollywood, California 91602

REDDING

Wm. O'Reilly, President
North State Lost Chord Club
2735 Radio Lane
Redding, California 96001

RIVERSIDE

Luther VanKirk, President
Nu Voice Club
11175 Foxdale Dr.
Desert Hot Springs, California 92240

SACRAMENTO

James R. Osborne, President
Forty-Niner Lost Chord Club
2517 S. Street, #10
Sacramento, California 95816

SAN DIEGO

Wm. Schenck, President
New Voice Club of San Diego County
3235 Bancroft Street
San Diego, California 92104

SAN FRANCISCO

Mario Pieretti, President
Lost Chord Club of Northern California
775 Parkway
S. San Francisco, California 94080

SAN JOSE

Preston Sanders, President
Chatter-Box Club
1201 Sycamore Terrace
Sunnyvale, California 94086

SANTA ANA

James R. Wedemann, President
Orange County Lost Chord Club
13381 Fairmont Way
Santa Ana, California 92705

SANTA MARIA

Louise Delp, President
Central Coast Laryngectomee Club
1201 East Guava Ave.
Lompoc, California 93436

VALLEJO

Alfred St. Germain, President
Second Voice Club of Northern
    California
115 Lemon Tree Circle
Vacaville, California 95688

COLORADO

DENVER

George H. Rogers, President
The Speakeasy, Inc.
3160 Wright Street
Denver, Colorado 80215

DENVER

L.C. Shannon, President
Lost Chord Club of Colorado
1573 S. Jamaica
Aurora, Colorado 80012

PUEBLO

Charles Ochs, President
Pueblo Lost Chord Club
615 Yale Place
Canon City, Colorado 80212

CONNECTICUT

BRIDGEPORT

Willis Laryney, President
New Voices Club of Greater Bridgeport
92 Roanoke Street
Fairfield, Connecticut 06430

DARIEN

Andrew Dattellic, President
New Voices Club of Southern Fairfield
  County
19 Nursery Road
Norwalk, Connecticut 06850

NEW BRITAIN

Barbara G. Smith, President
New Britain-Hartford Laryngectomee
  Club
190 Roxbury Road
New Britain, Connecticut 06053

NEW HAVEN

Dominick Primicerio, President
Lost Chord Club of New Haven
129 Hemingway Ave.
E. Haven, Connecticut 06512

NEW LONDON-NORWICH

Onofrio Amadeo, President
Eastern Connecticut New Voice Club
Norwich, Connecticut 06360

DELAWARE

WILMINGTON

Charles Yonkers, President
Delaware Laryngect Society
Bldg. 78, Clifton Park 3
Wilmington, Delaware 19802

DISTRICT OF COLUMBIA

WASHINGTON

Kenneth Lindersmith, President
Lost Chord Club of Washington
  Metropolitan Area
4000 Massachusetts Ave., N.W.
Washington, D.C. 20016

FLORIDA

CLEARWATER

Clarence Gillan, President
Sun Coast New Voice Club
10847 109th Lane, N.
Seminole, Florida 33540

DAYTONA BEACH

Raymond F. Ferraro, President
Volusia County New Voice Club
3815 S. Atlantic
Daytona Beach, Florida 32019

FT. LAUDERDALE

John McMahon, President
New Voice Club of Broward County
116 Lake Shore Drive
Hallandale, Florida 33009

FORT MYERS

Annie B. Wiggs, President
New Voice Club
2932 Central Ave.
Fort Myers, Florida 33901

JACKSONVILLE

R.L. Anderson, President
Jacksonville Laryngectomee Assoc.
6520 Shady Oak Dr.
Jacksonville, Florida 32211

PALM BEACH

B. Arnold, President
The Lost Chord Club of the Palm
 Beaches
117 Dolphin Road
Palm Beach, Florida 33480

PENSACOLA

Arthur Bond, President
Panhandle Chapter, F.L.A.
1831 Peyton Dr.
Pensacola, Florida 32503

ST. PETERSBURG

Clifford L. Shaw, President
St. Petersburg New Voice Club
705 Orangeview Dr.
Largo, Florida 33540

SARASOTA

George Barstow, President
Sunshine Nu Voice Club
16 Shady Lane
Bradenton, Florida 33505

GEORGIA

ATLANTA

Alfred Lawson
Greater Atlanta Voice Masters
6305 Tara Blvd.
Los C-31
Jonesboro, Georgia 30236

COLUMBUS

C.B. Mahaffey, President
The Gabbers Club
203 Waverly Way
La Grange, Georgia 30240

IDAHO

BOISE

Dean Rosecrans, President
New Voices of the Valley
P.O. Box 710
Nampa, Idaho 83651

ILLINOIS

AURORA

Cedric B. Ruch, President
Fox Valley Nu Voice Club
231 Sunset Avenue
Aurora, Illinois 60506

BELLEVILLE

Cecil Boyer, President
Nu Voice Club of St. Clair & Madison
 Counties
2902 Harvard
E. St. Louis, Illinois 62201

CENTRAL

Robert D. Edwards, President
New Voice Club of Central Illinois
700 Lincoln
Lincoln, Illinois 62656

CHICAGO

Daniel Tredici, President
Chicago Assoc. of Laryngectomees
821 W. 62nd St.
La Grange, Illinois 60525

Garni Booker, President
New Sounds Club
5346 S. Cornell
Chicago, Illinois 60615

Roger C. Nelson, President
New Voice Club
306 E. Wilson
Elmhurst, Illinois 60126

EVANSTON

Arthur W. Collins, President
North Shore Lost Chords
7340 N. Hoyne Ave.
Chicago, Illinois 60645

ROCKFORD

Ed O'Connor, President
Nu Voice Club of Rockford
1328 8th St.
Rockford, Illinois 61108

ROCK ISLAND

Thomas Inman, President
New Voice Club of Eastern Iowa &
  Western Illinois
3817 15th St. A
Moline, Illinois 61265

INDIANA

EVANSVILLE

George R. Holmes, President
1163 Covert Ave.
Evansville, Indiana 47714

FT. WAYNE

Don Ross, President
Nu Tones
Route 2
Churubusco, Indiana 46723

INDIANAPOLIS

John E. Dorsey, President
Hoosier Anamilo Club
5306 E. 9th St.
Indianapolis, Indiana 46219

LAFAYETTE

William Kaelin, President
Tippecanoe Lost Chord Club
RR 1
Rossville, Indiana 46065

MUNCIE

Charles W. Nelson, President
Lost Chord Club of Eastern Indiana
1204 W. Powers St.
Muncie, Indiana 47305

SOUTH BEND

Leland Easton, President
Michiana Nu Tones Club
213 Union St.
Osceola, Indiana 46561

TERRE HAUTE

Roy Divan, President
Nu Voice Club of Terre Haute
1030 Pine St.
Clinton, Indiana 47842

IOWA

SIOUX CITY

O.F. Huggenberger, President
Siouxland Lost Chord Club
Turin, Iowa

KANSAS

INDEPENDENCE

Clifford M. Funston, President
Sekan New Voice Club
P.O. Box 100
Independence, Kansas 67301

WICHITA

W.E. Krug, President
New Voice Club of Wichita
2265 Pattie
Wichita, Kansas 67211

KENTUCKY

LEXINGTON

Robert F. Watts, President
Blue Grass Lost Chord Club
1808 Old Paris Pike
Lexington, Kentucky 40505

LOUISVILLE

George Guelda, President
Kentuckiana Lost Chord Club
429 Oxford Pl.
Louisville, Kentucky 40207

OWENSBORO

O.L. Rickard, President
Owensboro Lost and Found Voice Club
R.R. 1–Box 291–A1
Bremen, Kentucky 42325

LOUISIANA

ALEXANDRIA

Charles B. Riffle, President
Louisiana Laryngectomee Association
2023 Marye St.
Alexandria, Louisiana 71301

NEW ORLEANS

Henry P. Gough, President
Crescent City New Voice Club
5619 Marshall Foch St.
New Orleans, Louisiana 70124

MAINE

PORTLAND

Lillian McKenney, President
The Nu Voice Club of Maine
15 Mayo St.
Portland, Maine 04101

WATERVILLE

Ernest Perrault, President
New Voice Club of Central Maine
6 Washington St.
Augusta, Maine 04330

MARYLAND

BALTIMORE

Wilmer Ausherman, President
510 Kent Road
Glen Burnie, Maryland 21061

CUMBERLAND

Roger Fazenbaker, President
Tri-State Lost Chord Club
304 Likens St.
Westernport, Maryland 21562

HAGERSTOWN

Robert S. Martin, Sr., President
Hagerstown Lost Chord Club
269 Parkview Dr.
Hagerstown, Maryland 21740

SILVER SPRING

George E. McMullen, President
Metro Maryland Laryngectomee Club
7008 23rd Pl.
Hyattsville, Maryland 20783

MASSACHUSETTS

BOSTON

John J. O'Hara, President
Boston Cured Cancer Club for
  Laryngectomees
117 Cowing St., W.
Roxbury, Massachusetts 02132

TAUNTON

Edward Machnik, President
Nu Voice Club of S.E. Massachusetts
57 South St., E.
Raynham, Massachusetts 02767

MICHIGAN

DETROIT

George Town, President
Anamilo Club of Detroit
26246 Clarita St.
Detroit, Michigan 48240

GRAND RAPIDS

Charlotte Myer, President
New Voice Club of Michigan
1236 Burke N.E.
Grand Rapids, Michigan 49505

KALAMAZOO

Harriet Laughlin, President
Lost Chord Club of Southwestern Mich.
2430 Charles Ave.
Kalamazoo, Michigan 49001

MARQUETTE

Ronald Richards, President
New Voice Club of the Upper
    Peninsula
1687 Larium
Calumet, Michigan 49913

MT. PLEASANT

Ed Wirsing, President
Central Michigan New Voice Club
1216 Townline Road
Auburn, Michigan 48611

MINNESOTA

DULUTH

Eugene Young, President
Vocalizers Club of Duluth
3546 Copley Road
Duluth, Minnesota 55811

MINNEAPOLIS

Franklin Dreissig, President
New Voice Club of Hennepin County
18930 Concord St.
Elk River, Minnesota 55330

ST. PAUL

John L. Cronk, President
Lost Chord Club of St. Paul
6 N.W. 8th St.
Buffalo, Minnesota 55313

MISSISSIPPI

JACKSON

Mrs. Knox Magee, President
Lost Chord Club of Central Mississippi
805 Meadowbrook Road
Jackson, Mississippi 39206

MISSOURI

COLUMBIA

Rosco Kikead, President
Nu Voice Club of Mid-Missouri
601 S. Allen
Centralia, Missouri 65240

JOPLIN

Lonnie Parrigon, President
Joplin Koam Speak E–Z Club
Scotts City, Missouri 65756

KANSAS CITY

Leland L. Nicoll, President
Heart of America Nu Voice Club
10209 Lowell
Overland Park, Kansas 66212

ST. JOSEPH

Claude Letts, President
Pony Express Nu Voice Club
505 Main St.
St. Joseph, Missouri 64501

ST. LOUIS

Chester Mumbower, President
Nu Voice Club of St. Louis
4840 Germainia St.
St. Louis, Missouri 63116

SEDALIA

Herbert Thee, President
West Central Missouri New Voice Club
Box 23
Dover, Missouri 64022

NEBRASKA

OMAHA

Laura Buckley, President
New Voice Club of Omaha
812 S. 19th St.
Omaha, Nebraska 68108

NEVADA

LAS VEGAS

Dominick Nuzzo, President
Vegas Voice Club
2900 S. Valley View
Las Vegas, Nevada 89102

NEW HAMPSHIRE

MANCHESTER

Ralph Dingee, President
Nu Voice Club of New Hampshire
625 S. Main St.
Nashua, New Hampshire 03060

NEW JERSEY

BERGENFIELD

Raymond A. Workman, President
Bergen County Laryngectomees
    Association, Inc.
189 Lexington Ave.
Cresskill, New Jersey 07626

COLLINGSWOOD

Harry McAllister, President
South Jersey Nu Voice Club
267 N. Broad St.
Penns Grove, New Jersey 08069

EAST ORANGE

Alfred Bellomo, President
North Jersey Nu Voices Assoc.
51 Sawyer Ave.
East Orange, New Jersey 07017

ELIZABETH

Bruce Morrison, President
Union County Gabbers
1110 W. Henry St.
Linden, New Jersey 07036

JERSEY CITY

Ernest H. Buntin, President
Echo Club of Hudson County
118 Webster Ave.
Jersey City, New Jersey 07307

MENLO PARK

John M. Rothwell, President
Middlesex County Chatter Box Group
208 Woodnor Ct.
New Brunswick, New Jersey 08902

PATERSON

Mrs. Stanley Eastman, President
Lost Chords of New Jersey
47–A Green Ave.
Westwood, New Jersey 07675

PLEASANTVILLE

Howard F.W. Taylor, President
Seashore Lost Chords
c/o ACS–5309 Atlantic Ave.
Ventnor, New Jersey 08406

RED BANK

Edward R. Saville, President
Garden State Nu Voice Club, Inc.
111 Van Brackle Road
Matawan, New Jersey 07747

TOMS RIVER

James Olsen, President
Ocean County Nu Voice Club
2250 Yorketowne Blvd.
Toms River, New Jersey 08753

NEW MEXICO

ALBUQUERQUE

Herman T. Trewer, President
615 Wellesley, N.E.
Albuquerque, New Mexico 87106

ROSWELL

Newton M. Tarlton, President
New Voice Club of Southern
   New Mexico
1614 S. Washington Ave.
Roswell, New Mexico 88201

NEW YORK

ALBANY

Agnes Goodman, President
Albany Lost Chord Club
P.O. Box 172
Albany, New York 12201

AMSTERDAM

Warren Ovitt, President
Fulmont Lost Chord Club
Ex. O'Neil Ave.
Johnstown, New York 12095

BAYSHORE, L.I.

Donald Zink, President
Sufco Laryngectomee Club
130 Lafayette Road
N. Babylon, New York 11704

BINGHAMTON

Joseph Zandy, President
Susquehanna County Lost Chord Club
3003 Magnolia Dr.
Endwell, New York 13760

BUFFALO

Edward Hartman, President
48 Courtland Ave.
Buffalo, New York 14215

CATSKILL

John Stay, President
Catskill Mountain Lost Chord Club
3 Raymond Dr.
Woodstock, New York 12498

CORNING—ELMIRA

Wm. H. Gibbons, President
Cor-el Lost Chord Club
Pultney St.
Corning, New York 14830

EAST MEADOW, L.I.

Donald Raye, President
Anamilo Speech Club of Nassau County
8 South Court
Hicksville, New York 11801

GLENS FALLS

Andrew DiCroce, President
North Country Laryngectomee Club
Beaty Road—RFD 2
Lake George, New York 12845

JAMESTOWN

Winton Stalvey, President
Chautauqua County Lost Chord Club
Bemus Point, New York 14712

NEWBURGH

Fred Vanzillotta, President
Mid-Hudson Lost Chord Club
42 Regency Dr.
Wappinger Falls, New York 12590

NEW YORK

Mario Bo, President
New Voice Club of Brooklyn
830 Greenwood Ave.
Brooklyn, New York 11218

Joseph Esquirol, President
Anamilo Club of New York
270 Jay St.
Brooklyn, New York 11201

George L. Walsh, President
Nu Voice Club of Queens
61–25 64th St.
Middle Village, New York 11379

Esther Brown, President
Nu Voices Club of Mount Sinai
    Hospital
2649 Eighth Ave.
New York, New York 10030

John Wilshaw, President
Bronx Nu Voices
2500 G Johnson Ave.
Riverdale, New York 10463

Chris Colizzi, President
Laryngectomy Club of Staten Island
191 Nevada Ave.
Staten Island, New York 10306

Sam A. Gregorio, President
Tru Talk Club of Staten Island
Box 487
Staten Island, New York 10314

PARISHVILLE

Lawrence R. Binan, President
Seaway Valley Lost Chord Club
Parishville, New York 13672

RHINEBECK

George Meehan, President
Rip Van Winkle Lost Chord Club
8 Newbold Dr.
Hyde Park, New York 12538

ROCHESTER

Raymond Statt, President
R. James Christie Lost Chord Club
52 Clifton Road
Clifton, New York 14431

SARATOGA SPRINGS

Joseph Smaldone, President
Saratoga Lost Chord Club
94 Ash St.
Saratoga Springs, New York 12866

SCHENECTADY

Louis Dicocco, President
Schenectady Lost Chord Club
72 Helderberg Ave.
Schenectady, New York 12306

SYRACUSE

Sam Desimone, President
Central New York Laryngectomee Club
118 Burdick Ave.
Syracuse, New York 13208

TROY

Basil Semenick, President
Trojan Nu Voice Club
73 First St.
Cohoes, New York 12047

UTICA

Henry Zuccaro, President
Lost Chord Club of Utica
287 W. Main St.
Little Falls, New York 13365

WATERTOWN

Lawrence McLean, President
St. Lawrence Valley New Voice Club
127 S. Hamilton St.
Watertown, New York 13601

WHITE PLAINS

Vincent Calabrese, President
Nu Voice Club of Westchester
4 Dogwood Dr.
Yorktown Heights, New York 10598

NORTH CAROLINA

CHARLOTTE

Leroy D. Foster, President
5259 Piedmont Ave.
Mt. Holly, North Carolina 28120

RALEIGH

Clayton Williams, President
North Carolina Lost Chord Club
P.O. Box 584
Burgaw, North Carolina 28425

WINSTON-SALEM

Jim Carter, President
Nu Voice Club of Winston-Salem
Rt. 4—2780 Evans Road
Winston-Salem, North Carolina 27107

OHIO

AKRON

Walter Park, President
Akron Lost Chord Club
867–144 Palmetto Avenue
Akron, Ohio 44306

BOWLING GREEN

Raymond Lechner, President
New Voice Club of Northwestern Ohio
387A Maple Ave., RFD #1
Castalia, Ohio 44824

CANTON

William Kline, President
Faber Drukenbrod New Voice Club
175 Oregon, N.W.
Louisville, Ohio 44641

CINCINNATI

Clyde Crawford, President
Lost Chord Club of Greater Cincinnati
RR #5—Box 372
Covington, Kentucky 41015

CLEVELAND

Julia L. Bobey, President
Fairview Lost Chord Club
14618 Rainbow Road
Cleveland, Ohio 44111

John McConnell, President
Cleveland Lost Chord Club
3731 West Park Road
Cleveland, Ohio 44111

COLUMBUS

John Worrell, President
Columbus Lost Chord Club
155 W. 5th Ave.
Columbus, Ohio 43201

DAYTON

Mr. Marion Chalecki, President
Miami Valley Lost Chord Club
643 Cushing Ave.
Kettering, Ohio 45429

KENT

Dick Whyte, President
Kent State Lost Chord Club
1575 Stratford Ave.
Kent, Ohio 44240

LORAIN

George Rosbrook, President
Lorain County Lost Chord Club
820 Rosewood
Elyria, Ohio 44035

MARIETTA

Priscilla Curtis, President
Mid-Ohio Valley Lost Chord Club
505 Chamberlain Dr.
Marietta, Ohio 45750

MARTINS FERRY

John Baughman, President
Nu Voice Club
Magnolia Lane
Bethlehem, West Virginia 26003

TOLEDO

George Swinehart, President
Laryngectomy Club of Toledo
316 Ellwood
Fostoria, Ohio 43604

YOUNGSTOWN

Edward Cliney, President
Mahoning Valley New Voice Club
3107 Rush Blvd.
Youngstown, Ohio 44502

ZANESVILLE

Orville McKibben, President
Zanesville Lost Chord Club
Rte. 3—Box 252
McConnelsville, Ohio 43756

OKLAHOMA

ENID

E.L. Moss, President
Northern Oklahoma Nu Voice Club
Billings, Oklahoma 74630

OKLAHOMA CITY

J.J. Martin, Jr., President
Sooner Nu Voice Club of Oklahoma
102 N.E. 11th
Moore, Oklahoma 73160

TULSA

Mrs. W.L. Taylor, President
New Voice Club of Tulsa
4511 S. Union
Tulsa, Oklahoma 74107

OREGON

PORTLAND

M.H. Hollyfield, President
New Voice Club of Oregon
6020 S.W. Luradel St.
Portland, Oregon 97219

PENNSYLVANIA

ALLENTOWN

Lawrence Beaulieu, President
Lost Chord Club of the Lehigh Valley
506 Jacobsburg Road
Nazareth, Pennsylvania 18064

ALTOONA

Walter Nisewonger, President
Central Pennsylvania Laryngectomee
    Club
1203 S. 27th St.
Altoona, Pennsylvania 16602

DANVILLE

Wm. VanBuskirk, President
Geisinger New Voice Club
213 S. High St.
Selinsgrove, Pennsylvania 17870

ERIE

Frank Fabin, President
Lost Chord Club of Erie
847 E. 21st
Erie, Pennsylvania 16503

HARRISBURG

Donald J. Beinhaur, Sr., President
New Voices of Capital City
4844 Erie Road
Harrisburg, Pennsylvania 17111

KINGSTON

Louis Zingarett, President
New Voice Club of Northeastern
    Pennsylvania
RD2—Box 7—Laflin Road
Wilkes-Barre, Pennsylvania 18702

LANCASTER

Harold H. Bowers, President
Red Rose Nu Voice Club
19 E. Frederick St.
Millersville, Pennsylvania 17551

NEW CASTLE

Andrew Kuzma, President and Vice-
President
Lost Chord Club of Midwestern
Pennsylvania
RD 6–Box 287
New Castle, Pennsylvania 16101

NORRISTOWN

Hollie Skidmore, President
Montgomery County Laryngectomees
Club
48 N. Richardson Ave.
Lansdale, Pennsylvania 19446

PHILADELPHIA

Leroy C. Berry, President
Philadelphia Laryngects
2538 N. Gratz St.
Philadelphia, Pennsylvania 19132

PITTSBURGH

Homer Lachman, President
Lost Chord Club of Pittsburgh
5430 Park Ave.
Bethel Park, Pennsylvania 15102

READING

James J. O'Neill, President
Nu Voice Club
251 Jameson St.
Reading, Pennsylvania 19601

UPPER DARBY

Esther Winters, President
Delco School for Laryngects
321 Sanford Road
Upper Darby, Pennsylvania 19082

WILLIAMSPORT

Ernie Brinson, President
Lycoming County New Voice Club
RD 1
Montgomery, Pennsylvania 17752

RHODE ISLAND

PROVIDENCE

Henry Simonetti, President
New Voice Club of Providence
66 Tappan St.
Providence, Rhode Island 02908

SOUTH CAROLINA

ANDERSON

Austin Elrod
The Piedmont Voice Club
Box 395
Anderson, South Carolina 29621

CHARLESTON

B.C. Lynes, President
New Voice Club of Charleston
3 Tenth Ave.
Charleston, South Carolina 29403

SPARTANBURG

Joann Weaver, President
Nu Voice Club
18 Beacon St.
Spartanburg, South Carolina 29301

SOUTH DAKOTA

VERMILLION

Vincent Jones, President
Nu Voice Club of South Dakota
804 North Indiana
Sioux Falls, South Dakota 57103

TENNESSEE

CHATTANOOGA

Thomas T. Wilson, President
Lost Chord Club of Chattanooga
5613 Clark Road
Harrison, Tennessee 37341

JACKSON

Lillian Vance, President
Lost Chord Club of Jackson
99 Everette St.
Jackson, Tennessee 38301

MEMPHIS

Franklin Ellis, President
Lost Chord Club of Memphis
4851 Hummingbird Lane
Memphis, Tennessee 38117

NASHVILLE

Leon Gerson, President
Lost Chord Club of Middle Tennessee
1913 Rosewood Valley Dr.
Brentwood, Tennessee 37027

TEXAS

AMARILLO

George Christian, President
Amarillo Lost Chord Club
1921 S. Highland
Amarillo, Texas 79103

BEAUMONT

C. Bert Grimes, President
Triangle Area Laryngectomee Klub
   (T.A.L.K)
2108 Jefferson
Nederland, Texas 77627

DALLAS

Frank Millar, Ph.D., President
Lost Chord Club of Dallas
7208 Wabash Ave.
Dallas, Texas 75214

FORT WORTH

Dee Thetford, President
Lost Chord Club of Forth Worth
4140 Wells Dr.
Fort Worth, Texas 76135

HOUSTON

John R. Hall, Jr., M.D., President
Houston Lost Chord Club
309 Ivy Lane
Dickinson, Texas 77539

LUBBOCK

Clyde A. Stovall, President
Lubbock Lost Chord Club
2902 69th St.
Lubbock, Texas 79413

ODESSA

Harry Wollner, President
Permian Basin Lost Chord Club
2726 N. Hancock
Odessa, Texas 79760

SAN ANTONIO

Joe Griggs, President
Lost Chord Club of San Antonio
6294 Deer Valley Dr.
San Antonio, Texas 78242

WICHITA FALLS

John Tucker, President
Lost Chord Club of Wichita Falls
3211 Kemp
Wichita Falls, Texas 76308

UTAH

SALT LAKE CITY

Joseph F. Potter, President
New Voices of Salt Lake City
251 S. Fourth E. #6
Salt Lake City, Utah 84111

VIRGINIA

BRISTOL

Beecher Jackson, President
Box 603
Honaker, Virginia 24260

CHARLOTTESVILLE

Godwin Golladay, President
320 Thompson St.
Staunton, Virginia 24401

LYNCHBURG

Wm. S. Osborne, President
Central Virginia Lost Chord Club
3100 Mayflower Dr.
Lynchburg, Virginia 24501

MERRIFIELD

Foster Mitchell, President
New Voice Club of Northern Virginia
11 North Sixth St.
Warrenton, Virginia 22186

NEWPORT NEWS

Howard Vaughn, President
Peninsula Association of
    Laryngectomees
P.O. Box 5269
Newport News, Virginia 23605

NORFOLK

C.L. Hershberger, President
Tidewater Lost Chord Club
3324 Hershridge Road
Virginia Beach, Virginia 23452

RICHMOND

George Grammer, President
Lost Chord Club of Richmond
2626 Parkside Ave.
Richmond, Virginia 23228

ROANOKE

Robert Ruff, President
The Lost Chord Club of South-
    western Virginia
3646 Greenland Ave., N.W.
Roanoke, Virginia 24012

WASHINGTON

PASCO

J.R. Guild, President
Southeastern Washington Laryn-
    gectomee Club
200 N. Underwood St.
Kennewick, Washington 99336

SEATTLE

Frank Novotny, President
Laryngectomee Club of Washington
    State
715 Tacoma St.
Kent, Washington 98031

SPOKANE

W.C. McLaughlin, President
Laryngectomee Club of the Inland
    Empire
So. 1708 S.E. Blvd.
Spokane, Washington 99207

TACOMA

William Ostrander, President
Lost Chord Club of Pierce County
7011 South M St.
Tacoma, Washington 98408

WEST VIRGINIA

CHARLESTON

Jack Spinks, President
Central West Virginia Lost Chord Club
2715 Washington Ave.
St. Albans, West Virginia 25177

HUNTINGTON

Harold Dillon, President
Tri-State Lost Chord Club
2057 Donald Ave.
Huntington, West Virginia 25701

WISCONSIN

GREEN BAY

Stanley Wallace, President
Green Bay Lost Chord Club
3216 S. Clay St.
Green Bay, Wisconsin 54304

MADISON

Paul Alfonsi, President
Lost Chord Club of Madison
5548 Century Ave.
Middletown, Wisconsin 53562

MILWAUKEE

Keith A. Schilling, President
New Voice Club of Milwaukee
1404 So. 87th St.
West Allis, Wisconsin 53214

OSHKOSH

William Demler, President
Fox River Valley Lost Chord Club
2226 W. 9th St.
Oshkosh, Wisconsin 54901

STEVENS POINT

Theodore Landowski, President
North Central Wisconsin Laryn-
    gectomee Club
2003 Burlich St.
Schofield, Wisconsin 54476

WAUKESHA

Robert A. Turzinski, President
Waukesha Lost Chord Club
18883 W. Gold Dr.
Muskego, Wisconsin 53150

International

AUSTRALIA

MELBOURNE

Kathleen Keighran, President
New Voice Assoc. of Victoria
12 Larwood St.
Windsor, Victoria 3181 Australia

SYDNEY, NEW SOUTH WALES

Ray Beness, President
Lost Chord Club of New South Wales
21 Margaret St.
Seven Hills 2147, NSW, Australia

BELGIUM

BRUSSELS

Paul Hauwaert, President
19, rue Ernest Solvay
1050 Brussels, Belgium

CANADA

ALBERTA

Calgary

Gertrude Paller, President
Calgary Lost Chord Club
3212 Richmond Road, S.W. #232
Calgary, Alberta, Canada T3E 4N4

BRITISH COLUMBIA

Vancouver

David Jock, President
Lost Chord Club of British Columbia
25523 Robertson Crs.
Aldergrove, B.C., Canada

Victoria

Seth Halton, President
Victoria Laryngectomee Club
747 Falkland Road
Victoria, B.C. V8S 4LP, Canada

MANITOBA

Winnipeg

Stanley Luby, President
Lost Chord Club of Manitoba
529 Doucet St.
Winnipeg, Man. R2J OM6, Canada

ONTARIO

St. Catherines

Wm. F. Stevenson, President
New Voice Club of the
　Niagara Region
337 Canboro Road, W.
Ridgeville, Ontario LOS 1MO, Canada

Toronto

John Hardy, President
Toronto Lost Chord Club
2800 Bloor St.
Etobicoke, Ontario, Canada

QUEBEC

Montreal

Pierre C. LeCault, President
Quebec Assoc. of Laryngectomees
7085 DeLanaudiere #1
Montreal, P.Q. H2E 1Y1, Canada

CHINA, REPUBLIC OF

TAIWAN

Taipei

P.F. Jung, M.D., President
Veterans General Hospital Laryngec-
　tomees Club
4, Lane 69, Kingshan St.
Taipei, Taiwan, R.O.C.

ENGLAND

LONDON

Attention: Miss V. Johns
The Swallo Club
Gray's Inn Road, W.C. 1
London, England

INDIA

BOMBAY

Dr. D.J. Jussawalla, M.S., F.R.C.S.,
　F.A.C.S., President
Indian Association of Laryngectomees
c/o Rehabilitation Centre, Indian
　Cancer Society
Chanchal Smruti–Dr. Ambekar Rd.
Bombay 400 031 India

ISRAEL

TEL AVIV

Mrs. A. Eban, President
Israel Laryngectomees
Israel Cancer Assoc.
91 Rehov Hahashmonaim St.
Tel Aviv, Israel 67011

JAMAICA

KINGSTON

Colin M. Fairweather, President
Laryngectomees Association of
　Jamaica
29 Tucker Ave.
Kingston 6, Jamaica, West Indies

JAPAN

KURASIKI CITY

Rev. Y. Yamamura, President
New Voice Club of Kurasiki
Amaki
Kurasiki City, Japan

TOKYO

Yuji Shigehara, President
Guinrei-Kai Incorporated Association
12–16 Fujimi Nichome
Chiyoda-Ku, Tokyo, Japan

NEW ZEALAND

AUCKLAND

R.H. Simmons, President
Kiwi Lost Chord Club
1 Achilles Cres-Davenport
Auckland, New Zealand

WELLINGTON

Mrs. F.G. Bell, President
Kiwi Lost Chord Club—Wellington
43 A Halswater Dr.—Churton Park
Wellington 4, New Zealand

SCOTLAND

GLASGOW

Peter S. Riddell, Secretary
"Theatre 5"
16 Nethercliffee Ave.
Netherlee
Glasglow, G44, Scotland

SOUTH AFRICA

CAPE TOWN

Mrs. G. Hilse, President
Cape Western Lost Chord Club
1 Athlone Ct.—Henley Road
Muizenberg, Cape, South Africa

NATAL

Durban

Hedley Glass, Chairman
The Lost Chord Club of Natal
20 Cullingworth Ave.—Sherwood
Durban 4001 Natal, South Africa

VENEZUELA

CARACAS

Mr. Jean Nouel, President
Venezuelan Laryngectomees Assoc.
Ave. Oriente 107–18
S. Bernardino, Caracas, Venezuela

THE AMERICAN CANCER SOCIETY, INC.

National Headquarters
777 Third Avenue
New York, New York 10017

Alabama Division, Inc.
2925 Central Avenue
Birmingham, Alabama 35209
(205) 879–2242

Alaska Division, Inc.
1343 G Street
Anchorage, Alaska 99501
(907) 277–8696

Arizona Division, Inc.
634 West Indian School Road
Phoenix, Arizona 85011
(602) 264–5861

Arkansas Division, Inc.
5520 West Markham Street
Little Rock, Arkansas 72203
(501) 664–3480–1–2

California Division, Inc.
731 Market Street
San Francisco, California 94103
(415) 777–1800

Colorado Division, Inc.
1809 East 18th Avenue
Denver, Colorado 80218
(303) 321–2464

Connecticut Division, Inc.
Professional Center
270 Amity Road
Woodbridge, Connecticut 06525
(203) 389–4571

Delaware Division, Inc.
Academy of Medicine Bldg.
1925 Lovering Avenue
Wilmington, Delaware 19806
(302) 654-6267

District of Columbia Division, Inc.
Universal Building, South
1825 Connecticut Avenue, N.W.
Washington, D.C. 20009
(202) 483-2600

Florida Division, Inc.
1001 South MacDill Avenue
Tampa, Florida 33609
(813) 253-0541

Georgia Division, Inc.
2025 Peachtree Road, N.E.
Suite 14
Atlanta, Georgia 30309
(404) 351-3650-1-2

Hawaii Division, Inc.
Community Services Center Bldg.
200 North Vineyard Boulevard
Honolulu, Hawaii 96817
(531) 1662-3-4-5

Idaho Division, Inc.
P.O. Box 5386
1609 Abbs Street
Boise, Idaho 83705
(208) 343-4609

Illinois Division, Inc.
37 South Wabash Avenue
Chicago, Illinois 60603
(312) 372-0472

Indiana Division, Inc.
2702 East 55th Place
Indianapolis, Indiana 46220
(317) 257-5326

Iowa Division, Inc.
P.O. Box 980
Mason City, Iowa 50401
(515) 423-0712

Kansas Division, Inc.
3003 Van Buren
Topeka, Kansas 66611
(913) 267-0131

Kentucky Division, Inc.
Medical Arts Bldg.
1169 Eastern Parkway
Louisville, Kentucky 40217
(502) 452-2676

Louisiana Division, Inc.
Masonic Temple Bldg., Room 810
333 St. Charles Avenue
New Orleans, Louisiana 70130
(504) 523-2029

Maine Division, Inc.
Federal and Greene Streets
Brunswick, Maine 04011
(207) 729-3339

Maryland Division, Inc.
200 East Joppa Road
Towson, Maryland 21204
(301) 828-8890

Massachusetts Division, Inc.
247 Commonwealth Avenue
Boston, Massachusetts 02116
(617) 267-2650

Michigan Division, Inc.
1205 East Saginaw Street
Lansing, Michigan 48906
(517) 371-2920

Minnesota Division, Inc.
2750 Park Avenue
Minneapolis, Minnesota 55407
(612) 871-2111

Mississippi Division, Inc.
345 North Mart Plaza
Jackson, Mississippi 39206
(601) 362-8874

Missouri Division, Inc.
P.O. Box 1066
715 Jefferson Street
Jefferson City, Missouri 65101
(314) 636-3195

Montana Division, Inc.
2115 Second Avenue North
Billings, Montana 59101
(406) 252-7111

Nebraska Division, Inc.
6910 Pacific Street, Suite 210
Omaha, Nebraska 68106
(402) 551-2422

Nevada Division, Inc.
4220 Maryland Parkway
Suite 105
Las Vegas, Nevada 89109
(702) 736-2999

New Hampshire Division, Inc.
22 Bridge Street
Manchester, New Hampshire 03101
(603) 669-3270

New Jersey Division, Inc.
2700 Route 22, P.O. Box 1220
Union, New Jersey 07083
(201) 687-2100

New Mexico Division, Inc.
205 San Pedro, N.E.
Albuquerque, New Mexico 87108
(505) 268-4501

New York State Division, Inc.
6725 Lyons Street
East Syracuse, New York 13057
(315) 437-7025

   Long Island Division, Inc.
   535 Broad Hollow Road
   (Route 110)
   Melville, New York 11746
   (516) 420-1111

   New York City Division, Inc.
   19 West 56th St.
   New York, New York 10019
   (212) 586-8700

   Queens Division, Inc.
   111-15 Queens Boulevard
   Forest Hills, New York 11375
   (212) 263-2224

   Westchester Division, Inc.
   107 Lake Avenue
   Tuckahoe, New York 10707
   (914) 793-3100

North Carolina Division, Inc.
P.O. Box 27624
222 North Person Street
Raleigh, North Carolina 27611
(919) 834-8463

North Dakota Division, Inc.
P.O. Box 426
Hotel Graver Annex Bldg.
115 Roberts Street
Fargo, North Dakota 58102
(701) 232-1385

Ohio Division, Inc.
453 Lincoln Bldg.
1367 East Sixth Street
Cleveland, Ohio 44114
(216) 771-6700

Oklahoma Division, Inc.
1312 Northwest 24th Street
Oklahoma City, Oklahoma 73106
(405) 525-3515

Oregon Division, Inc.
1530 S.W. Taylor Street
Portland, Oregon 97205
(503) 228-8331

Panama (Affiliate)
Canal Zone Cancer Committee
Drawer "A"
Balboa Heights, Canal Zone

Pennsylvania Division, Inc.
P.O. Box 4175
Harrisburg, Pennsylvania 17111
(717) 545-4215

   Philadelphia Division, Inc.
   21 South 12th Street
   Philadelphia, Pennsylvania 19107
   (215) 567-0559

Puerto Rico Division, Inc.
Avenue Domenech 257—Alto
Hato Rey, Puerto Rico 00918
(809) 765-2295

Rhode Island Division, Inc.
333 Grotto Avenue
Providence, Rhode Island 02906
(401) 831-6970

South Carolina Division, Inc.
4482 Fort Jackson Boulevard
Columbia, South Carolina 29209
(803) 787-5624

South Dakota Division, Inc.
700 South 4th Avenue
Sioux Falls, South Dakota 57104
(605) 336-0897

Tennessee Division, Inc.
2519 White Avenue
Nashville, Tennessee 37204
(615) 383-1710

Texas Division, Inc.
P.O. Box 9863
Austin, Texas 78766
(512) 345-4560

Utah Division, Inc.
610 East South Temple
Salt Lake City, Utah 84102
(801) 322-0431

Vermont Division, Inc.
13 Loomis Street, Drawer C
Montpelier, Vermont 05602
(802) 223-2348

Virginia Division, Inc.
3218 West Cary Street
P.O. Box 7288
Richmond, Virginia 23221
(804) 359-0208

Washington Division, Inc.
323 First Avenue West
Seattle, Washington 98119
(206) 284-8390

West Virginia Division, Inc.
325 Professional Building
Charleston, West Virginia 25301
(304) 344-3611

Wisconsin Division, Inc.
P.O. Box 1626
Madison, Wisconsin 53701
(608) 249-0487

Milwaukee Division, Inc.
6401 West Capitol Drive
Milwaukee, Wisconsin 53216
(414) 461-1100

Wyoming Division, Inc.
1118 Logan Avenue
Cheyenne, Wyoming 82001
(307) 638-3331

C

International
Directory
of Qualified
Oncologists
and Research
Specialists

GEOGRAPHICAL LISTING OF ONCOLOGISTS

How to use this section: the listing of oncologists and research specialists is broken down geographically, by state (or country) and city. Society memberships and specialities and certifications are given. One asterisk (*) before a name means that person is an M.D.; two asterisks (**) means that person is a D.D.S. As an example:

NEW YORK (212)

*Smith, John A. (AACE), *M/HEM*, 555–1212

The number following the name of the city is the area code for that region, and unless otherwise noted, all phone numbers in that city will begin with that area code. The use of the asterisk before the name is explained above. "AACE" is the society membership to which John Smith belongs (see the list following and the write-ups on each organization, which are found in Chapter 13.) "*M/HEM*" is the area of specialization or certification held by Smith (see list of those abbreviations following—in this case, it means that Smith is a specialist in Internal Medicine and Hematology). This is followed by the phone number.

Abbreviations for specialities and certifications used in this section are:

ANES	— anesthesiology
CRS	— colon and rectal surgery
CYT	— cytopathology
D	— dermatology
G	— gynecology
GE	— gastroenterology
GO	— gynecologic oncology
HEM	— hematology
HNS	— head and neck surgery
M	— internal medicine
MO	— medical oncology
MXF	— maxillofacial surgery
NM	— nuclear medicine
NS	— neurological surgery
O	— obstetrics
OG	— obstetrics and gynecology
ONC	— oncology
OP	— oral pathology
OS	— oral surgery
OT	— otolaryngology
PATH	— pathology
PD	— pediatrics
PLS	— plastic surgery
PM	— physical medicine and rehabilitation
PRM	— preventive medicine
PSYM	— psychiatric medicine
R	— radiology
RO	— radiation oncology
RT	— radiation therapy
S	— surgery
SO	— surgical oncology
TR	— therapeutic radiology
TS	— thoracic surgery
U	— urology
V	— virology
VETR	— veterinary radiology

Abbreviations for Society Memberships used in this section are:

AACE	— American Association for Cancer Education, Inc.
AACR	— American Association for Cancer Research
ARS	— American Radium Society, Inc.
ASCO	— American Society for Clinical Oncology, Inc.
ASHNS	— American Society for Head and Neck Surgery
ASTR	— American Society of Therapeutic Radiologists

SGO — Society of Gynecologic Oncologists
SHNS — Society of Head and Neck Surgeons
SSO — Society of Surgical Oncology, Inc.

United States of America

ALABAMA

BIRMINGHAM (205)

*Brascho, Donn (AACE, ASTR), *RO*,
934-5670
*Cooper, M.D. (AACR), *PD*, 934-3370
*Davis, Maxie (ASTR), *M*
*Dick, Donald A.L. (ASTR)
*Durant, J.R. (AACR, ASCO), *HEM/
ONC*, 934-5077
*Gams, R.A. (AACR, ASCO), *M/HEM/
ONC,* 934-2080
*Hammack, Wm. J. (ASCO), *M/HEM*,
933-8101
*Hicks, Julius N. (ASHNS), *OT*,
933-7431
*Maddox, Wm. (AACE, SHNS, SSO), *S*
**Martinez, Mario G., Jr. (AACE), *OP*,
934-3380
*Moreno, Hernan (AACE), *PD*,
934-5263
*Myers, G.H., Jr. (AACR, ASCO),
U/S, 934-4933
*Omura, George B. (ASCO), *M*,
934-2082
*Pretlow, T.G. (AACR), *PATH*,
934-4666
*Roth, Robert E. (ASTR), *RO*,
934-5770
*Salter, Merle M. (ASTR)
*Sherlock, Eugene C. (SHNS), *PLS*,
933-8841
*Shingleton, Hugh M. (SGO), *OG*,
934-3393
*Stevenson, Edward W. (ASHNS), *OT,*
591-6570

HUNTSVILLE

*Campbell, James E. (ASTR)

MOBILE (205)

*Peake, John D. (ARS), *R*, 433-3511

ALASKA

FAIRBANKS (907)

*Straatsma, Glen W. (ASCO), *M*,
452-2127

ARIZONA

PHOENIX (602)

*Brunner, John A. (ASCO), *M*,
258-4875
*Crisp, Wm. E. (SGO), *GO*, 258-8995
*Christianson, John F. (ASCO), *M*
*Foster, Robert E.L. (ARS), *R*,
258-3484
*Hilger, Martin T.J. (ASTR), *OT*
*Kalil, T.H. (ASTR)
*Murray, Ethelann (ASCO), *M*,
277-6611, ext. 3394
*Newton, Louis (ASCO), *M*, 258-4875
*Rossman, Kent J. (ASTR)
*Taggart, Charles H. (ARS, ASTR),
TR, 252-6611, ext. 3552
*Thoeny, Robert H. (ARS, ASTR),
RO, 252-6611
*Weinrach, Roy S. (ASCO), *M/HEM*,
257-1435

SCOTTSDALE (602)

*Defreitas, Gabriel F. (ARS, SHNS,
SSO), *S*
*Nash, Newman C. (ARS), *R*,
946-7223
*Simons, John N. (SHNS), *PLS*,
994-3996

SIERRA VISTA (602)

*Lenio, Paul T. (SHNS), *S*, 458-4614

TUCSON (602)

*Alberts, D.S. (AACR), *HEM/ONC*
Aristizabel, Silo Antonio (ASTR), *TR*,
    882-7236
*Boone, Max L.M. (ARS, ASCO,
    ASTR), *RT/R*, 882-7268
*Jones, Stephen E. (AACR, ASCO),
    M, 882-6372
*Mayer, Eric G. (ASCO), *R*, 882-7236
*Miller, Robert C. (ASCO), *RT/R*,
    882-7268
*Neubauer, Darwin W. (ASCO), *S*,
    325-2628
*Peacock, Earle E. (ASCO), *PLS/S*
*Russell, D.H. (AACR), 882-7495
*Salmon, Sydney E. (AACR, ASCO),
    M/HEM, 882-6372

ARKANSAS

FAYETTEVILLE (501)

*Nettleship A. (AACR), 443-3050

FT. SMITH (501)

*Broadwater, John R. (ASTR), *RT*,
    782-4092

JEFFERSON (501)

Wolff, G.L. (AACR), 536-6200

LITTLE ROCK (501)

*Barclay, David L. (SGO), *OG*,
    664-5000, ext. 265
*Berry, Daisilee H. (ASCO), *PD*,
    664-5000, ext. 520
*Caldwell, Fred T. (AACE)
Dalrymple, G.V. (AACR)
*Holoye, Paul (ASCO), *M*
*Suen, James Y. (SHNS), *OT/HNS*,
    664-4000

*Tranum, Billy Lynn (ASCO), *M*,
    664-5000, ext. 161
*Westbrook, Kent C. (AACE, SHNS),
    S, 664-5000

CALIFORNIA

ANAHEIM (714)

*Otis, Peter T. (ASCO), *M*, 991-4630

ARCATA (707)

*Winer, Melvin L. (ASCO), *M*,
    822-1797

BAKERSFIELD (805)

*Birsner, J.W. (ASCO), *R*, 327-3871
*Donovan, James F. (ASCO), 327-9393
*Gillin, Lloyd I. (ASTR)
*Lahiri, Sunril R. (AACR, ASCO), *M*,
    327-0988
*Tan, Donald C.S. (ASTR), *RO*,
    324-0607

BELVEDERE

*Meyler, Thomas S. (ASTR)

BELVERE (213)

*Pflueger, Otto (SHNS, SSO), *S*,
    435-4348

BERKELEY (415)

Dunn, J.E., Jr. (AACR)
*Purcell, Theodore R., *TR*, 845-7110

BEVERLY HILLS (213)

*Baker, Sol R. (ARS, ASTR), *TR*,
    553-0333
*Barton, Richard Thomas (ASCO),
    HNS/ONC, 276-7012
*Bierman, Howard R. (AACR, ASCO),
    HEM/ONC, 657-2110

Brower, A.B. (AACR), 273–5511
*Cutler, Max (ARS, SSO), *S*,
275–5177
*Field, John B. (AACR, ASCO), *M/ONC*, 278–0633
*Harpstreith, James L. (ASTR)
*Karlan, Mitchell S. (SHNS, SSO)
*Samuels, Arthur J. (ASCO), *M/HEM*, 657–2110
*Schenck, Samuel G. (ARS), *R*,
274–5457
*Schlemenson, Melvin (ARS), *S*,
276–6177
*Strum, S.B. (AACR, ASCO), *M*,
657–2110
*Sullivan, Robert (ASCO, SSO),
M/ONC, 553–8500
*Zuckerbraun, Lionel (SHNS), *S*,
274–5366

BURLINGAME (415)

*Johnson, Wm. C. (ASTR), *RT*,
687–4061 ext. 591

CARMEL

*Holley, David R. (ASTR)

CHICO

*Weinbaum, Jerome A. (SSO)

COSTA MESA

*Delaney, Charles A. (ASTR)

CULVER CITY (213)

*Bluming, A.Z. (AACR), 837–9115
*Plotkin, David (AACR, ASCO),
M/HEM/ONC, 837–9115
*Rosen, Peter Julian (ASCO), *M/HEM*, 837–9115

DAVIS (916)

*Andrews, Neil C. (ASCO), *M*,
752–0328

*Greenberg, Bernard R. (ASCO),
HEM/MO, 752–1333
*Raventos, Antolin (AACE, ARS,
ASCO, ASTR), *RT*, 752–1330
*Stowell, R.E. (AACR), *PATH*,
752–2086
Theilen, G.H. (AACR), 752–1398

DOWNEY (213)

*Holman, James H. (SHNS, SSO), *S*,
869–1514

DUARTE (213)

*Chillar, Ram K. (ASCO), *M*,
359–8111, ext. 408
*Jacobs, Melville L. (ARS, ASTR),
RT, 359–8111
*Javish, Joel (ASTR), *RT*, 359–8111
*Rappaport, Henry (AACR, ASCO),
PATH, 358–5519
*Solomon, Joel (AACR, ASCO), *M/HEM/MO*, 359–8111, ext. 405
Todd, C.W. (AACR), 359–8111

EL MACERO (916)

*Andrews, Neil C., (ASCO), *S*,
756–0209

ENCINO (213)

*Fink, Albert (ASCO), *M*, 788–1540
*Green, Jason I. (ASCO), *S*, 996–5606
*Horowitz, Morris (ASTR), *RT/NM*,
788–4400, ext. 88

FAIRFIELD (707)

*Reynolds, Ralph Duane (ASCO),
M/HEM/ONC, 438–3379

FOUNTAIN VALLEY (714)

*Desai, Rajendra (AACR, ASCO), *M*,
642–2591

*Flam, Marshall S. (ASCO), *M/HEM*, 233-0555
*Lau, B. Peck (ASTR), *RT*, 224-9451
*Moore, James E. III (ASCO), *RT/ONC*, 886-3311
*Morgan, Dix R. (ASTR)
*Prather, Charles E. (ASTR)

GLENDALE (213)

*Bogdon, Donald L. (ASCO), *M/HEM/ONC*, 247-5440
*Hum, Gilbert J. (ASCO), *HEM*, 247-5440

HILLSBOROUGH (415)

*Wurlitzer, Frederick P. (SHNS), *S/SO*, 347-4137

IRVINE (714)

Bostick, W.L. (AACR), 833-7207
Crocker, T.T. (AACR)
*Furnas, David (SHNS), *PLS/HNS*, 997-4300

LA JOLLA (714)

Bakay, B. (AACR), 452-4150
*Bernstein, Theodore C. (ASCO), *M*, 454-9336
Bethard, W.F. (AACR), 453-8250
Connor, J.D. (AACR)
Dixon, F.J. (AACR)
*Figueredo, Anita (SSO), *ONC*
*Seay, David G. (ASTR)
*Shimkin, Michael B. (AACR, ASCO), *M/PRM/ONC*, 452-3674
*Tannenbaum, A. (AACR), 459-5517
*Verity, Gordon L. (ARS, ASTR), *TR*, 748-2411, ext. 560

LA MESA (713)

*Abrams, Jack P. (ASTR), *RI*, 460-4920
*Lehmann, Quentin H. (ARS, ASTR)

LAFAYETTE

*Baker, Donald R. (ASTR)

LOMA LINDA (714)

Collins, Edwin M. (AACE)
*Godfrey, Thomas E. (AACE, ASCO), *MO*, 796-7311
*Kuhn, Irvin N. (ASCO), *HEM*, 824-0800
**Rick, Gordon M. (AACE), 796-7311
*Slater, James (ARS, ASCO, ASTR), *TR*, 796-7311, ext. 3283
*Thompson, Ralph J., Jr. (AACE, ASCO, SSO), *S*, 796-7311, ext. 2208
*Wong, Douglas S. (ASTR), *RO*, 796-7311, ext. 3901

LONG BEACH (213)

*Brook, Jack (AACR, ASCO), *M/HEM/ONC*, 498-1313, ext. 2321
*Chahbazian, Chahin (ARS, ASTR), *TR*, (303) 475-3275
*Cook, Galen B. (SHNS), *S*, (714) 846-9256
*Dworkin, David (ASCO), *M*, 437-0506
*Ellery, Sidney W. (ARS, SSO), *SO*, 437-0301
*Fass, Leroy (AACR, ASCO), *M/HEM*, 426-9442
*Hom, Lun W. (SHNS)
*Hyde, Leroy (ASCO), *M*, 499-1313, ext. 2233
*Keasbey, Louisa E. (SSO), *PATH*
*Kiely, Andrew A. (SHNS, SSO), *S/ONC*, 597-3364
*Liechti, Robert E. (SHNS), *ONC*
*Litman, Arthur G. (ASTR)
*Moore, Emory S. (ARS, SHNS, SSO), *SO*, 597-3364
*Nakai, George S. (AACR, ASCO), *M/HEM*, 498-1313, ext. 2674
*Richardson, Arthur P. (ASCO), *M/HEM*, 426-9442
*Stein, Justin J. (ARS, ASCO, ASTR, SSO), *RT/ONC*, 498-1313

*Steinfeld, Jesse L. (AACR, ASCO),
M/HEM, 498-1313, ext. 2305
*White, Irving L. (SHNS)

LOS ANGELES (213)

**Abrams, Albert M. (AACE)
*Acquarelli, Mario (ASHNS, SHNS),
OT, 670-3970
*Ashley, Franklin L. (SHNS), *PLS*,
277-6006
*Avedon, Melvin (ASCO), *M*,
657-1880
*Bailey, Wilbur (ARS)
*Bateman, Joseph R. (AACR, ASCO),
M/HEM/ONC, 748-3111, ext. 331
*Batzdorf U. (AACR), 825-5079
Benedict, W.F. (AACR), 663-3341
Beumer, John III (AACE)
*Bonorris, Jim (ASCO), *M/HEM*,
481-3948
*Braun, Ernest J. (ASTR), *RT*,
269-9131, ext. 375
*Calcaterra, Thomas C. (ASHNS),
OT, 825-6740
*Carnes, W.H. (AACR), *PATH*,
825-5648
*Chan, Paul Ying-Ming (ASCO, ASTR),
TR/ONC, 667-5841
**Cherrick, Henry (AACE), *OP*
Cline, M.J. (AACR)
Davis, H.A. (AACR)
*Disaia, Philip J. (ASCO, SGO)
*Dowswell, John W. (ASTR), *RT*,
269-9131, ext. 375
Dusault, Lucille (ASCO)
*Eilber, Frederick R. (AACR, ASCO),
S, 825-7081
Fahey, J.L. (AACR)
*Finck, Frank (SSO), *PATH*, 483-5750
*Frey, Harvey (ASTR), *TR*, 997-1522
Friedman, N.B. (AACR)
*Futoran, Robert J. (ARS)
*George, Frederick W., III (AACE,
ARS, ASTR, SSO), *RT*, 225-3115,
ext. 7-3008
*Gilbert, Harvey Alan (ASCO), *RT*,
667-5841

Golde, D.W. (AACR)
*Green, Nathan (ASTR), *TR*,
482-8111, ext. 436
*Griffiths, Cadvan O., Jr. (SHNS),
PLS/HNS, 477-5558
*Guiss, Lewis W. (AACE, AACR,
ARS, ASCO, SHNS, SSO), *S*,
483-2700
*Gwinn, John, *R/PD*, 663-3341
*Hall, Thomas C. (AACR, ASCO,
AACE, SSO), *S*, 226-4011
*Hammond, Denman (ASCO), *PD*,
335-1511, ext. 494
*Hammond, George D. (AACE, AACR,
ASCO) *PD*, 226-2008
*Haskell, Charles M. (AACR, ASCO),
M, 825-1608
*Hauskins, Larry A. (ASTR), *TR*,
825-6687
Hayes, E.F. (AACR)
*Hays, Daniel M. (AACE), *S*,
663-3341, ext. 2675
Higgins, G.R. (AACR)
Holmes, E.C. (AACR)
*Horn, Neal L. (ASTR)
Hyman, C.B. (AACR)
Irie, R.F. (AACR)
*Irwin, Lowell (AACR, ASCO), *MO*,
748-3111
*Kagan, Arthur R. (AACR, ARS,
ASCO, ASTR), *RT*, 389-2446
Karon, Myron (AACE, ASCO)
*Katz, Alfred (ASCO, SHNS),
HNS/S, 652-8992
*Kovacs, Ervin T. (ASCO), *HEM/S*,
657-2094
*Lagasse, Leo D. (SGO), *OG*, 825-5740
*Langdon, Edward A. (ASTR), *RT*,
825-6759
*Lebherz, Thomas (SGO), *OG*,
825-7155
*Lee, Yeu-Tsu N. (AACR, ASCO),
S, 226-7757
*McAllister, R.M. (AACR),
660-2450
*McKenna, Robert J. (ARS, ASCO,
SHNS, SSO), *S/RT*, 483-2700
*Meland, Orville N. (ARS)

*Melbye, Roy Wilbur (ASTR), *R*,
482-8111
**Melrose, Raymond J. (AACE), *OP*,
746-2826
*Miller, Alden H. (ASHNS, SHNS),
OT, 663-1211
*Moore, J. George (SGO), *G*, 825-5688
*Morrow, Charles Paul (ARS, ASCO),
GO
*Morton, Donald L. (ASCO, SHNS,
SSO), *S/TS*, 825-7951
*Mosher, Michael B. (ASCO), *M*,
657-1880
*Nolan, James F. (ASCO)
*Nussbaum, Herman (ASCO), *RT*,
667-5841
*O'Brien, R.L. (AACR), 226-2127
*Ortega, J.A. (AACR), 663-3341
*Parker, J.W. (AACR), 226-2121
*Penn, H.S. (AACR), 661-0048
*Perzik, Samuel L. (ARS, ASCO,
SHNS), *S/HNS*, 879-3363
*Rappaport, Herbert (ASCO),
M/HEM, 657-6131
*Rekers, Paul (ARS, SHNS, SSO),
S, 478-9858
*Riley, Cordell (AACE)
*Sadoff, Leonard (AACR, ASCO),
M, 667-5142
*Sahakian, George J. (ASCO), *M*,
839-4381
*Sakulsky, S. Barry (AACE, ASCO,
SHNS), *S/RT*, 483-2700
*Schwinn, Charles (SSO), *PATH*,
225-3115, ext. 7-9800
*Seeger, R.C. (AACR), 825-7525
*Sherwin, R.P. (AACR)
*Shore, N.A. (AACR), 660-2450
*Siegel, S.E. (AACR), 660-2450
*Siegler, R. (AACR), 639-8550
*Smith, Howard S. (ASTR), *TR*,
472-8916
*Smith, John Douglas (SHNS)
*Sparks, Frank C. (AACR, ASCO),
S, 825-7951
*Stolinsky, David C. (AACR, ASCO),
M/MO, 748-3111, ext. 331
Takasugi, M. (AACR), 825-7651

*Taub, Robert (ASCO), *M*, 657-1880
*Territo, M.C. (AACR), 825-7768
*Thompson, Ronald W. (ASCO, ASTR),
RT, 665-4241
*Townsend, Duane E. (SGO)
*VanLancker, J.L. (AACR), 825-6758
*Vonleden, Hans V. (ASHNS),
OT/HNS, 478-2100
Vredevoe, D.L. (AACR), 825-0816
*Ward, Paul H. (ASHNS), *OT*,
825-5179
*Weeks, Leroy R. (ASCO), *OG*,
731-8391
*Willis, Norman R. (ASTR)
*Wolever, Thomas H. (ARS, ASTR),
RT, 667-5841
*Zager, Warren J. (ASTR), *RT/NM*,
651-2200
*Zarem, Harvey A. (SHNS), *PS*,
825-5582

LOS GATOS

Sable, Morris (ASTR)

LYNWOOD (213)

*Miller, Charles J. (ARS, SHNS, SSO),
S/TR, 639-3890
*Zimmerman, Arthur S. (ASTR)

MARTINEZ (415)

*Samouhos, Emmanuel (ASTR), *R*,
228-6800, ext. 307

MENLO PARK

*Breslich, P. (AACR)
Freeman, G. (AACR)
*Zackheim, H.S. (AACR)

MERCED

*Say, C.C. (AACR)

MODESTO (209)

*Benak, Steve (ASTR), *TR*,
526-4500

MONTEBELLO (213)

*Tisman, G. (AACR), 724-6858

MONTE SERENO

*Howell, Roy K. (ASTR)

NEEDLES

O'Brien, Frederick (ARS)

NEWPORT BEACH (213)

*Sanderson, Roger S. (SHNS), *S,*
642-5411
*Turnbull, Frederick M. (ASHNS),
OT, 642-7630

NORTH RIDGE (213)

Greenblatt, M. (AACR)

OAKLAND (415)

*Englebrecht, Anthony H. (ASTR)
*Merrill, M. Donald (ARS, ASTR),
RT, 655-4000, ext. 434
*Odell, Rollin, W. Jr. (ARS, ASTR),
TR, 655-4000, ext. 434
*Schweitzer, Robert J. (ARS, SHNS,
SSO), *SO,* 451-8683
*Wurzel, John F. (SGO), *OG,* 639-2549

ORANGE (714)

*Armentrout, Steven A. (AACR,
ASCO), *HEM/ONC,* 633-9393,
ext. 746
*Copelan, Herschel (ASCO), *M/HEM,*
542-6711
*Recher, L. (AACR), 633-9393
*Slater, L.M. (AACR), *M/HEM*
*Vermuno, Halvor (ARS, ASCO,
ASTR), *RT/R,* 633-9393, ext. 277

OXNARD BEACH

*Sharp, Thomas R. (ASTR)

PALO ALTO (415)

*Arnold, Charles A. (ASCO), *M/ONC,*
321-4121
*Berliner, D.L. (AACR), 493-3200
*Fish, Victor J. (ASCO, ASTR), *RT/
NM,* 321-4121, ext. 291
*Wilbur, Jordan R. (ASCO), *PD,*
327-4800, ext. 222

PALO VERDES ESTATES (213)

*Beckstrand, Grant H. (ARS, SHNS,
SSO), *TR/SO,* 375-2809
*Dollinger, M.R. (AACR, ASCO), *M*

PALOS VERDES PEN. (213)

*Sutherland, Donald A. (ASCO),
M/HEM, 541-2266

PASADENA (213)

*Bullock, Weldon K. (SSO)
*Fister, H. Wm. (SHNS, SSO), *S,*
449-6606
Hall, T.C. (AACR)
*Helsper, James T. (ARS, ASCO,
SHNS, SSO), *S,* 449-3561
*Petro, Thomas A. (SSO), *MO,*
796-6144
*Sharp, George S. (ARS, SHNS, SSO),
S/ONC, 795-4343
*Vigario, Gordon (ASTR)

PRESIDIO (415)

*Corder, Michael P. (ASCO), *M,*
561-4386
*Flannery, Eugene P. (ASCO), *M/HEM,*
561-4386

RANCHO PALOS VERDES

*Feder, Bernard H. (ARS, ASTR)

RANCHO SANTA FE

*Hummon, Irvin F. (ARS, ASTR)

REDONDO BEACH (213)

*Scallon, Joseph E. (ARS, ASTR)
*Stuhlbarg, Jerome (ASTR), *TR*,
376-9474, ext. 500

REDWOOD CITY (415)

*Deffebach, Roy R. (ARS, ASTR),
RO, 369-5811
*Evans, A. McChesney (ASCO), *M*,
365-4321
*Natoli, Wm. J. (ARS), *OG,* 365-4321

RIVERSIDE (714)

*Hankins, Elmer (ARS, ASCO)
*Tourtellotte, Charles R. (ASCO),
M, 683-4891
*Wong, Francisco M. (ASCO), *HEM/
MO*, 683-6370
*Zimmermann, Kenneth W. (ASTR),
TR/NM, 683-6771

ROCHESTER (707)

*Speiser, Burton L. (ASTR), *RO*,
438-5640

ROLLING HILLS

*Small, Richard C. (ASTR)

SACRAMENTO (916)

*Andras, Ellis J. (ASTR), *TR*,
929-1870
*Doggett, R.L. (ARS, ASTR)
*Fisher, John J. (ASCO), *HEM/ONC*,
929-5891
*Hanks, Gerald E. (ARS, ASTR), *R*,
452-4818
*Ripple, Richard C. (ARS)
*Rowe, Jay F., Jr. (ASTR), *TR*
*Thomas, Neil F. (ASTR), *RT,*
929-1570

SAN BERNARDINO (714)

*Nies, Boyd A. (ASCO), *HEM/M*,
886-6806
*Skoog, Wm. A. (ASCO), *HEM*,
886-6806

SAN DIEGO (714)

*Barsky, Morley (ASHNS), *OT/S,*
583-0312
*Bone, Robert C. (ASHNS), *OT*,
453-7500, ext. 3405
*Callipari, Frank B. (ASCO), *S*,
291-6270
*Cantrell, Robert W. (ASHNS), *OT*,
233-2761
*Crews, Quintous E., Jr. (ASTR)
*Cudmore, John T. (ARS, ASCO,
SHNS, SSO), *S/RT*, 291-6270
*Eddy, Carl L. (ASTR), *RT*, 234-6410
*Groesbeck, H.P. (SSO, ARS, ASCO,
SHNS), *S/RT*, 291-6270
*Hankins, Franklin D. (ARS), *R*,
292-7601
*Kung, Faith H. (AACR, ASCO),
PD/HEM, 294-5880
*Lehar, Thomas J. (ASCO), *M*,
234-6261
*Levin, Howard Allen (ARS, ASCO),
M, 560-1661
*Lucas, Wm. E. (SGO), *GO*, 291-3330,
ext. 1285
*Newman Donald Richard (ASCO),
M, 234-6261
*Roland, Charles (ASTR), *TR*,
234-7341
*Saltzstein, Sidney L. (AACE, ASCO),
PATH, 294-5764
*Sanford, Frederic G. (ASTR)
*Von Essen, Carl F. (AACR, ASCO),
TR, 294-6727
*Weddle, Robert (ARS)
*Wepsic, H.T. (AACR), 755-2091

SAN FRANCISCO (415)

*Anlyan, A.J. (AACR, SHNS, SSO),
S, 775-1939

*Biskind, G.R. (AACR), 563–4550
*Bohannon, Richard (SSO), *M/HEM/
  ONC*, 668–0160
*Boles, Roger (ASHNS), *OT*, 668–1993
*Buschke, Franz (ARS, ASTR), *RO*,
  666–4815
*Cantril, Simeon T. (ARS, ASTR), *RT*
*Castro, Joseph R. (ARS, ASTR)
*Cohen, Richard (ASCO), *M/ONC/
  HEM*, 668–0160
*Dekelboum, Allen M. (ASHNS), *OT*,
  668–9655
*Dymott, Cleo Elaine (ASTR), *RO*,
  922–3823
Epstein, J.H. (AACR)
*Fu, Karen (ASTR)
*Galante, Maurice (ASCO, SHNS, SSO)
*Green, Jerold P. (ARS, ASTR)
*Jacobs, Edwin M. (AACE, AACR,
  ARS, ASCO, SSO), *M*, 666–1995
Kim, Y.S. (AACR)
*Kushner, Joseph H. (ASCO), *PD/
  HEM/ONC*, 752–7242
*Loder, Earl C. (ASTR), *TR*, 387–8700
*Mann, Steven G. (ASTR)
*Margolis, Lawrence W. (ASTR), *RT*
Meurk, Mary L. (ASTR, ARS)
*Newman, Harry (ASTR)
*Petrakis, N.L. (AACR), 666–2001
*Pollack, Robert S. (ARS, SHNS, SSO),
  S/ONC, 986–6565
**Roffinella, John P. (AACE)
*Rosenbaum, Ernest (ASCO), *M/HEM/
  ONC*, 567–5581
*Sheline, Glenn E. (ARS, ASTR), *TR*,
  666–4815
*Sherman, Robert S., Jr. (ARS, ASTR),
  R, 744–7139
*Silverberg, Ivan J. (ARS, ASCO), *M*,
  567–6000, ext. 546
*Silverman, Sol, Jr. (AACE), 666–1243
*Vaeth, Jerome M. (ARS, ASCO,
  ASTR, SSO), *RT*, 668–1000
*Wara, Wm. M. (ASTR)
*White, Laurens (AACR, ASCO), *M*,
  826–8778
*Wilson, C.B. (AACR) 666–1087
*Wood, David A. (AACE, SSO),
  PATH/ONC, 666–2201
Zippin, Calvin (AACE), 666–2331

SAN JOSE (415)

*Frenster, John H. (AACR, ASCO),
  M/HEM, 293–0262
*Guernsey, James M. (ARS), *S/TS*,
  (408) 293–0262
*Gunn, Walter G. (ARS, ASCO, ASTR),
  RT, (408) 426–1967
*Johnson, Gordon C. (ARS)
*Kraut, Joseph W. (ASTR), *RT*,
  (408) 293–0262

SAN JUAN CAPISTRANO

Garcia, H.G. (AACR)

SAN LUIS OBISPO (805)

*Hartman, John Robert (ASTR), *TR*,
  541–1200

SAN MATEO (415)

*Jegge, Gerard F. (SHNS, SSO), *S*,
  342–7276
*Quilici, John (ASCO), *M*, 342–7771

SANTA ANA (714)

*Crawford, Hugh H. (SHNS), *PLS*,
  558–3324

SANTA BARBARA (805)

*Erickson, Douglas W. (ASTR), *RT*,
  966–6121
*Love, Jesshill (ASTR, ASCO)
Masin, F. (AACR) 963–4358
*Medwid, Albert (ARS, SHNS, SSO),
  S/ONC, 962–8126
*Northrop, Mead F. (ASTR), *TR/NM*,
  966–6121
*Preston, F.W. (AACR), 964–9477
*Rowe, James W. (ASTR)
*Young, Barton R. (ARS)

SANTA CLARA (408)

*Yu, Kou-Ping (ASCO), *M*, 246–4000

SANTA MONICA (213)

*Avallone, Leopold T. (ASTR), *RT*,
451-1511, ext. 2235
*Silverstein, Melvin (AACR, ASCO), *S*,
394-2280
*Wagner, Donald E. (ASCO), *S*,
829-4505
*Weisenburger, Thomas H. (ASTR)
*Wilson, Wm. L. (AACE, AACR,
ASCO), *M*, 451-5995

SANTA ROSA (707)

*Hanahan, Ralph B. (ASTR), *RO*,
525-1150
*Kenney, John M. (AACR, SSO),
S/ONC, 546-5052
*Schroeder, Alan F. (ARS, ASTR),
RT, 456-1182

SAUSALITO

*Jack, George (ASTR)

SEPULVEDA (213)

*Hammond, Wm. G. (AACR, ASCO),
S, 894-2525

STANFORD (415)

*Bagshaw, Malcolm A. (ARS, ASTR),
RT, 321-1200, ext. 5650
*Donaldson, Sarah S. (ASTR)
*Earle, John D. (ARS, ASTR)
*Glatstein, Eli (ASCO, ASTR), *RT*,
497-5241
*Kaplan, Henry S. (ARS, ASCO,
ASTR), *RT*, 321-1200, ext. 5055
*Marsa, Gerald W. (ASTR), *RT*
*Nelsen, Thomas S. (SSO)
*Opler, S.R. (AACR), 364-0843
*Probert, John C. (ARS, ASTR), *RT*
*Rosenberg, Saul A. (ASCO), *M*,
497-5877
Tsuboi, K.K. (AACR), 497-6369

STOCKTON (209)

*Redalia, Richard B. (ASTR), *TR*,
466-4811
*Roeser, Erwin H. (SHNS), *S*

TORRANCE (213)

*Averbook, Beryl D. (SHNS), *S*,
378-8344
*Block, Jerome B. (ASCO), *M*
*Byfield, John E. (AACR, ASCO,
ASTR), *RT/R*, 328-2380
*Eichel, Berkley S. (ASHNS), *OT*,
534-3052
*Finkelstein, Jerry Z. (AACR, ASCO),
RT/R, 328-2380, ext. 1846
*Greenberg, Lowell H. (ASCO), *M/
HEM*, 289-1765
*Hemenway, Wm. G. (ASHNS), *OT*,
328-2380, ext. 1841
Imagawa, D.T. (AACR)
*Pilch, Yosef H. (AACE, ARS, ASCO,
SHNS), *S*, 328-2380, ext. 1380
*Robinson, Alfred G. (ASTR)
Siegler, R. (AACR)
*Wong, Stuart (ASCO), *M/HEM*,
373-8276

TRAVIS AFB (707)

*Reynolds, Ralph D. (ASCO), *M/
HEM/NM*, 438-3379
*Van Roy, Ronald L. (ASTR)

TUSTIN (714)

*Baughan, Marjorie A. (ASCO), *M*,
838-8151
*Lilly, Terry E., Jr. (ASCO), *S*,
838-6664
*Opfell, Richard W. (ASCO), *M/
HEM*, 838-8151
*Padova, James A. (ASCO), *M/HEM*,
838-8151
*Rappaport, Irving (SHNS, SSO),
PLS/HN, 544-0733
*Shiffman, Melvin A. (ASCO, SHNS,
SSO), *S*, 544-1720

UKIAH (707)

*Gordon, Hershel W. (ASCO),
PATH, 462-8221

UPLAND

Kelly, K.H. (AACR)

VACAVILLE (707)

*Peniston, Wm. H. (SHNS), *S*,
488-7137

VAN NUYS (213)

*Fingerhut, Aaron G. (ARS, ASTR),
RT, 997-1522
Gilbertsen, James D. (ASTR)

VENTURA (805)

*Parsa, Kooros (ASCO), *M/HEM*,
644-1848
*Schmela, Woodrow W. (ARS)

WALNUT CREEK (415)

*Attwood, Cyril J. (ASCO)
*Rozkalna, Baiba (ASCO), *M/HEM*,
933-3000, ext. 2298

WHITTIER (213)

*Fitzgerald, James P. (ASTR)
*Kurohara, Samuel S. (ASTR), *TR*,
698-0697

Colorado

COLORADO SPRINGS (303)

Herbert, Donald E. (ASTR)
*Kersey, Dudley H. (ASTR)
*Locke, Harry R. (ASCO), *M/HEM*,
473-4656
Marshall, John F. (ASTR)
*Mira, Hoaquin G. (ASTR)
*Schiller, John E. (ASTR), *RT*,
475-3275

DENVER (303)

*Aarestad, Norman (ASTR), *RT*,
292-0600, ext. 2410

*Berris, Robert F. (ASCO), *M*,
333-4876
*Brandenburg, Harmon P. (ARS)
*Chamoun, Chamoun D. (ASCO),
M, 534-4432
*Chau, Paul (ARS)
*DiBella, Nicholas J. (ASCO), *M*,
366-5311, ext. 26200
*Downing, Virginia (AACE, ASCO),
M, 233-6501
*English, Gerald M. (ASHNS), *OT*,
744-8222
Fennell, R.H., Jr. (AACR)
Fink, L.M. (AACR)
*Garfield, David (ASCO), *M/HEM*,
388-4876
*Hamilton, Paul K. (AACE, ASCO),
M/HEM, 388-4876
*Hays, Taru (ASCO), *PD*, 861-8888,
ext. 2321
*Holt, Charlene P. (AACE, ASCO),
PD/ONC
*Jennings, Robert L. (ARS, ASCO)
*Johnson, F.B. (ASTR)
*Kramish, David (SHNS), *S*,
388-6448
Kotin, P. (AACR)
*Kurnick, John A. (AACE, ASCO),
HEM/M, 394-8253
*Lackey, Robert W. (ARS, ASTR), *R*,
534-9011, ext. 2377
*Major, Francis (SGO), *GO*, 893-7658
*Minden, P. (AACR)
*Morfit, H.M. (SHNS)
*Nelson, Wm. R. (ARS, SHNS, SSO),
S, 222-1795
*Penniman, Raymond K. (ASTR)
*Pierce, G.B. (AACR, SSO), *PATH*
*Powell, Terry D. (ASTR), *RT*
*Ratzer, Erick R. (AACE, SHNS, SSO),
S, 394-7236
*Reiquam, Wm. C. (ASCO), *PATH*,
534-9011
*Reynolds, Weston (ARS)
*Robinson, Wm. A. (AACE), *HEM/
ONC*, 394-8253
*Silverberg, Steven G. (SSO), *S/PATH*,
394-8171

ENGLEWOOD (303)

*Cunningham, James K. (ASCO), *M*,
789-1851
*Sakamato, Arthur (AACR, ASCO),
M, 789-2323

FORT COLLINS (303)

*Gillette, Edward L. (ASTR), *VETR*,
491-6439
*Henson, Stanley W., Jr. (SHNS), *S*,
482-6456

SPIVACK (303)

*Huseby, Robert A. (ASCO), 233-6501

STERLING (303)

*Tennant, Edward E. (ARS, ASTR),
RT, 522-7100

CONNECTICUT

BETHEL

*Hall, Edward J. (SGO)

BRIDGEPORT (203)

*Corso, Philip F. (SHNS, SSO),
PLS/HNS, 366-5617
*Feldman, Morton G. (SHNS), *S/
HNS,* 336-2334

FAIRFIELD (203)

*Covey, Susan E. (ASTR), *RT*

FARMINGTON (203)

*Freymann, John G. (AACR, ASCO),
M, 677-4171
Sunderman, R.T. (AACR)
*Toomey, James M. (ASHNS), *OT*,
674-2480

GREENWICH (203)

*Rosenberg, Arthur H. (ASCO),
M/HEM, 661-9433

GUILFORD

*Braestrup, Carl B. (ARS)

HAMPTON (203)

*Sorenberger, Charles F. (ARS), *R*,
889-2049

HARTFORD (203)

*Foster, James H. (SSO), *S*, 524-2840
*Golub, Grant (ASCO), *M*, 249-6291
*Josel, Mark (ASCO), *M/HEM*,
525-5301
*Kandes, Martin J. (ASTR), *RT*,
524-2803
*Kiley, Robert F. (ASTR), *RT*,
524-2803
*Kuehn, Paul G. (SHNS, SSO), *S*,
524-5939
*Marsh, Spinks H. (ARS, ASTR), *RT*,
524-2803
*Martin, Robert S. (ASCO, SSO), *M*,
249-6291
*Wawro, Nestor W. (SHNS, SSO), *SO*,
246-4142
*White, Edward P. (SSO), *S*, 522-6664
*Williams, Henry M. (AACR, ASCO,
SSO), *M*, 249-6291

MANCHESTER

*Roberts, Douglas J. (ARS)

NEW BRITAIN (203)

*Owens, Guy (AACR, ASCO), *M*,
224-2634

NEW HAVEN (203)

*Bertino, Joseph R. (AACR, ASCO),
M, 436-2730
*Bobrow, S.N. (AACR), 562-6863
*Capizzi, Robert (AACR, ASCO),
M/MO, 436-4292
*Chen, Michael G. (ASTR), *TR*,
436-3195

Cole, J.W. (AACR)
*Collins, James T. (ASTR), *RT*
*Farber, Leonard R. (ASCO), *M/HEM*,
  562–6863
Finch, S.C. (AACR)
*Fischer, David S. (ASCO), *M/HEM*,
  624–6000
*Fischer, James J. (ARS, ASTR), *TR*,
  436–3195
Fischer, Rose J. (ASCO)
Goldenberg, I.S. (AACR)
*Hayes, Mark A. (SSO), *S*, 436–3438
*Knowlton, Arthur H. (ASTR), *RT*,
  432–4048
*Kohorn, Ernest I. (ARS, SGO), *PLS*
*Krizek, Thomas J. (SHNS), *PLS*,
  436–3436
*Marsh, John C. (AACR, ASCO),
  M/HEM, 436–8860
*Mitchell, Malcolm S. (AACR, ASCO),
  M, 436–8860
*Morris, John M. (SGO)
*Papac, Rose J. (AACR, ASCO), *M*,
  933–2561
*Polayes, Irving M. (SHNS), *PLS/HNS/
  MXF*, 776–3344
*Prosnitz, Leonard R. (ASCO, ASTR),
  RT/R, 436–4337
Schulz, Robert J. (ASTR)
*Shaw, Michael T. (AACR, ASCO),
  M, 436–8860
*Skeel, Roland T. (AACR, ASCO), *M*,
  436–8860
*Son, Yung H. (ARS, ASTR)
*Storer, Edward H. (AACE), *S*,
  933–2561
*Vera, Raul (AACE, ARS, ASTR), *TR*
Waters, L.L. (AACR)

NORWALK (203)

*Pool, John L. (ARS, SSO), *S/TS*,
  853–6868
*Schulman, Paul L. (ASCO), *M/HEM*,
  838–4131

ORANGE

*Whitcomb, Wayne P. (ASTR)

PORTLAND

*Silberstein, Allen B. (ASTR)

RIDGEFIELD

*Berger, David S. (ARS, ASTR)

SHARON

Craig, Howard (SSO)

STAMFORD (203)

*Bottiglieri, N.G. (ASCO), *M*, 325–3871
*Erichson, Robert B. (ASCO), *M/HEM*,
  325–2695
*Grann, Victor R. (ASCO), *M*,
  325–2695

STORRS (203)

Yang, Tsu-Ju T. (AACR), 486–4000

TORRINGTON (203)

*Epstein, Robert B. (AACE), *M*,
  666–6500, ext. 793
*MacDonald, Carlton A., Jr. (ASTR),
  TR, 482–9351

WATERBURY (203)

*Kaess, Kenneth R. (ARS)
*Ryan, Sylvester James (ASCO), *M*,
  756–8351

WEST HARTFORD

*Hall, Wendall, C. (ARS)

WEST HAVEN

*Hartman, Paul V. (ASTR)

WESTPORT (203)

*Biskind, M.S. (AACR), 227–6844

WOODBRIDGE

Capizzi, R.L. (AACR)

DELAWARE

HOCKESSIN (302)

*Meckelnburg, Robert L. (ASCO),
   M/NM, 994-5764

WILMINGTON (302)

*Cuccia, Carlo A. (ARS, ASTR), *RT,*
   428-4881
*Frelick, Robert W. (ASCO, SSO),
   M/NM, 652-3613
*Gledhill, Emerson Y. (ARS)
Laird, Edmund G. (SSO)
Lenaz, L. (AACR)
*Lippincott, Samuel W. (ARS), *R,*
   652-0841
*McInnes, George F. (SHNS, SSO),
   S, 428-2400
*Tilton, Donald C. (ASTR), *TR,*
   428-4881

DISTRICT OF COLUMBIA

WASHINGTON (202)

*Alford, T. Crandall (SHNS, SSO), *S*
*Alpert L.K. (AACR), 362-7744
*Andrews, J. Robert (AACE, AACR,
   ARS), *RT,* 483-6666, ext. 7345
*Bailar, J.C., III (AACR), 496-6317
*Blom, Johannes (ASCO), *M/HEM,*
   576-3131
*Bruno, Anthony M. (ASCO), *S,*
   223-4700
*Caulk, Ralph M. (ARS, ASTR)
*Cohen, Martin H. (AACR, ASCO),
   M, 483-6666, ext. 479
*Curreri, Anthony R. (AACE, ASCO,
   SSO), *S/TS,* (608) 262-2896
*Donn, Frederick Y. (SHNS, SSO),
   S/ONC, 946-7666
*Duvall, Charles (ASCO), *M/HEM,*
   223-3940
*Foye, Lawrence V., Jr. (ASCO), *M,*
   389-5071

Gillin, Michael T. (ASTR)
*Gould Ernest A. (SSO), *S,* 291-6100
*Henschke, Ulrich K. (ARS, ASTR,
   SSO), *RT,* 722-1400
*Hovey, Leslie M. (SHNS), *PLS*
*Jaques, Darrell A. (SHNS), *S,*
   576-2687
Jones, George W. (AACE, SSO)
*Keys, Henry M. (ASTR), *RT,*
   576-3575
*Klopp, Calvin T. (AACE, ARS,
   SHNS, SSO), *S*
*Leffall, LaSalle D., Jr. (AACE, ARS,
   SHNS, SSO), *S/SO,* 745-1446
*Leikin, Sanford (AACE, ASCO),
   HEM/ONC, 835-4170
*Lessin, Lawrence S. (ASCO), *M/HEM,*
   331-2939
*Letterman, Gordon S. (ASHNS,
   SHNS), *PLS,* 337-3535
*Lynch, John J. (ASCO), *ONC/M,*
   829-7888
*Maier, John G. (ARS, ASTR), *RT,*
   331-6454
*McFarland, James J. (ASHNS), *OT,*
   223-3560
*McGowan, Larry (ARS, SGO, SSO),
   OG, 331-6357
*Minna, J.D. (AACR), 389-7275
*Mirsky, Harold S. (ASCO), *M/HEM,*
   338-5050
*Mondzac, Allen (ASCO), *M/HEM,*
   223-5333
*Nelson, Warren J. (ASTR)
*Newman, Wm. (SSO), *PATH,*
   331-6383
*Ortega, L.G. (AACR), 389-7252
*Park, Robert (SGO), *OG,* 576-3442
*Patow, Warren E. (SGO), *OG*
**Peagler, Fredrick, *OP,* 636-6404
*Primack, Aron (ASCO), *M,* 829-7888
*Sabatini, Domenic E. (ASTR)
*Scheele, Leonard A. (SSO)
*Schneider, Roy L. (SHNS), *SO,*
   745-1406
*Schurter, Maxine A. (SHNS), *S,*
   337-3535
*Schwartz, Stanley (ASCO), *M/ONC,*
   829-7888

*Shnider, Bruce I. (AACE, ASCO),
  M/MO, 625-7582
*Shorb, Paul E. (AACE)
*Trible, Wm. M. (ASHNS, SHNS), OT,
  223-2676
Turner, W. (AACR)
West, W.L. (AACR)
*White, Jack E. (AACE, AACR, ARS,
  SHNS), S, 745-1406
*Whittington, Richard (ASCO), M/
  HEM, 389-5137
Woolley, G.W. (AACR)
Zahl, P.A. (AACR)

FLORIDA

BAY HARBOR ISLAND (305)

*Dickler, Emmanuel (ASTR), R,
  864-3532

BOCA RATON (305)

*Goodman, Alan N. (ASCO), M/HEM,
  395-1026
*Tamoney, Harry J., Jr. (SHNS, SSO),
  S/ONC, 395-8588

CORAL GABLES (305)

*Cloninger, Timothy E. (ASTR)
*Landy, Jerome (SHNS)
*Marquez, Antonio H. (ASCO), M,
  445-1504
*Snyder, Wm. (SSO), MO, 531-1146

DAYTONA BEACH (904)

*Kerman, Herbert D. (ARS, ASTR), R,
  255-4411
*Wolff, Alcuin D. (ASTR)

FORT LAUDERDALE (305)

*Buchanan, Wallace (ASTR)
*Fields, J. Allan (ASHNS), OT,
  523-0237
*Fonts, Ernesto A. (ASTR), TR,
  771-8000, ext. 7847
Jones, R.S. (AACR)

*Lang, Irving R. (ASCO), G, 771-9242
*Meadows, Paul M. (ASTR)
Nelson, Peter A. (ARS, SSO)
Russell, William O. (AACR)

FORT MYERS (813)

*Sayet, Ellen (ASCO), M, 332-2140

GAINESVILLE (904)

*Bloom, Gerald E. (AACE), PD
*Daly, James W. (ARS, SGO), OG,
  392-2890
*Million, Rodney R. (ASTR), TR,
  392-3161
*Noyes, Ward D. (ASCO), HEM/ONC,
  392-3301
*Thar, Timothy Lee (ASTR)

HOLLYWOOD (305)

*Kanner, Steven P. (AACE, ASCO), M,
  983-6307
*Klein, Rubin (AACE, ARS, ASTR),
  RT, 925-3301
*Teperson, H.I. (ARS)

JACKSONVILLE (904)

*Abramson, Neil (AACE, ASCO),
  M/HEM/MO, 733-6368
*Atkinson, Samuel C. (SSO), S,
  398-3222
*Castells, Jose (ASTR), RT, 358-3272,
  ext. 2240
*Joel, Robert V. (SSO), PATH
*Middlekauff, Robert K. (ASHNS),
  ·OT, 354-5491
*Phillips, Curtis M. (SHNS, SSO)
*Ridings, G. Ray (AACE, ARS, ASCO,
  ASTR), RT, 398-3511, 398-9444
*Rizk, Wade S. (ARS)
Sumner, Wilbur (SHNS, SSO)
*Williams, Ashbel C. (ARS, SHNS,
  SSO), S/ONC, 355-1481
*Zullo, Robert J. (ASCO, SSO), M,
  249-9229, 772-2201

KEY WEST (305)

*Knowlton, Isabel (ARS), *OG*, 294-2800

LAKE CITY (904)

*Beggs, John H. (SHNS), *S*, 752-1400

LAKELAND (813)

*Hutchinson, Troy H., II (ASHNS), *OT*, 682-1171
Kremer, W.B. (AACR)
Sokoloff, B.T. (AACR)
*Stone, John W. (ASHNS), *OT*, 682-1171

LIGHTHOUSE PT.

*Wehr, Wm. H. (ARS), *ONC*

MELBOURNE (305)

*Seelman, Robert C. (ASCO), *M*, 724-0122

MIAMI (305)

*Anderson, W.A.D. (AACE), *PATH*, 350-6219
*Averette, Harvy E. (AACE, SGO), *OG*, 371-9611, ext. 574
*Awad, Wm., Jr. (AACE)
*Broder, L.E. (AACR), 547-6909
*Chandler, J.R. (ASHNS, SHNS), *OT*, 371-9611, ext. 6101
*Charyulu, K.K. (AACE, ARS, ASCO, ASTR), *RT*, 324-1180
*Colsky, Jacob (ASCO), *M/MO*, 324-0040
*Davis, Harold E. (ARS), *R*, 444-3212
*Dembrow, Victor (SHNS, SSO), *S/ HNS*, 358-3433
*Egan, John W. (ASTR)
*Ford, John H., Jr. (AACE, SGO), *GO*, 325-6950
*Franzino, Arthur (ASCO), *M*, 371-1471
*Fuste, Ricardo R. (ASTR, SSO), *TR*

*Galluccio, Joseph R. (ARS), *R*, 854-4400
*Garciga, Carlos E. (ARS, ASTR)
*Gunn, Samuel A. (AACE), *CYT*, 350-6306
*Hananian, Juliet (ASCO), *PD*, 547-6091
Harrington, W.J. (AACR)
*Healey, John E., Jr. (AACE, SSO)
*Irvin, George L., III (AACE, SHNS), *S*, 377-2441, ext. 3441
*Ketcham, Alfred S. (AACR, ARS, ASCO, SHNS, SSO), *S*, 547-6364
*Kleinfield, George (ARS, SHNS, SSO), *S*, 947-5623
*Kung, Faith (AACE, ASCO), *PD/ HEM/ONC*, (714) 294-5880
*Lehfeldt, Richard W. (ASTR)
*Lessner, Howard E. (AACE, AACR, ASCO), *M*, 325-6129
*Linn, Bernard S. (SHNS), *S*, 377-2441, ext. 3663
*McKenzie, Doris (AACR, ASCO), *M*, 324-0040
*Millard, D.R., Jr. (SHNS), *PLS*
*Rosenberg, Eugene B. (AACR, ASCO), *M*, 674-2628
*Selawry, Oleg S. (AACR, ASCO), *M*, 547-6900
*Sims, Murry (SHNS), *S*, 371-4793
*Snyder, Gilbert B. (SHNS), *PLS*, 324-0536
*Sudarsanam, Anam (ASTR)
*Tejada, Francisco (AACR, ASCO), *M*, 547-6096
Vogel, C.L. (AACR)
*Vuksanovic, Mario M. (AACE, ARS, ASCO, ASTR), *RT/R*, 325-5691
Weinstein, G.D. (AACR)
Yunis, A.A. (AACR)
*Zavertnik, Joseph (SHNS, SSO), *HNS*, 371-4793
*Zubrod, C.G. (AACR)

MIAMI BEACH (305)

*Fix, Ivor (ARS, ASTR), *RT*, 532-3611, ext. 3425
*Fleming, R.M. (SSO), *S*, 538-5442

*Jacobson, Lawrence H. (ASTR)
*Levinson, Louis J. (ASTR)
*Nixon, Daniel D. (ASCO), *M/HEM/ ONC*, 531-0441
*Russin, David J. (ASCO), *S*, 532-5415
*Schneider, Jack J. (ARS), *RT*, 674-2650
*Shocket, Everett (ARS, SHNS, SSO), *S*
*Snyder, Wm. (ASCO), *M*, 531-1146

NAPLES

*Stewart, John S. (ARS)

NEW SMYRNA BEACH (904)

*Olson, Kenneth B. (AACE, ASCO, SSO), *M*, 427-7475

NOKOMIS

*Thomas, Merthyn A. (ARS)

NORTH MIAMI BEACH (305)

*Fieber, Mack H. (ASCO), *M*, 949-4259

ORLANDO (305)

*Browne, Kennedy W. (ASCO), *MO*, 425-4517
*Hadlock, Daniel C. (ASCO)

PALM BEACH

*Ackerman, Joseph L. (ARS, ASCO)

PENSACOLA (904)

*Amos, Eric H. (ASTR), *TR*, 432-1271
*Palmer, Robert C., Jr. (ASCO), *M/HEM*, 432-1271

PLANTATION

Karpas, C.M. (AACR)
*Mathews-Padow, Mildred L. (ASTR)
**Stern, Diane (AACE)

POMPANO BEACH (305)

*Gamble, James E. (ASHNS), *OT*, 942-6868
*Monson, Kenneth J. (ASTR)

ST. PETERSBURG (813)

*Beard, J.W. (AACR), 347-1881

SARASOTA (813)

Bralow, S.P. (AACR) 366-7282
*Silverstein, Herbert (ASHNS), *OT*, 366-9222
*Stephenson, Phillis A. (ASCO), *MO*, 958-5288
Stewart, Fred W. (SSO)

SOUTH MIAMI (305)

*Liebling, Martin E. (ASCO), *M/HEM/ ONC*, 665-6231
*Oren, Mark E. (ASCO), *M/HEM*, 595-2141

TALLAHASSEE (904)

*MacDonald, Jack Watt (ASCO), *HEM*, 878-4165
*Purcell, Dent W. (ASTR), *TR*, 599-5255

TAMPA (813)

*Alonso, Wm. A. (ASHNS), *OT/HNS*, 872-8794
*Barrett, O'Neill (ASCO), *M/HEM/ ONC*, 971-4500, ext. 557
*Boren, H.G. (AACR)
*Byvoet, P. (AACR)

*del Regato, Juan A. (ARS, ASTR), *TR*, 971-4500, ext. 459
*Farrior, Richard T. (ASHNS), *OT*, 251-1873
Garrett, C.T. (AACR)
*Hartmann, Robert C. (ASCO), *M/HEM*, 971-4500, ext. 136
*Holliday, James A. (ASHNS), *OT*, 872-8794
*Irvine, Donald W. (ASHNS), *OT*, 877-9428
*Jensen, Ralph (ASTR)
*Maxfield, Wm. S. (ARS, ASCO, ASTR), *RT/NM/ONC*, 971-6410, ext. 121
*Sanders, Harold L. (SHNS, SSO), *SO*, 253-0085
Sidransky, H. (AACR)
Wilkinson, D.S. (AACR)

W. PALM BEACH

*Van De Water, Malcolm S. (ASTR)
*Wimbush, Pennington R. (ARS, ASTR)

GEORGIA

ATLANTA (404)

*Birch, Herbert W. (SGO), *OG*
*Brown, Robert L. (AACE, ARS, SSO), *S*, 377-2472
*Franklin, Ernest (SGO)
Godwin, John T. (SHNS, SSO)
*Huger, Wm. E., Jr. (SHNS), *PLS*
*Huguley, Charles M., Jr. (AACE, ASCO), *M/HEM/ONC*, 377-2411, ext. 7714
*Jurkiewicz, Maurice J. (SHNS), *PLS*, 659-1660
*Kirchner, Arthur B. (ASTR)
*Leonard, James R. (ASHNS, SHNS), *OT/PLS/HNS*, 355-7897
*Letton, A. Hamblin (SSO), *S*, 525-8313
*McCord, Dale L. (ASTR)
*McLaren, John R. (ARS, ASTR), *R*, 377-2472, ext. 208

*Murray, Douglas R. (ARS, SSO), *NP*
*Olkowski, Zbigniew L. (ARS), 377-2472
*Perkinson, Neil G. (ARS, SHNS, SSO), *ONC*, 523-1333
*Phillips, Thomas W. (ASTR), *TR*, 892-4411, ext. 391
Powell, Ralph W. (SSO)
*Ragab, Abdelsalam H. (ASCO), *PD*, 659-1182
*Redd, Bryan L. (ARS, ASTR)
*Rivers, Shirley L. (ASCO), *M/HEM*, 874-1601
*Rosvoll, Randi V. (SSO)
*Schatten, Wm. E. (SHNS), *PLS*, 351-5315
*Thompson, John D. (SGO)
*Vasconez, Luis D. (SHNS), *PLS*, 377-9111
*Vogel, Charles L. (ASCO), *MO*, 659-1212, ext. 4327
*Vogler, Wm. (AACR, ASCO), *M/HEM/ONC*, 377-2411
*Wilkins, Sam A., Jr. (SHNS, SSO), *S/NP*, 377-2472
*Winokur, Stanley H. (ASCO), *M*, 688-1700

AUGUSTA (404)

*Brizel, Herbert E. (ARS, ASTR), *TR*, 724-0139
Engler, Harold (SSO)
*Fiveash, Arlie Eugene (ASTR)
*Gilman, Priscilla Ann (ASCO), *PD/HEM/ONC*, 924-7111, 828-3531
*Johnson, Robert H., Jr. (ARS, SHNS, SSO), *S*, 828-3396
**Kolas, Steve (AACE), 724-7111, ext. 8551
*Manganiello, L.O.J. (AACR), 738-0109
*Moores, Russell R. (AACE), *M/HEM*, 724-7111, ext. 8864
Soddard, L.D. (AACR)
*Sullivan, Daniel B. (SHNS, SSO), *ONC/S*, 724-7766

COLLEGE PARK

*Jones, Norman E. (ASTR)

COLUMBUS (404)

*Watson, John D., Jr. (ARS, ASTR),
  TR, 327-4515

EAST POINT (404)

Kubricht, Wm. S., Jr. (ASTR)
*Richter, Paul (ASCO), M/HEM,
  766-5657

HIAWASSEE (404)

*Bauer, Albert J. (ASTR), R,
  896-2610

LA GRANGE (404)

*Smith, Robert R. (SHNS, SSO), S,
  882-8664
*Wammock, Hoke (AACE, ARS, SHNS,
  SSO), S

MACON (912)

*Connell, H.C. (ASTR)
*Drew, Wilson D., III (ASTR), RT,
  742-1122

MARIETTA

*Lindsey, Mark M. (SGO)

SAVANNAH (912)

*Tanner, David E. (ASTR), R,
  355-3200
*West, John H. (ASCO), M,
  354-8722

STANFORD

*Goffinet, Don R. (ASTR)

HAWAII

HONOLULU (808)

*Batten, Grover H. (AACE, SHNS,
  SSO)
*Blaisdell, Richard K. (AACE), M/HEM,
  734-0221, ext. 363
*Condit, Paul T. (AACR, ASCO), MO,
  521-8737
Edynak, E.M. (AACR)
*Goldstein, Norman (AACR, ASCO),
  M, 538-7044
*Jim, Edward L. (ASHNS, SHNS), S,
  949-6116
*Keenan, John P. (AACE, ASCO),
  M/ONC, 521-6951
*Kokame, Glenn M. (AACR, ASCO),
  S, 845-2932
*Lau, Thomas K.L. (ASCO), M,
  533-4271
*McDowell, Frank (SHNS), PLS,
  531-0031
*Nishimura, E.T. (AACR), 948-8860
*Oda, Francis T. (ASCO), S,
  536-4431
*Oishi, Noboro (ASCO), M/HEM/
  ONC, 537-4880
*Tashima, Charles (ASCO), M,
  792-2817
*Uy, Quintin L. (ASCO), M,
  521-3008

KAILUA

*Boyer, Carl W., Jr. (ARS, ASTR)

IDAHO

BOISE (208)

*Burkholder, Maurice M. (ASCO),
  M, 344-1315
*Koons, C. Ronald (ASCO, ASTR),
  M/R/ONC, 345-1780
*Luce, James K. (AACR, ASCO),
  M, 345-1780
*Popma, Alfred M. (ARS, ASTR),
  R, 398-6000
*Smith, Charles E. (ASTR), RO,
  345-1780

POCATELLO (208)

*Haluska, Glenn M. (ASTR), *TR*, 232-6150

WEISER

Holton, C.P. (AACR)

ILLINOIS

ARGONNE

Fry, R.J.M. (AACR)
*Marinelli, Leonidas D. (ARS)

BERWYN

*Mrazek, Rudolph G. (AACE, SSO), *S*

BROOKFIELD

Pillai, Bhaskaran K. (ASTR)

BURLINGTON

*Bush, Irving (SSO), *U*

CHAMPAIGN

*Weissman, Irving (ARS)

CHICAGO (312)

*Ameen, Dean Mohammed (ASTR)
*Apostol, James V. (AACE, SHNS, SSO)
*Beck, Gerald (ASTR), *RT*, 649-2520
*Berlin, Nathaniel I. (AACR, ASCO), *M*, 649-8186
*Block, George E. (AACE, SHNS), *S*, 947-5605
*Brand, Wm. (ASTR), *RO*, 649-2524
*Breed, James E. (ARS, ASTR)
*Carroll, Walter W. (ARS)
*Chao, John J. (ARS, ASTR), *RT*, 842-4700
*Christou, Demetrios (ASTR)
*Cohen, Lionel (ASTR)

*Colman, Martin (ASTR)
*Cunningham, Myles P. (SHNS, SSO), *S*, 332-5058
*Das Gupta, Tapas K. (AACE, SHNS, SSO), *ONC*, 996-8438
*Davidsohn, Israel (AACE, AACR)
*Dederick, Margarida M. (AACR, ASCO), *PSYM*, 263-2637
Deihardt, F. (AACR)
DePeyster, F.A. (AACR)
*Desai, Dinesh V. (ASCO), *M/HEM*, 756-0100
*DeWys, Wm. D. (AACE, ASCO), *MO*, 649-8018
*Economou, Steven G. (AACE, SHNS, SSO), *S*, 226-3647
El-Domeiri, A.A. (AACR)
*Ezdinli, Ediz Z. (AACR, ASCO), *M*, 542-2724
Falk, L.A., Jr. (AACR)
*Ferenzi, George W. (ASCO), *M/HEM*, 581-2322
*Griem, Melvin L. (ARS, ASTR)
*Gross, Alvin (ASTR)
*Gynn, Thomas N. (ASCO), *M*, 664-5400
*Hahneman, Betty M. (ASCO), *M/HEM/ONC*, 542-2322
*Hendrickson, Frank R. (ARS, ASTR, SSO), *RT*, 942-5755
*Hindo, Walid A. (ASTR)
*Holinger, Paul H. (ASHNS), *OT*, 944-2972
Huggins, C. (AACR)
*Hugo, Norman E. (SHNS), *PLS*, 943-1614
*Hutchison, George B. (AACE, ASTR)
*Isaacs, Bertha L. (ASCO), *M/HEM*, 664-5400
Jacobson, L.O. (AACR)
*Kartha, Ponnunni K. (ASTR), *TR*, 942-5751
*Kearney, John J. (ARS)
*Khan, Fazlur R. (ASTR), *TR*, 878-8700, ext. 104
*Kirsten, Werner (AACE, AACR)
*Kline, Thornton C., Jr. (ASTR)
*Knospe, Wm. H. (ASCO), *M*, 942-5982

*Kolb, Leonard H. (AACE, AACR, ASCO), *S*, 641-2275
*Lee, Myung S. (ASTR)
*Loewy, Arthur (ASHNS), *OT*, 372-8543
*Louis, John (ASCO), *HEM*, 238-4410
*Lutterbeck, Eugene F. (ARS)
*Magalotti, Marion F. (ARS, ASTR), *RT/NM*
*Marks, James E. (ASTR)
*Mayer, Andrew (AACE, SSO)
*Mayorca, G. (AACR), 996-7473
*McDonald, G.O. (AACR), 384-4411
*McGrew, E.A. (AACR), 328-7682
**Medak, Herman (AACE)
*Millburn, Lowell F. (ASTR), *RO*
*Miree, James Jr. (ASTR), *R*, 664-6600, ext. 395
*Moran, Edgar M. (AACR, ASCO), *M/HEM*, 947-5012
*Mrazek, R.G. (AACE, AACR, SSO), *S*
*Nevinny, Hans B. (AACE, AACR, ASCO), *M*, 878-8700, ext. 171
Ovadia, Jacques (ASTR)
*Oyasu, R. (AACR), 649-3213
*Perez-Tamayo, Ruheri (ARS, ASTR), *RT*
*Perlia, Charles (AACR, ASCO, SSO), *M/MO*, 942-5906
*Perrin, Ward E. (AACE), *M,* 363-6800
*Renaud, Oliver V. (SHNS, SSO), *ONC/S*, 922-3201
*Robson, Martin C. (SHNS), *PLS*, 947-6965
*Sassoon, Harry (ASTR)
*Schmitz, Robert L. (AACE), *S/ONC*, 842-4700, ext. 505
Schreiber, H. (AACR)
Schweppe, J.S. (AACR)
*Shah, Mir. J. (ASTR), *TR*, 791-2510
*Shapiro, Charles M. (ASCO), *M/HEM*, 236-6730
*Sheth, Devdas N. (ASTR)
*Shirazi, Syed J.H. (ASTR)
*Sisson, George A. (SHNS, SSO)
*Skolnik, Emanuel M. (ASHNS), *OT/HNS*, 996-6905

*Slayton, Robert E. (ASCO), *M*, 942-5909
*Smith, Charles J. (SGO), *OG*, 567-2490
*Sobroff, Burton J. (ASHNS), *OT*, 332-0313
*Southwick, Harry W. (AACE, SHNS, SSO), *S*, 226-3647
**Stuteville, Orion H. (AACE)
Swerdlow, Martin (AACE)
*Taylor, Samuel G., III (AACR, ARS, ASCO, ASTR)
*Tenta, Louis T. (ASHNS), *OT*, 561-7348
*Thomas, Sydney F. (ASTR), *R*
*Tio, Liep T. (ASTR)
*Townsend, Darryl E.R. (ARS), *OG*, 996-7430
*Ultmann, John E. (ASCO), *HEM/M*, 947-6386
Vesselinovitch, S.D. (AACR)
*Wilbanks, George D., Jr. (ASCO, SGO), *OG*, 942-6380
Williams-Ashman, H.G. (AACR)
*Wissier, Robert (AACE)
Wolfe, L.G. (AACR)
*Wolter, Janet (AACR, ASCO), *M*, 942-5908
Yang, N.C. (AACR)

DE KALB

*Wiley, Darrell B. (SHNS), *S*

DECATUR (217)

*Locke, G. Richard (ASTR), *RT*, 877-8121

DES PLAINES (312)

*Britton, George T. (AACE), 298-7030

ELGIN (312)

*Morton, Douglas R. (ARS, SHNS, SSO), *S*, 741-3677

ELMHURST (312)

*Turner, James E. (ASTR), *R*,
833-1400

EVANSTON (312)

*Garces, Rafael M. (ASTR), *RT/NM*,
492-6520
Heller, P. (AACR)
*Scanlon, Edward F. (SHNS, SSO),
SO, 492-2000
Sebestyen, Paul S. (ASTR)

GRANITE CITY (618)

*Safdar, Shabbir H. (AACR, ASCO),
M/HEM, 876-1500

HARWOOD HEIGHTS

*Smoron, Geoffrey L. (ASTR)

HIGHLAND PARK

Schwartz, S.O. (AACR)

HINES (312)

*Eells, Richard W. (ASTR), *RT*,
261-6700
*Reyes, Efraim L. (ASTR)
Spencer, H. (AACR)
*Stefani, Stefano (ARS, ASCO,
ASTR), *RT/R*, 343-7200, ext. 2170

LAGRANGE

Tomisek, A.J. (AACR)

LAKE FOREST

Louis, J. (AACR)

LOMBARD (312)

*McCombs, Rollin K. (ASTR)
*Mehta, Yashbir (ARS, ASTR),
696-5490

MAYWOOD (312)

*Alconcia, Elpidio Y. (ASTR), *S/TR*,
531-3931
*Gatti, Wm. M. (ASHNS), *OT*,
531-3184
*Masterson, John G. (SGO), *OG*
**Toto, Patrick D. (AACE), *OP*

MOLINE

*Rathe, John (ASTR)

MORTON GROVE

*Ausman, Robert K. (AACR, ASCO),
S, 965-4700

NORTHBROOK

Goodheart, C.R. (AACR)

OAK PARK

*Grigg, E.R.N. (ARS), *R/NM*,
794-5649

PARK RIDGE (312)

*Abbate, Joseph S. (ASTR)
*Phillips, Richard L. (ARS, ASTR), *RT*,
696-2210, ext. 1674
*Staley, Charles J. (SHNS), *S*, 696-2201

PEORIA (309)

*Otten, John W. (SHNS), *S*, 674-1322
*Roberts, Stuart (ASCO, SSO), *S*,
673-5247
*Weigensberg, Irving J. (ARS, ASTR),
RT, 685-5623

RIVER FOREST (312)

*Liebner, Edwin (ARS, ASTR), *RT*,
966-6960
*Sinha, Birendra Kumar (SHNS),
S/ONC, 771-7590

ROCKFORD (815)

*Gilberti, Joseph J. (ASCO), *M*,
968-0051

SKOKIE (312)

*Isaacs, John H. (SGO, SSO), *O/G*,
673-3530

SPRINGFIELD (217)

*Myers, Phillip W. (ASHNS), *OT*,
522-8824
*Roddick, John W., Jr. (SGO, SSO),
O/G, 525-7502
*Stokes, Michael F. (ASTR), *RT*,
544-6464, ext. 537
*Stutz, Alan J. (ASTR)

URBANA (217)

*Neucks, Howard C. (ASTR), *R/RT*,
337-3311

WILLMETTE (312)

*Lochman, David J. (ARS, ASTR), *TR*,
883-6520

INDIANA

BLOOMINGTON (812)

*Robison, Roger F. (ASCO), *M/HEM*,
336-0119
Taylor, M.W. (AACR)

BLUFFTON (219)

*Graf, Russell, E. (ASTR), *R*,
824-3500

EVANSVILLE (812)

*Follis, Clifton Gene (ASTR), *TR*,
479-4429
*Hayes, Thomas P. (ASTR), *TR*,
426-3366

FORT WAYNE (219)

Gastineau, David C. (ASTR)
*Giffin, Charles S. (ASHNS), *OT*,
743-8117

INDIANAPOLIS (317)

*Baehner, Robert L. (ASCO), *PD*,
264-8784
*Bennett, James E. (SHNS), *PS*,
264-8106
*Bond, W.H. (AACR), 264-8346
Cavins, J.A. (AACR), 257-1049
*Dillon, John F. (ASTR), *RT*
Epstein, Sheldon M. (AACR)
*Geisler, Hans E. (SGO), *GO*,
359-4309
*Hornback, Ned. B. (ASTR)
*Johnson, Thomas W. (ASHNS), *OT*,
923-5441
*Katterjohn, James C. (ARS, ASTR,
SSO), *R*, 846-0600
*Lingeman, Raleigh E. (ASHNS), *OT*,
264-3582
*Morton, Joseph L. (ARS), *TR*,
741-3677
*Robbins, Lewis C. (SSO), *M*,
924-8494
*Rogers, Robert E. (SGO), *OG*
*Rohn, Robert (AACE, AACR,
ASCO)
Wagle, S.R. (AACR)
Weber, G. (AACR)
*Wong, Howard H. (ASTR)

KOKOMO (317)

*Tignor, Sterling P. (SHNS), *S*,
453-0802

IOWA

AMES (515)

*Blackburn, Charles M. (ASCO),
M/HEM, 292-2523

CEDAR RAPIDS (319)

*Hass, Curtis A. (ARS, ASTR), *R*, 366–5265

DES MOINES (515)

*Kaung, David T. (ASCO), *M/HEM*, 255–2173
*Maher, Louis L. (ASTR)
*Senty, Roger (AACE)
Song, J. (AACR)

GRIMES

Ross, C.A. (AACR)

IOWA CITY (319)

*Berg, John (SSO), *PATH*, 338–8159
*Brunk, S. Fred (AACE, ASCO), *M*, 356–2727
*Buchsbaum, Herbert J. (SGO), *OG*, 356–2294
*Burns, C. Patrick (AACR, ASCO), *M*, 356–2038
Corder, M.P. (AACR)
*Krause, Charles J. (ASHNS), *OT*, 356–3574
*Latourette, Howard B. (AACE, AACR, ARS, ASTR), *RT*, 356–2253
*Lawton, Richard L. (AACR, ASCO), *S*, 356–2003
Spector, A.A. (AACR)
*Tewfik, Hamed H. (ASTR), *TR*, 356–2253

SIOUX CITY (712)

*Leafstedt, Stuart W. (SHNS), *S/HNS/SO*, 252–3211
*Marriott, Charles M. (ASTR), *TR*, 279–2011

WATERLOO (319)

*Guthrie, Robert T. (ASTR), *TR*, 291–3473

KANSAS

HALSTEAD

*Welch, Jack (SHNS)

KANSAS CITY (913)

*Barth, R.F. (AACR), 831–5396
Dean, Richard D. (ASTR)
*Hartman, Gerald V. (ASTR), *RT*, 831–6815
*Hoogstraten, Barth (AACR, ASCO), *M*, 831–6028
*Humphrey, Loren J. (AACE, ASTR), *S*, 831–6101
*Jewell, Wm. R. (AACE, SHNS), *S*, 831–6112
*Larsen, Wm. (AACE), *M/HEM*, 831–6031
*Masters, Francis W. (SHNS), *PLS*, 831–6142
*Morrison, Richard A. (ASTR), *RT*, 831–6815
*Robison, David W. (SHNS), *S*
Schloerb, P.R. (AACR)
*Stephens, Ronald (ASCO), *M*, 831–6029
*Throne, Bennie J. (ASTR)

LEAWOOD

Laren, W.E. (AACR)

PRAIRIE VILLAGE

*Masterson, Byron Jack (SGO)

TOPEKA (913)

*Travis, John W. (ASTR), *TR*, 234–3451

WICHITA (316)

*Baumann, Paul A. (ASTR), *RT*, 685–2151
*Garfinkel, Lester S. (ASCO), *M/HEM*, 684–5213

*Hynes, Henry E. (ASCO), *M*,
262-3362
*Moore, Dennis Frederick (ASCO),
M/HEM, 267-6944
*Winchell, H.H. Forsyth (ASTR), *RT*,
262-6711, ext. 127

KENTUCKY

ASHLAND

*Roth, Oliver R. (ARS), *R*

FORT KNOX

*Tumbusch, Wilfred T. (SHNS)

LEXINGTON (606)

*Aliva, Jose A. (ASTR), *TR*
Chipps, H.D. (AACR), 278-1691
*Cronin, John D. (ASCO), *M*,
269-4568
*Harris, Walter D. (ASHNS), *OT*
*Maruyama, Yosh (AACR, ARS,
ASTR), *TR*, 233-5108
*Meeker, Wm. R., Jr. (AACE, AACR,
ASCO), *SO*, 233-6121
*Moore, Andrew M. (SHNS), *PLS*,
252-4406
**Rovin, Sheldon (AACE)
*Smith, Ralph A., Jr. (ASTR)
Sydnor, K.L. (AACR)
*Van Nagell, J.R., Jr. (AACR, ASCO),
G, 233-5553
*Vider, Manuel (ASTR), *RT/NM*,
233-6380

LOUISVILLE (502)

*Arena, Paul J. (ASCO), *M*, 897-0228
*Birkhead, Ben M. (ASTR)
*Burzynski, Norbert J. (AACE), *M*,
583-6681
*Conley, Joe (ASTR)
*Farnsley, Wesley (ARS, ASTR), *RT*,
637-8221
*Gray, Laman A. (SGO, SSO), *OG*,
587-0767

*Jacobson, Ahren (ASTR), *R*,
582-2211, ext. 541
*Knutson, Carl O. (AACE, SHNS), *S*,
582-2211, ext. 529
*Lowenbraun, Stanley (ASCO), *M*,
282-3735
*Makk, Laszlo (SSO)
*Moore, Condict (AACE, ARS, SHNS,
SSO), *S*, 582-2211, ext. 510
*Mullins, Fitzhugh (SHNS, SSO), *SO*,
585-4727
*Polk, Hiram C., Jr. (AACE, SSO), *S*,
583-5220
*Scott, Ralph M. (AACE, ARS, ASTR),
TR, 582-2211, ext. 541
*Tobin, Daniel A. (ASCO, ASTR),
TR/RO, 582-2211, ext. 541
*Utley, Joelia F. (ASTR)
Wallace, J.H. (AACR)
*Weiner, Leonard J. (SHNS), *PLS*

WINCHESTER

*Allen, Albert L. (ARS)

LOUISIANA

BATON ROUGE

*Joiner, D. Wayne (ASTR), *TR*

HOUMA

*Weatherall, Thomas J., Jr. (ASTR)

LAFAYETTE (318)

*Kraemer, Eugene A. (ASTR), *TR*
*Romagosa, Jerome J. (ASTR), *R*,
234-5261

METAIRE (504)

*Cohn, Isidore, Jr. (SSO), *S*,
527-8241

MONROE

*Green, Allan E., Jr. (ARS)

NEW ORLEANS (504)

*Bush, David J. (ASTR), *TR*,
   837-3000
*Cairns, Adrian B., Jr. (ASHNS), *OT*,
   486-5729
*Carter, Rebeca Devilene (ASCO), *S*,
   588-5351
Cohen, I., Jr. (AACR)
*Crapanzano, Joseph T. (SGO)
Dunlap, C.E. (AACR)
Gottieb, A.A. (AACR)
*Krementz, Edward T. (AACE, AACR,
   ASCO, SSO), *SO*, 588-5351
*Krupp, Philip J., Jr. (SGO), *GO*,
   588-5217
*Kuebler, Walter J. (ASCO, ASTR),
   RT/R, 899-3441, ext. 229
*Merlin, Carl S. (ASTR), *TR*,
   486-7483
*Mickal, Abe (SGO), *OG*, 527-8141
*Nelson, Norman C. (SHNS), *S*
*Ochsner, Seymour F. (ARS, ASTR)
**Odenheimer, Kurt John S. (AACE),
   OP, 947-9961, ext. 251
*Owens, Arthur (SHNS)
*Porter, George H. III (ASCO, SSO),
   HEM/MO, 834-7070, ext. 5671
*Ryan, R.F. (AACE, AACR, SHNS),
   PLS, 588-5347
*Segaloff, Albert (AACR, ASCO, SSO),
   M, 837-3000, ext. 5800
*Stuckey, Walter J. (AACE, ASCO),
   M/HEM/ONC, 588-5482
*Tabb, Harold G. (ASHNS), *OT*,
   588-5451
*Taylor, B. Gray (SHNS, SSO), *SO*,
   524-0811, ext. 334
*Tornyos, Karl (ASCO), *M/HEM*,
   534-0811
*Torres, Jose E. (SGO), *OG*, 527-8141
*Welsh, Ronald A. (AACE), *PATH*,
   527-5643

SHREVEPORT (318)

*Carroll, Wynton H. (ARS), *R*,
   422-1149

*Hendrick, John A. (SHNS), *S/HNS*,
   221-8521
*Quinn, Harold J., Jr. (ASHNS), *OT*,
   424-6686
Uzman, B.G. (AACR)

MAINE

AUBURN (207)

*Branch, C.F. (AACR), 782-7119

BAR HARBOR (207)

*Meier, H. (AACR), 288-3373
*Murphy, E.D. (AACR), 288-3721

CARIBOU (207)

*Siddiqui, Saleem A. (ASCO), *M*,
   498-8855

FAIRFIELD (207)

*Pratt, Loring W. (ASHNS), *OT*,
   453-6641

PORTLAND (207)

*Carroll, Ronald J. (AACE)
*Hahnemann, Howard J. (ASTR)
*Lowry, Wm. S. (ASTR)
*Phelps, Hugh M. (ASTR), *TR*,
   871-2276

SANFORD

*Ogden, Ralph T. (ARS)

WATERVILLE (207)

*Beckerman, Stanley C. (ASCO),
   M/MO, 873-4011

MARYLAND

ANNAPOLIS (301)

*Jones, Bryant L. (ASCO), *M*,
   757-4501

BALTIMORE (301)

*Abeloff, Martin (ASCO), *M*, 955-3300
*Allen, Willard M. (ARS)
*Anderson, Paul (AACR, ASCO), *M*, 955-3303
*Baker, E.R. (SHNS)
*Bang, F.B. (AACR), 955-3459
**Beckerman, Todd (AACE), *OP*, 528-7936
*Bell, James E. (AACE)
*Berman, Harry L. (ARS, ASTR), *R*, 367-7800, ext. 8767
*Brandes, D. (AACR), 323-4892
*Burke, Philip J. (AACR, ASCO), *M*, 955-3300
*Chambers, Robert G. (ARS, SHNS, SSO), *HNS*, 728-3645
Colvin, O.M. (AACR)
Elias, E.G. (AACR)
Firminger, H.I. (AACR)
Frost, J.K. (AACR)
Goodman, L.E. (AACR)
*Hazra, Tapan A. (ARS, ASTR), *TR*, 955-5622
*Hoopes, John E. (SHNS), *PLS*, 955-6431
*Inalsingh, Carol H.A. (ASTR), *RT*, 955-5622
*James, E. (ARS)
*Julian, Conrad G. (SGO)
Kessler, I.I. (AACR)
*Lenhard, Raymond E., Jr. (AACR, ASCO), *M*, 955-3300
ʻLevi, John Anthony (AACR, ASCO), *M*, 528-7394
Lewison, E.F. (AACR)
*Mardinwz, M.R., Jr. (AACR), 821-5660
*Order, Stanley E. (ARS, ASCO, ASTR), *RT*, 955-5622
*Owens, Albert H., Jr. (AACR, ASCO), *M*, 955-3300
*Peeples, Wm. J. (ASTR), *RT*
*Potchen, E. James (ARS), *R/NM*, 955-5757
*Prempree, Thongbliew (ASTR)
*Ramsey, Harold (SHNS, SSO), *SO*, 338-1100, ext. 268

*Santos, George W. (AACR, ASCO), *M*, 342-5400, ext. 1291
*Sanwalani, Shankar C. (ASTR)
Scott, W.W. (AACR)
Seligmann, A.A. (AACR)
*Sensenbrenner, Lyle L. (AACR, ASCO), 342-5400, ext. 1292
*Serpick, Arthur A. (AACR, ASCO), *M/HEM*, 685-0411
*Slawson, Robert G. (ASTR), *RT*, 528-6080
Sutherland, J.C. (AACR)
*Tepper, Marcos (ASTR)
Ts'o, P.O.P. (AACR)
Ulfohn, A. (AACR)
*Walker, Michael D. (ASCO), *NS*, 528-7518
*Weiner, Seymour (ASTR)
*Wiernik, Peter H. (AACR. ASCO), *M/PD*, 528-7912
Witten, B. (AACR)
*Woodruff, J. Donald (SGO), *OG*
*Woods, Alan C., Jr. (SHNS)

BELTSVILLE (301)

Baig, Mahmoodullah (ASCO), *M/MO*, 937-1467

BETHESDA (301)

*Appella, E. (AACR), 496-4549
Bailar, John C. (AACE)
*Beazley, Robert M. (SHNS), *S*, 496-1436
*Bender, R.A. (AACR), 476-4916
*Bono, V.H., Jr. (AACR), 496-3268
*Brace, Kirkland C. (ASTR)
*Brereton, H.D. (AACR), 496-5457
*Bull, Joan M.C. (ASCO), *M/ONC*, 496-4252
Cantarow, A. (AACR)
*Carbone, Paul P. (AACR, ASCO), *M/MO*, 496-4251
*Carter, Stephen K. (AACR, ASCO), *M*, 496-1196
*Chabner, Bruce Allan (AACR, ASCO), *M*, 496-4116

*Chretien, Paul B. (ARS, SHNS, SSO), S, 496-1574
Chu, E.W. (AACR), 496-6355
Cooney, D.A. (AACR)
**Corio, Russell L. (AACE)
Curreri, A.R. (AACR)
*Defries, Hugh (ASHNS, SHNS), OT, 295-0024
*Demoss, Ernest V. (SHNS, SSO), SO, 496-4001
*DeVita, Vincent (ASCO), M/HEM/ONC, 496-4291
*Edwards, Margaret H. (AACE)
*Egan, James W. (ASCO), M, 530-2244
*Fink, Diane J. (AACE, AACR, ASCO), M, 427-7996
Fink, M.A. (AACR)
*Fraumeni, Joseph F., Jr. (AACR, ASCO), M, 496-4947
Gallagher, R.E. (AACR)
Gallo, R.C. (AACR)
Gazdar, A.F. (AACR)
*Graw, Robert G., Jr. (AACR, ASCO), PD, 496-4514
Gullino, P.M. (AACR)
Haenszel, W.M. (AACR)
*Halterman, Roger H. (ASCO), M, 299-2743
Hampar, B. (AACR)
Harris, C.C. (AACR)
*Heller, J. R. (AACR, SSO), 496-1932
Herberman, R.B. (AACR)
*Herzig, Geoffrey P. (ASCO), M, 496-4514
*Hoye, Robert C. (ARS, ASCO, SHNS, SSO), S
Huebner, R.J. (AACR)
*Johnson, Ralph E. (ARS, ASTR), TR/ONC, 496-5457
Laquer, G.L. (AACR)
*Leventhal, Brigid Gray (AACR, ASCO), PD, 496-5007
*Levine, A.S. (ASCO), PD/HEM, 496-1543
Levine, P.H. (AACR)
*Levis, W.R. (AACR)
Lingeman, C.H. (AACR)

Love, R. (AACR)
*MaGrath, Ian Trevor (ASCO, ASCR), M, 496-1543
*McIntire, K.R. (AACR), 496-3310
*Mercado, Raul (ARS, ASTR), R, 427-7477
*Mider, G. Burroughs (SSO), PATH
*Mironescu, S. (AACR), 530-6040
*Mushinski, J.F. (AACR), 496-5260
*Newell, Guy Rene, Jr. (AACR, ASCO), M, 496-3505
*O'Conor, G.T. (AACR), 496-1933
*Perry, Seymour (ASCO), M/HEM/ONC, 496-2500
*Pomeroy, Thomas C. (ASCO, ASTR), TR/R, 496-5457
*Potter, M. (AACR), 496-2777
*Rabson, A.S. (AACR), 496-4346
*Rhim, J.S. (AACR), 654-3400
*Saffiotti, U. (AACR), 496-5591
*Schein, Philip S. (AACR, ASCO), M/ONC/HEM, 496-4916
*Schoenberg, B.S. (AACR), 496-1611
*Sears, Mary A. (AACR, ASCO), M, 496-6718
*Shackney, Stanley E. (AACR, ASCO), M, 496-2163
*Slavik, Milan (AACR, ASCO), M, 496-1196
*Sloan, Margaret H. (AACE, ASCO, SSO), 427-8081
*Spatz, M. (AACR) 496-6231
*Sporn, M.B. (AACR) 496-5391
*Stephenson, Richard (SSO)
*Stewart, Sarah (SSO)
*Stromberg, K. (AACR), 496-6970
Taylor, D.J. (AACR), 496-6718
*Terry, W.D. (AACR), 496-5461
*Thomas, L.B. (AACR, SSO), PATH, 496-3185
*Thompson, E.I. (AACR), 496-4561
*Ting, C.C. (AACR), 496-2343
*Tormey, Douglass C. (AACR, ASCO), M, 496-1547
Uphoff, D.E. (AACR), 496-1232
Venditti, J.M. (AACR), 427-7334
Vernon, M.L. (AACR), 654-3400
*Vollmer, E.P. (AACR)

*Waalkes, P.T. (AACR, ASCO)
Weisburger, E.K. (AACR), 496-5688
White, F.R. (AACR), 427-7328
*Whitlock, J.P. (AACR), 496-6934
Whitmire, C.E. (AACR), 654-3400
*Wilson, S.H. (AACR), 496-2745
Wood, H.B., Jr. (AACR), 427-7390
Woodman, R.J. (AACR), 654-3400
*Wu, A.M.T. (AACR), 881-5600
Yamamoto, R.S. (AACR), 496-4366
Yang, S.S. (AACR), 496-4366
*Yarbro, John W. (AACE, ASCO,
  SSO), *M*, 496-7427
Young, D.M. (AACR), 496-5433
*Yuspa, S.H. (AACR), 496-5211
*Ziegler, John L. (AACR, ASCO),
  M, 456-4256

CHEVY CHASE (202)

*Mostofi, F.K. (AACR), 576-2961

COLUMBIA

Reuber, M.D. (AACR)

FREDERICK (301)

*Bates, R.R. (AACR) 663-3162

HEMPSTEAD (301)

*Cox, Everard F. (AACE, SHNS, SSO),
  S, 239-8276

IJAMSVILLE

Waravdekar, Vaman S. (AACR)

KENSINGTON (301)

*Lee, Lyndon E., Jr. (ASCO), *S*,
  942-5875
Wallen, W.C. (AACR)

LAUREL (301)

*Matias, Pedro I. (ASCO), *M*, 725-5600

POTOMAC (301)

*Halterman, Roger H. (AACR, ASCO),
  M, 299-2743
*Young, Robert C. (AACR, ASCO),
  M/HEM, 299-4782

ROCKVILLE (301)

*Baker, C.G. (AACR), 443-6237
*Ross, Wm. L., Jr. (SSO)
Stewart, H.L. (AACR)
Ting, R.C.Y. (AACR)
Vadlamudi, S. (AACR)
*Waalkes, Phillip T. (ASCO)
*Whittington, Richard (ASCO),
  M/HEM, 389-5137
Wyckoff, Harold O. (ASTR)

SILVER SPRINGS (301)

Amoroso, Wm. L. (SHNS, SSO), *S*,
  681-7775
Dennis, Lewis H. (AACR, ASCO)
Gold, G. Lennard (AACR, ASCO)
*Levin, Edgar (ASCO), *M/HEM*,
  588-2525

MASSACHUSETTS

ARLINGTON (617)

*Charrette, Edmond E. (AACE, ASCO),
  M/MO, 648-4343

BELMONT (617)

*Mueller, H. Peter (ARS), *R*, 484-3194

BOSTON (617)

*Abelson, H. (AACR)
*Abrams, H.L. (AACR)
*Aisenberg, Alan C. (AACR, ASCO), *M*,
  726-3677
*Alarcon, R.A. (AACR) 734-7000
Alpert, E. (AACR) 726-3766
*Amick, Robert M. (ASCO), *M/ONC*,
  522-5359

*Anglem, Thomas (SHNS, SSO), *S*, 277-8490

*Baker, Wm. H. (AACR, ASCO), *M*, 742-1337

*Beck, W.S. (AACR) 726-3760

*Belli, James (ASTR)

*Berman, L.D. (AACR), 232-9500

*Biano, Giacomino (AACR, ASCO), *ONC/HEM*, 734-6000, ext. 3389

*Binder, Sheldon C. (SHNS), *S*, 482-3800

*Bloedorn, Fernando (ARS, ASTR), *TR*, 482-2800, ext. 2501

*Boyer, Arthur Lonnie (ASTR)

Bucker, N.L.R. (AACR)

*Buell, D.N. (AACR) 734-6000

*Burstein, N.A. (AACR) 734-4400

*Cady, Blake (SHNS, SSO), *S*, 262-4900, ext. 218

*Camitta, Bruce M. (AACR, ASCO), *PD*, 734-6000

*Carey, Robert W. (ASCO), *M/ONC/HEM*, 525-2515

*Cassady, James Robert (ASCO, ASTR), *RT*, 734-3300, ext. 355

Chaffey, John T. (ASTR), *TR*, 734-8000

Chawla, Prem L. (ASCO), *M/HEM*, 872-4301

Choi, Chan H. (ASTR)

Chu, Ann M. (ASTR)

*Cohen, Joseph L. (AACE, ASCO), *M*, 522-8400

*Costanza, Mary E. (AACR, ASCO), *M*, 482-2800, ext. 2638

*Cummings, Charles W. (ASHNS, SHNS), *OT*, 523-0280

*Dealy, James Bond, Jr. (ARS), *R*, 522-8110, ext. 365

Deckers, P.J. (AACR)

Diamandopoulos, G.T. (AACR)

*Elkort, Richard J. (AACE)

*Evjy, Jack T. (AACE, ASCO), *M*, 262-4200, ext. 5821

*Feldman, Merrill I. (ASTR), *TR*, 252-4200, ext. 5772

*Finkel, Harvey E. (ASCO), *M/HEM*, 262-4200, ext. 5821

*Frei, Emil, III (ASCO, SSO), *M*, 734-6000

*Gallitano, Alphonse (AACE, ASCO), *SO*, 894-0097

*Galvin, James M. (ASTR)

Gates, O. (AACR)

*Geiser, Clementina F. (AACR, ASCO), *PD-ONC*, 734-6000

Goitein, Michael (ASTR) 726-8153

Goldhaber, P. (AACR)

*Goodman, Robert L. (ASCO), *RT*, 734-4400, ext. 2345

*Guralnick, Walter C. (AACE)

*Harris, Melvyn H. (AACE)

*Hegener, Diane H. (ASCO, ASTR), *RT/R*

*Hellman, Samuel P. (AACR, ARS, ASCO, ASTR), *RT*, 734-3300, ext. 355

Henshaw, E.C. (AACR)

*Herbst, Arthur L. (SGO), *OG*

Hiatt, H.H. (AACR)

*Hoar, Carl S., Jr. (SHNS), *S*, 227-2463

*Jaffe, Norman (AACR, ASCO), *PD*, 734-6000

Kasdon, S.C. (AACR)

*Kaufman, Sheldon (ASCO), *MO*, 726-8689

*Kelley, Rita M. (AACR, ASCO), *M*, 726-2000

*King, George D. (ASHNS), *OT/PLS*, 262-4900

Knox, W.E. (AACR)

*Kondi, Edward S. (AACE, ASCO), *S*, 262-4200, ext. 5893

Krant, M.J. (AACR), *MO*, 522-8400

*Levene, Martin B. (ARS, ASTR), *RT*, 734-4400, ext. 234

Li, Frederick P. (AACR, ASCO), *M*, 734-6000, ext. 3137

Lisco, H. (AACR)

Little, J.B. (AACR)

*Lofgren, Robert H. (ASHNS), *OT*, 523-0280

*Malt, R.A. (AACR) 726-2821

*Mannick, J.A. (AACR)

*Marchant, Douglas J. (ARS, SGO)
*Marck, Abraham (ASTR), *RT*
*McLaughlin, A.P., III (AACR)
  734-8000
*Mendiondo, Oscar A. (ASTR), *TR*,
  726-3080
*Merrill, Keith, Jr. (AACE, ASTR)
*Miller, Daniel (ASHNS), *OT*,
  232-3432
*Mitchell, George W., Jr. (SGO),
  OG
*Moloney, Wm. C. (AACR, ASCO),
  M/HEM, 734-5112
*Moolten, F.L. (AACR) (205) 917-3442
*Montgomery, Wm. W. (ASHNS), *OT*,
  523-7900
*Mozden, Peter J. (AACE, ASCO),
  S/ONC, 262-4200, ext. 5506
*Mukherji, Bijay (AACR, ASCO), *M*,
  482-2800, ext. 2638
*Munzenrider, John E. (ASTR), *TR*,
  482-2800, ext. 2501
*Murray, Joseph E. (SHNS), *PLS*,
  734-6000
*Nardi, George L. (SSO)
*Nathan, David G. (AACR, ASCO),
  PD, 734-6000, ext. 3471
*Nathanson, Larry (AACE, AACR,
  ASCO, SSO), *M*, 482-2800,
  ext. 2638
Necheles, Thomas F. (ASCO), *PD*,
  482-2800, ext. 2253
*Oberfield, Richard A. (AACE, AACR,
  ASCO, SSO), *M/ONC*, 262-4900,
  ext. 454
*Piro, Anthony J. (AACR, ASCO,
  ASTR), *M/RT*, 734-3300, ext. 355
*Prout, George R., Jr. (SSO), *U*,
  726-3010
*Reynolds, Charles T. (SHNS, SSO),
  S/ONC, 277-0715
*Rogers, Wm. P., Jr. (SHNS, SSO),
  S, 523-3812
*Rudders, Richard A. (ASCO),
  HEM/M, 482-2800
*Rutenburg, Alexander M. (AACE),
  S, 262-4200, ext. 6305
*Ryser, H.J.P. (AACR) 262-4200

*Salzman, Ferdinand A. (ARS, ASTR),
  RT, 264-4900, ext. 376
*Scher, C.D. (AACR) 734-6000
*Schilling, Albert (AACR, ASCO),
  M, 262-4200, ext. 5675
*Schulz, Milford D. (ARS, ASCO,
  ASTR), *RT*, 726-3082
*Scott, J.F. (AACR) 726-3673
*Scully, Robert E. (SCO), *PATH*,
  696-6526
*Sewall, Warren (ASTR)
*Shipley, W.U. (AACR, ASTR),
  726-8153
**Shklar, Gerald (AACE)
*Skarin, Arthur (AACR, ASCO),
  M/HEM/ONC, 734-6000, ext. 3381
*Smith, R.W. (AACR)
*Straus, Marc J. (AACR, ASCO), *M*,
  262-4200, ext. 5331
*Strome, Marshall (ASHNS), *OT*,
  734-4492
*Strong, M.S. (ASHNS, SHNS), *OT*,
  424-5526
*Suit, Herman D. (ARS, ASTR)
*Taft, E.B. (AACR) 726-3653
*Tepper, Joel (ASTR)
*Tevethia, S.S. (AACR) 423-4600
*Ucmakli, Alptekin (ASTR), *TR*,
  482-2800, ext. 2501
*Ulfelder, Howard (SGO), *S/G*,
  726-3001
*Vallee, B.L. (AACR)
*Vaughn, Charles (SHNS)
*Wallach, D.F.H. (AACR) 482-2800
*Wang, Chiu-Chen (ARS, ASTR),
  RT, 726-3081
*Warren, S. (AACR) 734-7000
*Watkins, Elton, Jr. (AACR, ASCO), *S*
  277-8777
*Weiner, R.S. (AACR) 734-6000
*Whelton, James (SSO), *OG/ONC*,
  782-7000
*Wotiz, H.H. (AACR) 262-4200
*Yankee, Ronald A. (AACR, ASCO),
  M, 734-6000, ext. 3145
*Yerganian, G. (AACR) 739-1100
*Zamcheck, Norman (AACR, ASCO),
  GE/M, 536-4746

BREWSTER

*Daland, Ernest M. (SHNS), *S*

BRIGHTON

*O'Brien, Richard G. (ASCO)

BROOKLINE (617)

*Goldstein, Michael (ASCO), *M*,
  232-6350
*Griffiths, Charles T. (ASCO, SGO),
  G, 734-6200
*Knapp, Robert C. (ARS, ASCO), *OG*,
  734-6763
*Lenson, Norman (SSO)
*Nelson, Diana F. (ASTR)
*Parsons, Langdon (SSO)
*Rutenberg, A.M. (AACR), *S*,
  262-4200, ext. 6305
*Schwartz, R.S. (AACR)

CAMBRIDGE (617)

Homburger, F. (AACR)
Kensler, R.M. (AACR)
Trump, John G. (ARS) 253-2592
Wodinsky, I. (AACR)
Wogan, G.N. (AACR)
*Wolfort, Francis G. (SHNS),
  PLS/S, 734-3372
Yesair, D.W. (AACR)

CONCORD (617)

*Barrie, Joseph R. (SSO), *S*,
  369-4468

DEDHAM (617)

*De Loca, Arthur L., Jr. (ASCO),
  M, 329-1400

FALL RIVER (617)

*Derechin, Michael M. (ASCO),
  M, 676-3411

GLOUCESTER

*O'Donnell, Walter E. (SSO)

HINGHAM (617)

*Samaha, Richard J. (ASCO), *M*,
  749-5275

JAMAICA PLAIN (617)

Geiser, C.F. (AACR, ASCO), *PD*,
  734-6000
*Krant, Melvin J. (AACE, ASCO),
  MO, 522-8400
*Ross, Winifred M. (ARS, ASTR),
  OG/TR

LONGMEADOW (413)

*Lewin, Isaac (AACR, ASCO),
  M/MO, 567-0738

LYNN (617)

*Bargoot, Ferris John, Jr. (ASTR), *TR*,
  598-5100, ext. 352
*Tobin, Lester H. (ASCO), *M/ONC*,
  599-5860
*Willett, Bernard L. (SSO)

MILTON (617)

*Toch, R. (AACR) 698-0717

NATICK (617)

*Jao, John Y.C. (ASCO), *M/MO*,
  655-5577
Wharton, D.R.A. (AACR)

NEEDHAM (617)

*Lawrence, Knowles B. (SHNS), *S*,
  444-1541
*Lokich, Jacob J. (ASCO), *M/HEM*,
  449-1183

NEWTON (617)

*Choi, Ock Soon (ASCO), *M*,
  527–4872
*Weiss, Donald R. (ASTR)

NEWTON LOWER FL. (617)

*Garcelon, Gerald G. (SHNS), *S*,
  527–3450

NORTHBOROUGH

Greenfield, R.E., Jr. (AACR)

PORTLAND

*Briggs, Russell C. (ASTR)

REHOBOTH

Werthessen, N.T. (AACR)

SPRINGFIELD (413)

*DeConti, Ronald C. (AACR, ASCO),
  M, 787–3368
*Hoovis, Marvin L. (AACE, AACR,
  ASCO), *M/MO*, 878–3676
*Stein, Robert A. (ASTR)
*Stevens, Walton E. (ARS, ASTR),
  R/TR

WALPOLE (617)

Apffel, C.A. (AACR)
*Stolbach, Leo L. (AACE, AACR,
  ASCO), *M*, 762–6837
*Yatsuhashi, Masao (AACE)

WELLESLEY (617)

*Bloomer, Wm. D. (ASTR), *RT*,
  734–3300
*Stetson, Charles G. (ARS, ASTR,
  SSO)
*Weber, Eric T. (ASTR)

WEST NEWTON (617)

*Towbin, A. (AACR) 527–5850

WESTON (617)

*Canellos, George P. (AACR, ASCO),
  M, 237–1835

WORCESTER (617)

*Friedell, Gilbert H. (AACR, ASCO,
  SSO), *PATH*, 798–6044
*Gacek, Richard R. (ASHNS), *OT*,
  856–3111
*Meltzer, Adolph (SSO), *S*, 752–5470
*Zamansky, Marshall J. (ASHNS), *OT*,
  791–6305

MICHIGAN

ALLEN PARK (313)

*Thornhill, Joseph E. (ASTR)
*Weaver, Arthur W. (SHNS), *S/HNS*,
  832–2444

ANN ARBOR (313)

*Aye, Maung S. (ASTR), *TR*, 764–3270
*Beierwaltes, W.H. (AACR) 764–1302
*Bull, Frances E. (ASCO), *M/HEM-ONC*
  764–2217
*Campos, Jose L. (ASTR)
**Courtney, Richard M. (AACE),
  OP, 764–1535
*Dabich, Lyubica (ASCO), *M/HEM*,
  764–8103
*Fayos, Juan V. (ARS, ASCO, ASTR),
  TR, 764–3272
*Heyn, Ruth M. (ASCO), *M/HEM*,
  764–7126
*Hiss, Ronald Graham (ASCO), *M*,
  763–0200
*Kass, Lawrence (ASCO), *M*, 764–2217
**Kerr, Donald A. (AACE)
*Lampe, Isadore (ARS, ASTR)
*Lim, Chiu-Guat (ASCO), *M*, 663–0476
*Morley, George W. (SGO), *OG*,
  764–8125
*Penner, John A. (ASCO), *M*, 764–2237
*Pollard, H. Marvin (SSO), *M/GE*,
  764–4166
Pratt, W.B. (AACR)

**Rowe, Nathaniel H. (AACE), *OP*,
763-0145
*Votaw, May L. (ASCO), *M/HEM*,
764-8105
Wu, C. (AACR)
*Zarafonetis, Chris J. (ASCO), *M/HEM*,
764-8100

BAY CITY (517)

*Grigg, John W. (ASHNS), *OT*,
892-3541

BIRMINGHAM

*Corrigan, Kenneth E. (ASTR)

DEARBORN (313)

*Berkas, Ernest M. (SHNS), *S*,
565-7710
*Signori, Enrique E. (ASCO), *M/HEM*,
277-7800

DETROIT (313)

*Albert, S. (AACR) 833-0710
*Al-Saraf, Muhyi (ASCO), *M*,
494-6232
*Arenas, Bueno Ildefonso (ASTR)
*Baker, Laurence H. (AACE),
494-6418
*Beekhuls, G. Jan (ASHNS), *OT*,
872-1350
*Binns, Philip M. (ASHNS), *HNS*
*Block, Melvin A. (SHNS), *S*, 876-3031
*Boles, Murray (ASTR), *TR*, 876-1021
*Boyce, Charles R. (SGO), *OG*,
494-7286
*Brennan, Michael J. (AACR, ASCO,
SSO), *M/ONC*, 833-0710
*Brownlee, Robert W. (ASCO), *HEM*,
876-1841
*Chang, Hang Soon (ASTR), *TR*,
272-6000
*Considine, Basil, Jr. (ASTR)
*Cook, Carla A. (ASTR), *RT*, 876-1021
*Cook, James C. (ARS, ASTR), *TR*,
494-8401

*Dickson, Basil R. (ARS)
*Drukker, Bruce H. (ASCO), *G*,
876-2464
*Fisher, George (ASCO), *M/HEM*,
963-4313
*France, Charles J. (SHNS, SSO), *S*
*Gatesi, Roman A. (ASCO), *M/NM*,
876-1848
*Gulick, Arthur E. (ASTR)
Harkness, Stuart F. (AACE)
*Hasley, Clyde K. (ARS), *R*,
823-3389
Izbicki, Ronald (ASCO), *M*, 494-6234
*Kambouris, Angleos (SSO)
*Kopple, Eugene A. (ASTR), *RO/TR*,
869-1200, ext. 402
*Krabbenhoft, Kenneth L. (ARS)
*Leucutia, Train (ASTR)
*Mattes, Max W. (ARS), *R*, 273-4582
*Perrotta, Augustine L. (ASCO),
M/HEM, 869-1080
*Perry, Harold (ARS, ASTR), *TR*,
272-6000, ext. 8591
*Rachmaninoff, Nikolai (SSO)
*Reed, Melvin (AACR, ASCO), *M*,
494-6232
*Royer, Richard R. (ASHNS), *OT*,
885-6800
*Ruble, Paul E. (ASCO), *M*, 494-8213
*Saltzstein, Harry C. (SHNS, SSO)
*Scheer, Alan Clark (ARS, ASTR),
TR, 965-1200
*Sexon-Porte, Maria E. (ASCO), *M*,
494-6232
*Sherman, Alfred I. (ARS, SGO), *OG*
*Singhakowinta, A. (ASCO), *M*,
831-1111
*Sorock, Milton (SHNS)
*Stobbe, Godfrey D. (SSO), *PATH*,
494-6313
Talley, Robert W. (AACR, ASCO),
M/ONC, 876-1846
*Vaitkevicius, V.K. (AACE, AACR,
ASCO, SSO), *M/ONC*, 494-6204
*Vandenberg, Henry John, Jr. (SHNS,
SSO), *S*, 833-3680
*White, Joel E. (ASTR), *TR*, 876-1021
*Zack, Burton Jay (SHNS), *S*,
272-4670

EAST DETROIT (313)

*Betanzos, Guillermo (ASCO), *M/ONC*, 779-3400

EAST LANSING (517)

*Dimitrov, N.V. (AACR, ASCO), *M*, 355-1855
*Welsch, C.W. (AACR) 353-4549

FLINT (313)

*Dodds, Max (SHNS, SSO), *S*, 234-5663
*Dwyer, Wm. F. (SSO)
*Kelly, James E. (ASCO), *M*, 373-4303
*Phillips, Alan F. (ARS, ASTR), *RT*, 232-1161, ext. 405

FRANKLIN

*Wang, Chun-Heng H. (ASTR), *TR*

GRAND RAPIDS (616)

*Borst, James R. (ASCO), *M*, 949-5260
*Gillies, Robert W. (ASTR)
*Helmus, Christian (ASHNS), *OT/HNS*, 459-4514
*Jubert, Andre V. (AACE, ASCO), *S*, 774-6384
*Moorehead, Edward L. II (AACE, ASCO), *M/MO*, 949-5260
*San Diego, Emiliana L. (ASCO) 949-5260

GROSSE POINTE (313)

*Burrows, John H. (ASCO), *M*, 885-5932
*Coello, Eudoro (ASCO), *M*, 855-5932
*O'Bryan, Robert M. (ASCO), *M*, 881-4385

HIGHLAND PARK (313)

*DeMattia, Michael D. (AACE, ASCO), *M*, 869-1080
*Opipari, Michael I. (ASCO), *M/MO*, 869-1080

JACKSON (601)

*Shands, Wilbourn C. (SHNS, SSO) 948-1411

KALAMAZOO (616)

*Antemann, Richard W. (ASTR)
*Crest, Clarence P. (ARS)
*Dolan, James R. (ASTR), *TR*, 381-5412
*Hildreth, R.C. (ARS)
*Simons, Charles S. (ASTR) 381-2920
*Tucker, Wm. (ASCO), *M/ONC*, 382-4062
*Wechter, W.J. (AACR) 385-7100

MONROE

Pinkus, H. (AACR)

OAK PARK

Lattin, Paul B. (ASTR)
*Erich, John B. (SHNS)

ROYAL OAK

*Bloor, Robert J. (ARS, ASCO, ASTR), *RT*, 549-7000, ext. 467
*Mahrt, Delmar H. (ASTR), *TR*, 549-7000
*Poulik, M.D. (AACR) 549-7000

SAGINAW

*Campbell, Lloyd A. (ASCO)

SOUTHFIELD (313)

*Chen, Shek (ARS, ASTR), *R*, 414-3321

*Vaughn, Clarence (ASCO), *M*,
424-3341
*Wilner, Freeman M. (ASCO), *HEM*,
358-5560
*Young, Shun S. (SHNS), *S/HNS*,
557-5717

MINNESOTA

DULUTH

Lenta, M.P. (AACR)

EDINA (612)

*O'Brien, Wm. A. (ASCO), *M/HEM/
ONC/NM*, 941-2453

MINNEAPOLIS (612)

*Allen, David W. (AACR, ASCO),
M/HEM/ONC, 725-6767
*Arhelger, Stuart W. (SHNS)
*Benjamin, Robert B. (SHNS),
S/HNS, 927-3180
*Bloomfield, Clara S. (AACR, ASCO),
M, 373-4320
*Brown, John H. (ASCO), *MO*,
927-3248
*Brunning, R.D. (AACR) 373-8557
*Fallon, Virgil T. (ASTR)
*Farley, Harrison H. (SHNS), *S*
*Fortuny, Ignacio E. (AACR, ASCO),
M, 373-4309
*Fraley, E.E. (AACR)
Frantz, I.D., Jr. (AACR)
*Goudsmit, Arnoldus (ASCO), *M*,
725-6767, ext. 6440
*Grage, Theodor B. (AACE, ASCO,
SHNS), *S*, 373-4308
*Green, Robert A. (ASCO), *M*,
927-3123
Gutmann, H.R. (AACR), *R*, 579-8494
Halberg, F. (AACR)
Hebbel, R. (AACR)
*Hedrick, Wm. L. (ASCO), *M*,
339-9786

*Hoffman, Neil Robert (ASCO),
M/ONC, 333-7215
*Jones, Thomas K. (ASTR), *TR*,
373-8680
*Kelly, John (ASTR), *R*, (218)
335-6595
*Kennedy, B.J. (AACE, AACR, ASCO,
SSO), *M/ONC*, 373-4303
Kersey, J.H. (AACR)
*Kiang, David Teh-Ming (AACR,
ASCO), *M/ONC*, 373-5870
*Kremen, Arnold J. (SHNS), *S*,
335-7851
*Kuisk, Hans (ASTR), *TR*, 725-6767,
ext. 6504
Levitan, Alexander Allen (ASCO),
MO, 788-9749
*Levitt, Seymour H. (ARS, ASTR),
TR, 373-8680
*Mathog, Robert H. (ASHNS), *OT*,
373-8846
*McKhann, C.F. (AACR), *S*, 373-7733
*McQuarrie, Donald G. (SHNS), *S*,
725-6767, ext. 6460
*Mosser, Donn G. (ASTR), *RO*,
335-6595
*Murray, Charles L. (ASCO), *MO*,
927-3123
*Nesbit, Mark E., Jr. (AACE, ASCO),
PD, 373-4318
*Prem, Ronald A. (SGO), *GO*, 373-8854
*Reynolds, James F. (ASCO), *M*,
941-3473
*Schwartz, S. (AACR) 376-3690
*Sher, N.A. (AACR) 373-5393
*Simmons, Richard L. (AACR, ASCO),
S, 373-8196
*Singher, Lawrence J. (ASCO), *PD*,
825-1626
*Smith, David G. (ASTR), *TR*
*Theologides, Athanasios (AACR,
ASCO, *M*, 373-4315
**Vickers, Robert (AACE), *OP*,
373-4858
*Vince, R. (AACR) 373-2185
*Vosika, G.J. (AACR), *M*,
373-4309
*Wattenburg, L.W. (AACR) 373-2808

ROCHESTER (507)

*Ahmann, David L. (AACR, ASCO), *MO/M*, 288-9386
*Beahrs, Oliver H. (SHNS, SSO), *HNS/S* 282-2511
*Bisel, Harry F. (AACE, AACR, ASCO, SSO), *MO*, 282-2511
*Burgert, E. Omer, Jr. (AACR, ASCO), *PD/HEM/ONC*, 282-2511
*Carr, David T. (SSO)
*Childs, Donald S., Jr. (AACR, ARS, ASCO, ASTR), *RT*, 282-2511
*Colby, Malcolm Y., Jr. (ARS, ASTR), *TR*
Creagan, E.T. (AACR)
*Cupps, Roger E. (ASTR)
*Decker, David G. (ARS, SGO), *OG*, 282-2511, ext. 2033
*Desanto, Lawrence W. (ASHNS), *OT*, 282-2511
*Devine, Kenneth D. (SHNS), *HNS*, 282-2511
Eagan, Robert T. (AACR, ASCO), *M*, 282-2511
*Edmonson, John H. (AACR, ASCO)
*Fricke, Robert E. (ARS, ASTR), *M/MO*, 282-2511
Gilchrist, Gerald S. (ASCO), *PD*, 282-2511
Go, V.L. (AACR)
*Hahn, Richard G. (ASCO), *M*, 282-2511
*Hayles, Alvin B. (SHNS), *PD*, 282-2511
*Holbrook, Margaret A. (ASTR), *TR*, 282-2511
*Jorgensen, Edward O. (ASCO), *OG*, 282-2511
*Kiely, Joseph M. (AACR, ASCO), *HEM/ONC*, 282-2511
*Kyle, Robert A. (AACR, ASCO), *M/HEM*, 282-2511
*Lee, Robert E. (ARS, ASTR), *R*
*Maldonado, Jorge (AACR, ASCO), *M/HEM*, 282-2511
*Malkasian, George (ARS)
*Masson, James K. (SHNS), *PLS*, 282-2511
*Moertel, Charles G. (ASCO)

O'Connell, Michael J. (ASCO), *M*, 282-2511, ext. 3903
*Pritchard, D.J. (AACR), *ONC*
*Reitemeier, Richard J. (ASCO), *M/GE*, 282-2511
*Remine, Wm. H. (SHNS), *S*, 282-2511
*Ritts, R.E., Jr. (AACR) 282-2511
*Scanlon, Paul W. (AACR, ARS, ASCO, ASTR), *TR*, 282-2511
*Schutt, Allan J. (AACR, ASCO), *M/GE/ONC*, 282-2511
*Silverstein, Murray N. (AACR, ASCO), *M/HEM*, 282-2511
*Symmonds, Richard E. (SGO), *OG*, 282-2511
*Van Herik, Martin (ARS, ASTR), *TR*, 282-2511
*Williams, Marvin (ARS, ASTR), *R*, 289-6424
*Williams, Tiffany J. (SGO), *OG*, 282-2511
*Woolner, Lewis B. (SHNS), *PATH*, 282-2511

ST. PAUL (612)

*Hilger, Jerome A. (ASHNS), *OT*, 645-0691
*Lerner, Irving J. (ASCO), *M*, 229-2378
*Taddeini, Luigi (ASCO), *M*
*Veinbergs, Arnolds (ASTR), *RT*, 291-3111
*Ytredal, Duane O. (ASTR), *TR* ·

MISSISSIPPI

HATTIESBURG (601)

*Owen, David McIntosh (ASCO), *M*, 544-0511

JACKSON (601)

*Boronow, Richard C. (ARS, SGO, SSO), *OG*, 362-4411
*Deraps, Gordon D. (AACE), *M/HEM-ONC*, 362-4411, ext. 2551
*Evers, Carl G. (AACE)
**Finch, Robert R. (AACE), *OP*
*Hickman, B.T. (ARS, ASTR)

*Jabaley, Michael E. (SHNS), *PLS*,
362–4411, ext. 2366
*Lockey, Myron W. (ASHNS), *OT*,
362–8663
*Morrison, Francis S. (AACE, ASCO),
M, 362–4411
Randall, C.C. (AACR)
Williams, W.L. (AACR)

KESSLER AFB (601)

*Spigel, Stuart Charles (ASCO),
M/ONC, 377–6362

MISSOURI

COLUMBIA (314)

*Amlinger, Philip R. (ASTR), *TR*
*Candy, Nestor Rabe (ASTR), *R*
Carolla, Robert Louis (ASCO), *M*,
882–6163
*Corwin, Louis A., Jr. (ASTR),
VETR, 882–2846
*Donegan, Wm. L. (AACE, SHNS)
Farrell, C. (AACR)
*Glass, Robert L. (SHNS)
*Harris, Hugh S., Jr. (SHNS), *S*,
449–6466
*Henry, Patrick H. (AACR, ASCO),
M/HEM-ONC, 882–6163
Hopps, H.C. (AACR)
*Mengel, Charles L. (ASTR)
*Paig, Camilo U. (ASTR), *TR*,
443–3103
*Perez-Mesa, Carlos (ASTR)
*Schewe, Elmer J., Jr. (SHNS), *S*,
443–8773
*Spratt, John S., Jr. (SHNS, SSO), *SO*,
443–3101, ext. 274
*Thomson, James M., Jr. (ARS, ASTR),
TR
Watson, F.R. (AACR) 443–3103
Wood, R. (AACR) 882–2229

CREVE COEUR

*Kumar, Bharath (ASTR)

FARMINGTON

*Hoye, Robert C. (ASCO, ARS, SSO,
SHNS), *S*, 756–6751

KANSAS CITY (816)

*Beckloff, Gerald L. (ASCO) 761–2500
*Berry, Neill (SHNS, SSO), *S*
*Cowan, George A. (AACE, ASTR)
Hall, L. Raymond (AACE), *M*,
283–2000
*Miles, George O. (SHNS, SSO), *S*,
931–4443
*Rector, Joe Lee, Jr. (ASTR), *RT*,
932–2572
*Smith, Arthur B. (ARS), *R*, 523–2400

KIRKSVILLE

Rohweder, Claus A. (AACE), *M*

ST. ANN

*Sudholt, Alfred F. (ARS)

ST. LOUIS (314)

*Ackerman, Lauren V. (ASTR), *PATH*
*Allen, Wm. E. (ASTR), *R*, 533–8554
*Arneson, Axel N. (ARS), *G*,
367–0353
*Butcher, Harvey R. (AACE), *S*,
367–5235
*Cavanagh, Dennis (SGO), *OG*
Costello, C.J. (AACR)
*Donaldson, Robert C. (SHNS), *S*,
652–4100
*Fryer, Minot P. (SHNS), *PLS*,
367–6060
Goldstein, M.N. (AACR)
Herzig, G.P. (AACR)
*Hill, George J., II (AACE, ASCR,
ASCO), *S*, 367–6400
*Keltner, Raymond M. (AACE)
Korba, Alvin (ASTR), *RO*, 454–3481
*Land, Vita J. (AACE, ASCO), *HEM-
ONC*, 367–6880
*Lee, Fransiska A. (ASTR)

*Loeb, Virgil, Jr. (AACR, ASCO), *MO*, 832-9836
*Marvin, Camel H. (SGO), *OG*, 367-1401
*McElfresh, Arthur E. (ASCO), *PD*, 865-2288
Madel, E.M. (AACR)
*Mill, Wm. B. (ASTR), *TR*
*Montazee, Sam (ARS), *OG*, 872-9135
*Ogura, Joseph H. (ARS, SHNS, SSO), *OT*, 454-2426
Oliver, George D., Jr. (ASTR)
*Paletta, Francis X. (SHNS), *S*
*Perez, Carlos A. (AACR, ARS, ASCO, ASTR, SSO), *RT*, 367-6400, ext. 3381
*Philpott, Gordon W. (AACE, AACR, ASCO)
Pinkerton, H. (AACR)
*Powers, Wm. E. (AACR, ARS, ASCO, ASTR, SSO), *RT*, 367-9333
*Presant, Cary A. (AACR, ASCO), *ONC-HEM*, 367-8060
**Pullon, Peter A. (AACE), *OP*, 361-1040
*Ratkin, Gary A. (ASCO), *M/HEM*, 361-7786
Razek, A.A. (AACR)
*Sessions, Donald G. (ASHNS) *OT*, 454-2426
*Shapleigh, John (ASCO), *M/HEM*
*Spector, Gershon J. (ASHNS), *OT/HNS,* 454-2426
Ter Pogossian, Michel M. (ARS) 367-6400, ext. 3596
Tolmach, L.J. (AACR)
Valeriote, F.A. (AACE, AACR, ASTR) 367-5676
*Verde, Dominio J. (AACE, ARS, SGO, SHNS), *S*, 367-8400
*Vietti, Teresa J. (AACE, AACR, (ASCO), *PD/HEM-ONC*, 367-6880, ext. 318
*Walz, Bruce J. (ASTR), *TR*
*Willman, Vallee (AACE)
*Wray, Robert C., Jr. (SHNS), *PLS*, 454-3455
*Zeffren, Joel Lester (ASCO), *M*, 427-2424

*Zivnuska, Frederick R. (ASTR), *RT*, 454-3481

SPRINGFIELD

*Sala, Jose (ARS, ASTR)

MONTANA

BILLINGS (406)

*Deigert, Frederick A. (ASCO, ASTR), *RT/R*, 248-6871

NEVADA

RENO (702)

*Miercort, Roger D. (ASTR), *RT/R*, 785-5192

NEBRASKA

LINCOLN

*Frazer, Maurice D. (ARS)
*McGreer, John T. (ASTR)
**Waggener, Donald T. (AACE), *RT*

OMAHA (402)

*Davis, John B. (SHNS), *S*, 551-5251
*Dettman, Prentiss M. (ARS, ASTR)
*Dowell, Dawson A. (ARS)
*Foley, John F. (AACE, AACR, ASCO), *M*, 541-4802
*Frank, Albert (ASTR)
*Hunt, Howard B. (AACE, ARS, ASTR), *R*
*Karrer, F. William (SHNS), *S*, 393-6363
*Kelley, James F. (ARS)
*Kessinger, Margaret Anne (ASCO), *MO*, 541-4813
*Lemon, Henry M. (AACE, AACR, ASCO, SSO), *M/ONC*, 541-4810
*Lynch, Henry T. (AACE, AACR, ASCO), *M*, 536-2942
**Marley, John F. (AACE) 536-3045

*Miller, Daniel M. (AACE, AACR, ARS, ASCO, SSO), *S/ONC*, 558–4850
*Organ, Claude H., Jr. (SHNS), *S*, 348–2256
Schenken, J.R. (AACR)
*Shahbazian, Arman A. (ASTR)
*Shubik, Phillipe (AACE)
*Tollman, Perry J. (AACE)
Toth, B. (AACR)
*Waggener, Ronald T. (ARS, ASTR), *RT*
*Yonkers, Anthony J. (ASHNS), *OT/MXF*, 541–4433
*Zastera, Jack (ASTR)

NEW HAMPSHIRE

CONCORD

*Eberhart, Warren F. (SHNS, SSO), *S/HNS*

HANOVER (603)

*Crichlow, Robert (ARS, ASCO), *S/ONC*, 643–4000
*Eaton, Walter L., Jr. (ASCO, ASTR), *RT*, 643–4000
*Forcier, R. Jackson (ASCO), *M*, 643–4000
*Lane, Frank W., Jr. (ARS, ASTR, SSO), *RT*, 643–4000
*Lipowski, Barbara Y. (ASCO), *HEM*, 643–5519
*Maurer, L. Herbert (AACE, ASCO), *M/ONC*, 643–4000
*Tulloh, Marchant E. (ASTR), *RT*, 643–4665
Yager, J.D., Jr. (AACR)

MANCHESTER (603)

*Powel Smith, Cyril John (ARS, ASCO, ASTR), *TR*, 669–5300
*Yudicky, Stanley W. (SSO), *S/ONC*, 625–5912

MIRROR LAKE (603)

*Smedel, Magnus I. (ARS), *R*, 569–2412

NORTHWOOD (603)

*Schlang, Henry A. (ASCO), *M*, 942–8384

NEW JERSEY

ATLANTIC CITY (609)

*Ellenbogen, Leonard S. (ARS), *R*, 345–5947
*Stella, Joseph G. (ASTR)
*Wilner, Daniel (SSO, ARS)

CAMDEN

*Denk, Mary W. (ASTR)

CHERRY HILL (215)

*Bellet, Robert E. (ASCO), *MO*, 722–1900
*Glassburn, John R. (ASTR)
*McDonnell, Wm. V. (AACE), *S*
*Schatanoff, David (ASTR)
*Siegel, Norman H. (ASCO), *MO/HEM*, 795–0747

COLONIA

Klausner, C. (AACR)

DOVER

*Buznitsky, Arnold (ASTR)

EAST ORANGE (201)

*Auerbach, O. (AACR) 676–1000
*Mallams, John T. (AACE, ARS, ASTR), *TR*
**Mashberg, Arthur (AACE), *OS*, 676–1000, ext. 541

EDGEWATER

*Lenz, Maurice (ASTR)

ELIZABETH (201)

*Forsberg, Roy T. (SSO), *ONC/S/RT*,
351-7600
*Knauer, Warren (SHNS, SSO),*ONC*,
351-7600
*Mastroianni, Frank (SSO), *ONC/S*,
351-7600
*Wuester, Wm. O. (ARS, SSO), *ONC*,
351-7600

ENGLEWOOD (201)

*Forte, Francis A. (ASCO), *ONC/HEM*,
568-5250
*Jacox, Harold W. (ARS, ASTR), *RT*
*Klein, Richard (ASCO), *M/HEM-ONC*,
568-5250
*Koven, Bernard J. (AACE, ASCO),
M/MO, 567-7767
*Meyers, Edward A. (ASHNS), *OT*,
567-1616

HACKENSACK (201)

**Balden, E. (AACE)
*Knight, Wm. T. (ARS)
*Medrek, Theodore J. (AACR, ASCO),
M, 939-9000, ext. 2027

HADDONFIELD (609)

*Stambaugh, John E., Jr. (AACR,
ASCO), *M*, 428-8866

HARVEY CEDARS

*Yahrus, Wm. P. (SSO)

HIGHLAND PARK (201)

*Moolten, Sylvan E. (ASCO),
PATH/M, 249-2244
Wase, A.W. (AACR)

HILLSIDE (201)

*Chodosh, Paul L. (ASHNS), *OT*,
354-0112

IRVINGTON (201)

*Santoro, Eliswa J. (AACE, ASCO), *S*,
273-1300

LEONIA (201)

*Klauber, Leo D. (SSO), *S*,
947-2492

LIVINGSTON (201)

*Hutter, Robert V.P. (AACE, ASCO,
SHNS, SSO), *PATH*, 992-2787
*Sanfilippo, Louis J. (ARS, ASTR),
TR/RT/NM, 445-8877
*Shapiro, Myron J. (ASHNS), *OT*,
994-1660

LONG BRANCH (201)

*Glover, John R. (ASTR)
*Tepper, Erwin (ASTR), *RT*,
229-3611, ext. 515

MADISON

Smith, W.E. (AACR)

MAPLEWOOD

*Fram, Edward D. (ASTR)

MARGATE

*Bradley, Robert A. (ARS)

MENDHAM (201)

*Phillips, Ralph F. (ARS, ASTR), *RT*,
543-4957

METUCHEN (201)

*Moolten, Sylvan E. (ASCO), *PATH/M*, 249-2244

MILLBURN (201)

*Winn, Rodger J. (ASCO), *M*, 379-3678

MONTVALE

*Ruegsegger, James M. (ASCO), *M*

MORRISTOWN (201)

*Holland, Thomas R. (ASCO), *M*, 391-3121
*Scher, Allan J. (ASTR), *RT*, 538-4500, ext. 352
*Tilney, Robert W., Jr. (ARS, SHNS, SSO), *HNS*, 538-5787

NEW BRUNSWICK

*Haas, Alexander A. (ASTR)

NEWARK (201)

*Briody, Bernard (AACE) 877-4483
*Cohen, Frederick B. (ASCO), *M/ONC*, 923-6000
*Hirschberg, D.E. (AACE)
Kaminetzky, H.A. (AACR)
Kirschner, M.A. (AACR)
*Koeck, George P. (ARS, ASTR), *RT*
*Lippman, Alan J. (ASCO), *M/ONC*, 926-7230
*Mallams, J.T. (AACR), *R*, 456-4820
*Marcus, Stanley S. (ASTR)
*Rush, Benjamin F., Jr. (AACE, AACR, ASCO, SHNS, SSO), *SO*, 877-4435
*Swaminathan, Anangur P. (AACE), *ONC*, 643-8800, ext. 2549
Walters, T.R. (AACR)

NEWTON (201)

*Lucas, John C., Jr., (ARS, SSO), *S/ONC*, 383-7000

NUTLEY (201)

Levin, W.M. (AACR)
*Miller, Edward (AACR, ASCO), *M*, 235-2977

OAK RIDGE

*Brothers, James, III (SSO)

OCEAN CITY

*Lehman, J.S. (ARS)

PARK RIDGE (201)

*Rubenstein, Stuart (ASCO), *M/ONC*, 391-7799

PATERSON

*Gallo, James S. (ARS)
Rubin, A.D. (AACR)

PISCATAWAY (201)

*Norris, Donald G. (ASCO), *PD*, 564-4287
*Schlesinger, R.W. (AACR)

PLAINFIELD (201)

*Lynn, Robert (ASCO), *HEM/ONC*, 754-0400
*Sharett, Terrence E. (ASTR), *TR*

PRINCETON (609)

*Rothberg, Harvey D. (ASCO), *M*, 924-9300

RAHWAY

Zimmerman, M. (AACR)

RED BANK (201)

*Dedick, Andrew P., Jr. (ARS), *R*, 747-1429

RIDGEWOOD

Swarm, R.L. (AACR)

SHORT HILLS (201)

*Hudock, John J. (AACE, SSO), *SO*, 376-2858
*Riva, Humbert L. (SGO), *G*, 376-4201

SOMERVILLE (201)

*Adler, Howard Ervi (ASCO), *R*, 725-1291
*Miller, Brewster S. (ARS, SSO), 725-4000, ext. 490

SOUTH ORANGE

*Miller, Wade N. (SSO)

SPARTA (201)

**Kurtz, J. Phillip (AACE), *OS*, 736-4983

TEANECK (201)

*Palazzo, Wm. L. (ARS), *R*, 837-7116
*Rosin, Henry D. (ASHNS), *HNS*, 837-2174

TENAFLY

*Collier, Fred C. (ARS)

TOMS RIVER

Harris, C. (AACR)

UPPER MONTCLAIR

*Carella, Richard J. (ASTR)

WEST PATERSON

*O'Donnell, Thomas (ASTR)

WILLINGBORO (609)

*Zeidner, Steven R. (ASTR), *RT*, 871-6818

NEW MEXICO

ALBUQUERQUE (505)

*Doberneck, Raymond C. (SHNS), *S*, 265-4411, ext. 2264
*Grossman, Jack W. (ARS), *R*, 296-3591
*Hilgers, Robert D. (SSO)
*Kligerman, Morton M. (AACR, ARS, ASCO, ASTR, SHNS), *RO*, 227-3631
*Sternhagen, Charles J. (ASTR)
*Young, Alma L. (AACE)

KIRTLAND AFB

*West, Gary W. (ASTR)

LOS ALAMOS (505)

*Boone, I.J.U. (AACR) 662-5556
Tobey, R.A. (AACR)

SANTA FE

*Repass, Paul E. (ARS)

NEW YORK

ALBANY (518)

*Cunningham, Thomas J. (AACR, ASCO), *M*, 445-5037
*Eckert, Charles (AACE)
*Elliott, Ray A. (SHNS), *PLS*, 472-9148
*Etkin, Sidney I. (ARS), *R*, 462-0423
*Hoffmeister, F.S. (SHNS), *PLS*
*Horton, John (AACE, ASCO), *MO*, 445-5037
*Sponzo, Robert W. (AACR, ASCO), *M*, 445-5037
*Walsh, Thomas S., Jr. (SHNS, SSO), *S*, 462-1721
Wright, A.W. (AACR)

AMHERST

*Calamel, Peter M. (SHNS)

APO NEW YORK

*Kemmerer, Wm. T. (AACE), S

BAY SHORE (516)

*Feuerstein, Benjamin L. (ARS), TR,
859-3043

BINGHAMTON (607)

*Adams, Andrew B. (ASTR), R/RO,
729-6521
*Grinberg, Raul (ASCO), M,
797-7627
*Vargha, Zia (ASTR), RT

BRONX (212)

*Adam, Yehuda G. (AACE, ASCO,
SHNS, SSO), S/SO-HNS
*Bases, R.E. (AACR) 430-2219
*Blum, Isaac (AACE), S
*Botstein, Charles (ARS, ASTR), R,
920-4361
*Brimberg, Arthur (ASTR), RT,
653-3000
*Cook, Wm. A. (AACE), TS, 430-8721
*Dilorenzo, James C. (SSO)
*Elias, Kurt (ASCO), M/ONC,
920-5286
*Ghossein, Nemetallah A. (AACE,
ASTR), R, 430-2922
*Gray, John (AACE)
Gross, L. (AACR)
*Kaplan, Barry H. (AACE, AACR,
ASCO), M/MO, 430-2015
*Koss, Leopold G. (SSO)
*Markham, Mark J. (ASCO), M/HEM/
ONC, 920-4071
*Markman, H.D. (AACE)
*Muggia, Franko M. (AACR, ASCO),
M, 430-8585
*Ochs, A. Daniel (ASTR), RT/NM.
294-5085
*Rosen, Richard G. (SHNS), S,
920-5411
*Rosen, Samuel M. (AACE)

*Roswit, Bernard (ARS, ASTR), TR,
584-9000, ext. 418
*Silver, Carl E. (SHNS), HNS, 920-4308
Steeves, R.A. (AACR)
*Wolf, Julius (ASCO), M, 584-9010
Zimmerman, H.M. (AACR)

BRONXVILLE (914)

*Goodner, John T. (ARS, SHNS, SSO),
TS, 793-1084

BROOKLYN (212)

*Alfonso, Antonio E. (AACE), S/SO,
270-1372
*Appelbaum, Jerome (ASCO), M,
783-4484
*Arlen, Myron (SHNS, SSO)
**Bassiur, Martin (AACE), OS,
946-6600
*Bochetto, Joseph F., Jr. (SHNS, SSO),
S, 622-9357
*Bohorquez, Joseph (ARS, ASTR), RT,
270-1593
*Boyce, John (SGO), OG, 270-1364
*Camiel, Mortimer R. (ARS), R,
270-1580
*Chamberlain, W. Edward (ARS)
*Cifarelli, Frank (SSO), TS, 638-0818
Freund, H. Robert (SHNS), S, 875-3244
*Gardner, Bernard (AACE, ASCO,
SSO), S/SO, 270-1955
*Gonzalez, Mario (ASTR), R
*Harris, Alvin H. (SHNS), PLS,
875-0746
Harshaw, David H., Jr. (AACE, ARS)
*Hayes, James J. (ARS), U, 833-2420
*Herbsman, Horace (AACE), S/SO,
270-1954
*Kaplan, Gustave (ASCO), R,
854-5066
*Khafif, Rene A. (SHNS), SO/HNS,
284-0338
*Leichter, David (ASCO), M, 240-1163
*Leone, Nicholas T. (ASCO), HEM-
ONC, 622-8549
*Lerner, Robert (SHNS), S, 789-0303
Lindner, A. (AACR)

*Livingston, Saul F. (SSO)
*Luomanen, Raymond K.J. (SSO),
 TS, 238-0238
*Meyer, L.M. (AACR), *HEM*, 836-6600
*Mule, Joseph E. (SSO), *S/ONC*,
 467-7000
*Nelson, James H., Jr. (AACE, SGO),
 OG, 270-2057
*Nicastri, Anthony D. (SSO), *PATH*,
 270-1668
*Rafla, Demetrious Sameer (ARS,
 ASTR, SSO), *RT*, 780-3127
*Saltzman, Eric I. (SHNS), *HNS*,
 240-5432
*Strauss, Hyman (ARS), *OG*,
 282-0303
*Turner, Sophie S. (AACE, ASTR),
 TR, 796-1801
*Zeff, Seymour D. (AACE)

BUFFALO (716)

*Abdel-Dayem, Hussein M. (ASTR)
*Ambrus, Clara M. (ASCO), *PD/HEM*,
 845-5731
*Ambrus, Julian (ASCO), *HEM*,
 845-5731
*Barlow, Joseph J. (ASCO, SGO),
 G/ONC, 845-5784
Carter, W.A. (AACR)
*Chen, Tah Yee (ASTR), *RT*,
 845-2300
*Cooper, Richard G. (ASCO), *M*,
 886-3400
Cudkowicz, G. (AACR)
*Dao, Thomas L. (AACR, ASCO)
Dobson, R.L. (AACR)
Dougherty, T.J. (AACR)
*Douglass, Harold O., Jr. (AACR,
 ASCO), *S*, 845-3253
*Ellison, Rose Ruth (AACR, ASCO),
 M/ONC, 894-1212
*Evans, James T. (ASCO), *S*, 845-3243
*Freeman, Arnold (ASCO), *PD-ONC*,
 845-2334
*Friedman, Moshe (AACR, ASCO,
 ASTR), *RT*, 845-3283
*Gailani, Salman D. (ASCO), *M*,
 845-5898

Gomez, German A. (ASCO), *M*,
 845-5787
*Greene, George W., Jr. (AACE)
*Haar, Jean George (ASHNS, SHNS),
 HNS, 882-1023
*Han, Tin (AACR, ASCO), *M*,
 845-3303
*Henderson, Edward S. (AACR,
 ASCO), *M*, 845-3221
*Higby, Donald J. (ASCO), *M*,
 845-3221
Horoszewicz, J.S. (AACR)
*Hreshchyshyn, Myroslaw M. (SGO),
 OG, 845-6554
Jones, R., Jr. (AACR)
*Kaufman, Jerome H. (ASCO), *MO*,
 688-6883
*Laor, Yehuda G. (ASTR), *RT/NM*,
 845-6446
*Lore, John M. (ASHNS, SHNS, SSO,
 ARS), *OT/HNS*, 862-2000
*Marchetta, F.C. (AACR, SHNS), *S*,
 845-3158
*Mihich, E. (AACR), 845-5860
*Minowada, J. (AACR), 845-5847
*Mittleman, Arnold (AACR, ASCO),
 S, 845-3243
*Moayeri, Housang (ASCO), *M*,
 845-3114
*Murphy, Gerald P. (SSO), *U*, 845-5770
*Nadler, Sigmond H. (AACE, ASCO),
 S, 689-8244
*Nemoto, Takuma (AACR, ASCO),
 S, 845-5899
Osman, Gamal E.M. (ASTR), *R*,
 845-3235
*Panahon, Alvin H. (ASTR), *TR*,
 845-3296
Pickren, J.W. (AACR)
*Piver, M. Steven (ASCO, ARS, SGO),
 G/ONC, 845-3110
*Plager, John Everett (AACR, ASCO),
 M, 845-3349
*Preisler, Harvey D. (AACR, ASCO),
 M, 845-3352
*Rao, Ardor R. (ASTR), *TR*
*Rosner, Dutzu (ASCO), *S*, 845-5847
*Sako, Kumao (AACR, SHNS), *S*,
 845-3158

Sandberg, A.A. (AACR)
*Schmidt, Martha C. (ASTR), *R*
*Shah, Narendra K. (ASTR), *RT*,
845-3296
*Shatkin, Samuel (SHNS), *PLS/HNS*
*Shedd, Donald P. (SHNS), *HNS*,
845-3278
*Shimaoka, Katsutaro (AACR,
ASCO), *MO*, 845-5787
*Sinks, Lucius F. (AACR, ASCO),
PD-ONC, 845-2333
Sokal, J.E. (AACR)
Sproul, E.E. (AACR)
*Stutzman, Leon (AACR, ASCO),
M/MO, 845-5787
*Takita, Hiroshi (AACR, ASCO), *TS*,
845-2300
Tidwell, T.J. (AACR), *RT*, 792-3400
Tritsch, G.L. (AACR)
Tunis, M. (AACR)
Vincent, R.G. (AACR)
*Vongtama, Vitune (ARS, ASTR), *R*
*Wallace, H. James (AACE, ASCO),
M/ONC, 845-5946
Wang, Jaw J. (ASCO), *PD-ONC*,
845-2335
Weinfeld, H. (AACR)
Wenner, C.E. (AACR)
Zakrzewski, S.F. (AACR)

CARMEL

*Driver, James R. (ARS)

CASTLETON (518)

Hosley, Henry F. (ASCO), *M/ONC*,
732-7211

CHEEKTOWAGA

*Kim, Taik Hwan (ASTR)

COLD SPRINGS

Watson, J.D. (AACR)

COOPERSTOWN (607)

*Olson, John E. (SHNS), *S/HNS/SO*,
547-6444

CUBA (716)

*Martin, Wm. P. (SSO), *R*,
366-1111
*Suh, Kenneth (ASCO), *M*,
908-2434

EAST AURORA (716)

*Costa, Giovanni (ASCO), *M*,
652-4404

EAST MEADOW (516)

*Archambeau, John O. (ASTR), *TR*,
542-3527
*Au, Shiu Cheong (ASTR), *R*
*Miller, Sherwood P. (ASCO), *M*,
546-6211
*Pochedly, Carl E. (AACR, ASCO),
PD/HEM/ONC, 542-3336

ELIZABETHTOWN (518)

*Savel, Herbert (ASCO), *M*, 873-2221

ELMHURST

*Goldman, Leonard B. (ARS)

FAR ROCKAWAY (212)

*Brenner, Seymour (ASTR), *RT*,
945-7100, ext. 320

FLUSHING (212)

*Sanfilippo, Paul J. (ARS), *RT/NM*,
445-8877

FOREST HILLS (212)

*Caracciolo, Pasqualino R. (ASHNS,
SHNS), *HNS*, 657-1155

*Medina, Antonio (ARS)
*Olshin, Seymour (ASCO), *M*,
263-7766

FREEPORT (516)

*Pariser, Sanford (ASCO), *M/HEM-
ONC*, 389-0790

GARDEN CITY (516)

*Butler, Frank S. (ARS, SSO)
*Rasweiler, Calvin L. (SHNS), *HNS*,
248-4242

GREAT NECK (516)

*Attie, Joseph N. (SHNS), *HNS*,
487-2212
Greenberg, J. (AACR)

HEMPSTEAD (516)

*Akbiyik, Nejat H. (ASTR), *R*
*Guild, Carlton J. (ASCO), *M/GE/MO*,
489-8444

HUNTINGTON (516)

*Benninghoff, David (ARS, ASTR),
RO, 351-2295
Kuschner, M. (AACR)

JAMAICA (212)

*Cortes, Engracio P. (ASCO), *M*,
990-2727
*Levy, Robert N. (ASCO), *HEM*,
441-4100

JERICHO (516)

*Ritter, Seymour D. (ASCO), *M*,
433-9230

JOHNSON CITY (716)

*Gajwani, B. (ASCO), *M*, 845-5898

LONG BEACH (516)

*Mackenzie, A.R. (SSO), *U*, 431-0240

LONG ISLAND CITY

*Tenzel, Wm. V. (ARS)

MANHASSET (516)

*Alexander, Leslie L. (ARS, ASTR),
RO, 562-2233
*Loring, Marvin F. (ARS, ASTR),
RO, 562-2232
*Rogers, Charles E. (AACE, ARS,
SHNS, SSO), *S*

MERRICK (516)

Miller, Sherwood P. (ASCO), *M/HEM*,
546-6211

MINEOLA (516)

*Li, M.C. (AACR, ASCO, SSO), *M/MO*,
742-4200
*Mandel, Perry R. (ARS, ASTR), *R*,
742-4200, ext. 462
*Saxe, Bruce I. (ASTR), *R/RT*,
742-4200, ext. 462

MT. VERNON

*Roach, Lawrence C. (ASTR)

NEW HYDE PARK (212)

*Aral, Isamettin (ARS, ASTR), *RT*,
343-6700, ext. 2444
*Cole, Andrew T. (ASCO), *SU*,
343-6700, ext. 2773
**Eisenbud, Leon (AACE),
437-6700
Feinstein, Michael (ASCO), *M*,
441-4100
*Lanzkowsky, Philip (AACR, ASCO),
PD/HEM, 343-6700, ext. 2431
*Rai, Kanti Roop (AACR, ASCO),
HEM-ONC, 343-6700, ext. 2457

*Sawitsky, Arthur (AACR, ASCO), *M/HEM-ONC*, 343-6700, ext. 2426

*Booher, Robert J. (SSO)
*Greenwald, Edward S. (ARS, ASCO), *M/ONC*, 632-2124
*Mahoney, Wm. (SHNS), *S/HNS*, 636-3373
*Williams, John R. (ASHNS), *OT/HNS*, 636-0104

*Adair, Frank E. (ARS, SSO)
*Ager, Phyllis J. (ASCO, ASTR), *RT*, 879-3000, ext. 2253
*Agostino, Domenico V. (ARS)
*Albert, R.E. (AACR), 679-3200
*Angers, John W. (ASCO), *M*, 684-4422
*Ariel, Irving M. (AACR, ARS, ASCO), *S*, 683-8212, 532-4060
*Arje, Sidney L. (AACE, SGO, SSO), *OG*, 371-2900
*Ashikari, Rof Hiroyuki (SSO), *S*, 879-3000
*Bank, A. (AACR), 579-4186
*Barber, Hugh R. (AACE, ARS, ASCO, SSO, SGO), *OG*, 734-6555
*Barnes, W.A. (AACR), 737-2050
*Barsa, Jean M. (ASTR)
*Batata, Mostafa Ali El (ASTR), *TR*
*Beattie, Edward J., Jr. (ARS, ASCO, SSO), *S*, 879-3000
*Becker, F.F. (AACR), 679-3200
*Benjamin, Fred J. (ASTR)
*Bentivegna, Saverio S. (AACE), *S*, 876-5500, ext. 303
*Biller, Hugh F. (ASHNS), *HNS*, 650-6141
*Black, M.M. (AACR), 876-5500
*Boland, John (ARS, ASCO, ASTR, SSO), *RT*, 876-1000, ext. 8170
*Bowden, Lemuel (ARS, ASCO, SSO), *S*, 535-3323
*Brandon, Donald E. (ASCO), *M*, 838-4130

*Breed, Charles N. (SSO), *S*, 734-5107
*Brockunier, Alfred (SSO), *G/ONC*, 535-9447
*Bronstein, Eugene (ARS, ASTR, SSO), *R*
*Bruckner, H.W. (AACR)
*Burchenal, Joseph H. (AACR, ASCO, SSO), *M/PD*, 794-7590
*Byrne, Rudolfo (ASTR), *RO*, 774-5538
*Cahan, Wm. G. (ARS, SSO), *TS*, 737-4734
*Caron, Arthur S. (SSO), *S*, 686-0297
*Catlin, Daniel (ARS, SHNS, SSO), *HNS*, 879-3000
*Chang, Chu-Huai (ARS, ASTR), *R*, 579-2944
*Chinn, May E. (SSO) 662-7575
*Chong, Claude Y. (ARS, ASTR), *R*
*Choy, Daniel S.J. (ASCO), *M*, 535-6040
*Chu, F.C.H. (ARS, ASCO, ASTR), *RT*, 879-3000
*Clark, Donald G.C. (ARS, ASCO, SSO), *S*, 535-7335, ext. 2477
*Clarkson, Bayard D. (AACR, ASCO), *MO/HEM*
Claude, A. (AACR)
*Cliffton, Eugene (AACE)
*Cohen, Carmel J. (SGO), *OG*
*Cohen, Seymour M. (ASCO), *M/HEM*, 249-9141
*Colman, Morton (ASCO), *M/HEM*, 861-1383
*Conley, John J. (ASHNS, SHNS), *HNS*, 787-3066
*Conte, Alexander J. (ARS, ASCO, ASHNS, SHNS, SSO), *S/TS/OS*, 688-8666
*Cooper, Jay S. (ASTR), *TR*, 679-3200, ext. 2626
*Cornell, George N. (ASCO, SSO), *S*, 289-3530
*Currie, Violante E. (ASCO), *M*, 879-3000, ext. 2634
*Cuttner, Janet (AACR, ASCO), *M/HEM*, 650-6481
*D'Anglo, Giulio J. (ARS, ASCO, ASTR), *RT*, 879-3000

*Daly, John (SSO), *S*
*Daniel, William W. (SSO), *S*
*DeBellis, Robert (ASCO), *M/HEM-ONC*, 579-5353
*Deddish, Michael R. (SSO), *S*, 879-6569
Defendi, V. (AACR)
DeHarven, E. (AACR)
*DeJager, Robert L. (ASCO), *M*, 879-3000
*De Palo, Angelo J. (SSO), *S*, 535-2711
*Dickinson, Jeanne R. (ARS)
*Dietz, J.H., Jr. (SSO), *PM/S*, 879-3000
*Dowling, Monroe D., Jr. (AACR, ASCO), *M*, 861-3856
*Dvoskin, Samuel (ASCO), *M*
Edgcomb, J.H. (AACR)
*Edmunds, Robert T. (ASCO), *S*, 870-6291
*Ellis, Frank (ASTR), *R*
*Exelby, Philip R. (SSO), *S*
*Fahey, Thomas J., Jr. (SSO), *S*
*Farina, Anthony T. (ASTR), *R*
*Farr, Hollon W. (SHNS, SSO), *S*, 744-1646
*Feind, Carl (ASCO, SHNS), *S/HNS*, 579-5569
*Feinstein, Jeffrey J. (ASTR), *R*
*Fingerhut, Bruno (ACR, ASCO), *U,* 928-5093
*Finkbeiner, John A. (ARS, ASCO, SSO), *M/MO*, 744-5719
*Fitzgerald, Patrick J. (SSO), *S*
*Foote, Frank W. (SSO), *S*
*Fortner, Joseph (ARS, SSO), *S*, 879-3000, ext. 2873
*Fracchia, Alfred A. (SSO), *S*
*Francis, Kenneth C. (SSO), *S*
*Franklin, John E. (SSO), *S*
*Freid, Jacob R. (ARS, ASCO, ASTR), *R*
*Frick, Henry C., II (ARS, ASCO, SGO, SSO), *OG*, 579-1897
*Friedman, Eugene W. (ASCO, SHNS, SSO), *S/HNS*, 737-8757
*Friedmann, Asa B. (ARS, ASCO)
*Fuller, L.G. Anthony (ASTR), *RO*, 879-3000
Furth, J. (AACR)

*Gee, Timothy (ASCO), *M/MO*, 879-3000, ext. 2955
*Gelhorn, A. (AACR), *S*
*Geller, Wm. (ARS, ASCO, SSO), *M/MO*, 861-8844
*Gerold, Frank P. (SHNS, SSO), *HNS*, 794-1513
*Ghavimi, Fereshteh (ASCO), *PD*, 879-3000, ext. 3079
*Golbey, Robert B. (AACR, ASCO), *M*, 879-3000
*Goldberg, Arthur I. (AACR, ASCO), *M/HEM/ONC*, 535-3648
*Goldiner, Paul L. (SSO), *ANES*, 879-3000, ext. 3394
*Golomb, Frederick M. (AACR, ASCO, SHNS), *S*, 679-3200
*Good, Robert A. (AACR, ASCO), *PATH/PD*, 879-3000
*Grabstald, Harry (ARS, ASCO, SSO), *U*, 988-0233
Graf, L. (AACR)
*Greenspan, Ezra M. (AACR, ASCO), *M/MO*, 289-1765
*Grossbard, Lionel (ASCO), *HEM/ONC*, 579-5291
*Grossi, Carlo E. (AACE, ASCO, SSO), *S/ONC*, 988-7337
*Gumport, Stephen (AACE, AACR, ASCO, SSO), *S*, 679-3200
Gusberg, S.B. (AACR, SGO), *OG*, 650-6555
*Guttmann, Ruth J. (ARS, ASTR, SSO), *R*, 579-8494
*Haagensen, Cushman D. (SSO)
*Habif, David V. (ASCO), *S*, 579-5525
*Haghbin, Mahroo (AACR, ASCO), *PD,* 879-3000
*Hahn, Eric W. (ASTR), *TR*
*Hajdu, Steven I. (SSO), *PATH*
*Hardy, Mark A. (AACE), *S*, 579-4072
*Harris, Matthew N. (ASCO, SSO), *SO*, 679-3200, ext. 3901
*Harrold, Charles C., Jr. (SHNS, SSO), *HNS*, 737-4630
Heiman, H.I. (AACR)
Hellman, L. (AACR)
*Helson, Lawrence (AACR, ASCO), *PD-ONC*, 879-3000, ext. 2558

*Henschke, Gisela F. (ASTR), *TR*, 620-1689

*Herrmann, Julian B. (ARS, SSO), *ONC*, 879-1999

*Hersh, Joseph H. (ASHNS), *OT*

*Hersvovic, Arnold M. (ASTR), *TR*, 879-3000

*Herter, Frederic P. (ASCO), *S*, 579-1848

*Hertz, Ralph E.L. (SSO), *S*, 988-8007

*Higinbotham, Norman (SSO), *S*

*Hilaris, Basil S. (ARS, ASCO, ASTR), *RT*, 879-3000

*Hirshaut, Yashar (AACR, ASCO), *M*, 861-1799

Hoffman, J. (AACR)

*Holland, James F. (AACR, ASCO), *M*, 348-5855

*Holleb, Arthur I. (AACE, AACR, ARS, ASCO, SSO), *S*, 371-2900

*Hopfan, Seymour (ARS, ASTR), *RT*, 879-3000, ext. 3004

*Horowitz, Ira A. (ASTR), *RT*, 544-6750

*Houde, Raymond W. (SSO), *S*

*Howland, Wm. S. (SSO) *ANES*, 879-3000

*Huh, Sun H. (ASTR), *TR*

*Huvos, Andrew G. (SSO), *S*

*Hyman, George A. (AACR, ASCO), *M/HEM-ONC*, 737-4400

*Hyman, Julian (ASCO), *M/HEM-ONC*, 737-4400

Ioachim, H.L. (AACR)

*Johnston, Barbara (ASCO), *M*, 677-1818

*Jordan, Michael J. (SSO), *S*

*Ju, David M. (SHNS), *PLS*

*Kabakow, Bernard (AACR, ASCO), *M*, 477-2220

*Karpas, C.M. (AACE)

*Kaufman, Richard J. (AACR, ASCO, SSO), *M*, 879-3000

*Kelley, Charles D. (ASTR), *TR*

*Kelly, John A. (ARS, SSO)

*Kim, Jae Ho (ASTR), *TR*

Kopf, A.W. (AACR)

*Krakoff, Irwin H. (AACR, ASCO, SSO), *M/MO*, 879-3000

*Lacher, Mortimer J. (AACR, ASCO, SSO), *M/ONC-HEM*, 879-3000

*Ladue, John S. (SSO), *S*

*Lane, Stanley L. (ASHNS, SSO), *HNS*, 734-1484

*Larsen, Martha (SSO), *M*, 576-6131

*Lattes, R. (AACR), 579-3758

*Laughlin, John S. (ARS, ASTR), *R*

*Leaming, Robert H. (ARS, SHNS, SSO), *R*, 861-9050

*Lee, Burton (AACR, ASCO, SSO), *M*, 879-3000

*Leis, Henry P., Jr. (AACE, ASCO), *S*, 427-2131

*Lepley, James B. (SHNS), *MXF*, 879-3000

Lesnick, Gerson (ASCO), *S*, 879-1910

*Lewis, John L., Jr. (SGO, SSO), *OG*, 879-3000, ext. 2751

*Lewis, John S. (ASHNS, SSO), *S*

*Lieberman, Philip H. (SSO), *PATH*, 879-3000

*Liegner, Leonard M. (ARS, ASTR, SSO), *RO*, 870-6767

Lipkin, G. (AACR)

Lipkin, M. (AACR)

*Loseke, Lucile E. (SSO), *S*

Luhby, A. (AACR)

*Macfee, Wm. F. (SHNS)

*Madden, Robert E. (AACE, AACR, ASCO, SSO), *TS*, 876-5500, ext. 307

*Magill, Gordon B. (AACR, ASCO), *MO*, 879-3000, ext. 2654

*Marcove, Ralph (SSO), *OS*, 535-2514

*Marino, John M. (AACE)

*Marks, P. A. (AACR), 579-3807

*Marquardt, H.W. (AACR), 879-3000

*Martin, Hayes (SSO), *S*

*Martini, Neal (ARS, SSO)

*Mason, R.P. (AACR), 867-3700

*Mcpeak, Charles J. (ARS, SHNS, SSO), *S*, 734-4450

*Meister, A. (AACR), 472-6212

*Melamed, Myron R. (SSO), *PATH*, 879-3000

*Merriam, George R., Jr. (ARS)

*Mersheimer, Walter L. (AACE)

*Miller, Daniel G. (ASCO, SGO), *M/MO*, 683-1000

*Miller, Denis R. (AACR), *PD*,
(402) 558-4850
*Miller, Theodore R. (ARS, SHNS,
SSO), *S*, 532-4060
*Molander, David W. (AACR, ARS,
ASCO, SSO), *M*, 532-0550
*Moore, Oliver S. (SHNS, SSO)
*Muggia, Franco (ASCO), *M*,
430-8585
*Munnell, Equinn W. (SGO, SSO),
OG
*Murphy, M. Lois (AACR, ASCO,
SSO), *PD/ONC*, 879-3000
*Myers, Warren P.L. (AACR, ASCO,
SSO), *M/MO*, 879-3000, ext. 2665
*Nealon, Thomas F., Jr. (ARS, SSO),
S/TS, 243-1314
*Newall, Joseph (ARS, ASCO, ASTR),
RO, 679-3200, ext. 2623
*Nieburgs, H.E. (AACR)
*Nisce, Lourdes Z. (ASTR), *RT*,
879-3000, ext. 2240
*Nobler, Myron P. (ARS, ASTR),
RT/R, 673-3000, ext. 2841
*Nussbaum, Moses (SHNS),
HNS, 734-1140
*Ochoa, Manuel, Jr. (AACR, ASCO),
M, 879-3000
*Oettgen, Herbert F. (AACR, ASCO),
M, 879-3000
*Ohnuma, Takao (AACR, ASCO), *M*,
650-6664
*Old, L.J. (AACR), 879-3138
*Oropeza, Ruben (SHNS, SSO), *S*
Orris, L. (AACR)
Osserman, E.F. (AACR)
*Paglia, Michael A. (SSO), *S*, 288-3948
*Patel, Vinubhsi C. (ASTR)
*Pearlman, A.W. (ARS)
*Perlberg, Harry J., Jr. (ASTR), *R*
*Pickett, Elisabeth (SSO), *S/U*,
737-6010
*Pierce, Virginia K. (SSO), *G*
*Pierson, John C. (ARS)
*Pinsky, Carl M. (AACR, ASCO), *M*,
879-3000
Popper, H. (AACR)
Post, J. (AACR)

*Pressman, Peter I. (ASCO), *S*,
249-8040
Prince, A.M. (AACR)
Puthawala, Ajmel S. (ASTR)
*Quan, Stuart H.Q. (ARS, SSO), *S*,
535-6164
Quimby, Edith H. (ARS, SSO)
*Rankow, Robin M. (SHNS)
*Ratner, Lynn H. (ASCO), *M*, 249-8752
*Rauscher, Frank J., Jr. (AACR,
ASCO)
*Rausen, Aaron R. (AACR, ASCO),
PD-HEM, 673-3000, ext. 2251
*Richart, Ralph M. (SGO), *PATH*,
579-3531
*Robbins, Guy F. (AACR, ARS, ASCO,
SSO), *S*, 879-3000
*Rosen, Gerald (AACR, ASCO), *PD*,
879-3000
*Rosen, Paul P. (SSO), *PATH*
Rossi, Harald (ARS)
*Rothenberg, Sheldon P. (AACR,
ASCO), *M/HEM*, 876-5500, ext. 446
*Rotman, Marvin (ASCO, ASTR),
R/RT, 876-5500, ext. 835
*Rottino, Anthony (AACR, ASCO),
620-1642
*Rubinfeld, Sidney (ARS, ASCO,
ASTR), *TR*, 679-3200
*Sage, Harold (AACE, AACR, ASCO),
S, 679-3200
*Sahagian, Edward Alex (ASCO), *M*,
986-1000, ext. 8448
*Sall, Sanford (AACE, SGO), *GO*,
831-0444
*Schetlin, Charles F. (SHNS), *S*
*Schottenfeld, David (AACR, SSO),
M/MO, 879-3000, ext. 2643
*Schwartz, Arthur E. (ASCO), *S*,
737-8757
*Schwartz, M. Stephen (ASCO), *M*,
838-0980
*Schwarz, George (ARS, ASTR), *R*
*Schweizer, Olga (SSO), *ANES*,
879-3000
*Selby, Henry M. (SSO)
*Shapiro, Wm. R. (AACR, ASCO),
879-3000, ext. 2462

*Sherlock, Paul (ASCO, SSO), *M/GE*, 879-3000
*Sherman, Robert S. (SSO), 744-7139
*Silver, Richard T. (ASCO), *M/HEM*, 472-6140
*Silverstone, Sidney (ARS, ASCO, ASTR), *M/RT*
*Simon, Norman (ARS, ASCO, ASTR), *RT*, 744-5538
Sitarz, A.L. (AACR)
*Smith, Frank R. (ARS, SSO)
*Smith, Julius (SHNS, SSO), *R*, 879-3000
*Snyder, Ruth E. (SSO), *R*, 879-4488
*Solis, Mario H. (ASTR), *TR*
Sommers, S.C. (AACR)
*Spiegelman, Sol (ARS)
*Spiro, Ronald (ASCO), *S*, 879-3000 ext. 2713
Stearnberg, S.S. (AACR)
*Stearns, Maus W., Jr. (SSO), *S* 288-0011
Stevens, J.J. (AACR)
**Stoll, John B., (SHNS), 879-3000, ext. 2366
*Strax, Philip (ASCO, SSO), *R*, 369-2720
*Strong, Elliot W. (ARS, SHNS, SSO), *HNO*, 879-3808
Stutman, O. (AACR)
*Sykes, Marguerite P. (AACR, ASCO, SSO), *M*, 879-3000
Tallat, L. (AACR)
*Tan, Charlotte T.C. (AACR, ASCO, SSO), *PD-ONC*, 879-3000
*Taylor, Howard C., Jr. (ARS, SSO), *G*, 838-4972
Tennant, J.R. (AACR)
*Thiessen, Eugene U. (ASCO), *S*, 753-2211
*Thomas, Lewis (ASCO), *M*, 879-3000
*Tollefsen, H. Randall (ARS, SHNS, SSO), *HNS*, 737-0042
*Tretter, Patricia (ASTR), *R/RT*, 579-2611
Troll, W. (AACR)
Tsien, K.C. (ARS)
*Turnbull, Alan (SSO)

*Twombly, Gray H. (AACR, ARS, ASCO, SSO), *G*, 753-2211
*Urban, J.A. (AACR, ARS, SSO), *S/ONC*, 744-1766
*Vallejo, Alvaro (ASCO, ASTR), *RT*, 879-3000
*Vanamee, Parker (SSO)
Van Duren, B.L. (AACR)
*Veenema, Ralph J. (ASCO), *U*, 579-8557
*Vialotti, Charles P. (ASTR), *TR*
*Vieta, John D. (SSO), *S/ONC*, 879-6616
Vivona, S. (AACR)
*Vogel, James M. (ASCO), *M/HEM-ONC*, 369-4250
*Volk, Herbert (AACE, AACR, ASCO, SSO), *S*, 430-8001
Wainfan, E. (AACR)
Wallerstein, H. (AACR)
Wanebo, H.J. (AACR)
*Wasserman, Louis R. (AACR, ASCO), *M/HEM*, 876-1000, ext. 6029
*Watson, Robin C. (SSO), *R*, 879-3000
*Watson, Wm. L. (ARS, SSO)
Waxman, S. (AACR)
*Weiner, Martin J. (ASCO), *MO/M*, 369-5522
*Whiteley, Horace (SSO), *S*, 861-0874
*Whitmore, Willet F. (ARS, SSO)
Wienstein, I.B. (AACR)
*Winawer, Sidney J. (SSO), *M/GE*, 879-3017
*Wolff, James A. (AACR, ASCO), *PD/HEM*, 579-1882
*Wollner, Norma (AACR, ASCO), *PD*, 879-3000, ext. 2306
Wolman, S.R. (AACR)
Wood, G. Congdon (AACE), 371-2900
Woodard, H.Q. (AACR)
*Wright, Jane C. (AACR, ASCO), 876-5500, ext. 804
Wynder, E.L. (AACR)
*Yagoda, Alan (ASCO), *M*, 879-3000, ext. 2651
*Young, Charles W. (AACR, ASCO), *M*, 879-3000, ext. 2857
Zedeck, M.S. (AACR)

**Zegarelli, Edward V. (AACE), 579–1985

NORTH BELLMORE

Schick, M. (AACR)

NORTH TARRYTOWN

**Zegarelli, David J. (AACE)

OLD WESTBURY (516)

*Li, Min Chiu (ASCO, SSO), *M/MO*, 742–4200

PEARL RIVER (914)

*Masur, Charles J. (ASCO), 735–5000, ext. 3642
Wallace, R.E. (AACR)

PITTSFORD

*Belgrad, Richard (ASTR), *TR*

PLAINVIEW (516)

*Crampton, Ray (AACE, SSO), *S*, 248–3788

PORT WASHINGTON (516)

*Cudmore, Ruth J. (SSO)
*Tomao, Frank A. (ASCO), *M*, 767–0122

ROCHESTER (716)

*Bakemeier, Richard F. (AACE, AACR, ASCO), *M*, 275–5537
*Bennett, John M. (AACE, AACR, ASCO), *MO*, 275–3923
*Cooper, Robert A. (AACE)
*Craver, Wm. L. (SSO)
Folsch, E. (AACR)
Hare, J.D. (AACR)
*Lewis, Charles L. (ASTR), *RT*, 266–4000

Lichtman, M.A. (AACR)
*Maxwell, Walter T. (SHNS), *S/HNS*, 454–6754
*McCormack, Robert M. (SHNS), *PLS*, 271–8896
*Morgan, H.R. (AACR), 275–4531
*Paterson, Eileen (ASTR), *RT*, 338–4032
*Patterson, W. Bradford (AACE, AACR, ASCO), *PD/S*, 275–2737
*Poulter, Glin A. (ASTR), *RT*
*Powers, Francis M., Jr. (ASTR)
*Rubin, Jerome (AACE, ASG)
*Rudolph, Jerome H. (AACE, ASCO), *OG*, 275–3208
*Salamone, Raymond P. (SSO), *S/ONC*, 232–5352
*Salazar, Omar M. (ASTR), *RO*, 275–5625
*Savlov, Edwin D. (ASCO, SSO), *S/ONC*, 271–3300
*Schmale, Arthur H. (AACE), 275–3588
*Sherman, Charles D., Jr. (AACE, ARS, SHNS, SSO), *S*, 473–7172
*Sischy, Benjamin (ARS, ASCO, ASTR), *RT*, 473–2200, ext. 280
*Sobel, Sidney H. (ASCO, ASTR), *TR*, 473–2200
Wittliff, J.L. (AACR)

ROCKVILLE CENTER (516)

*Berlanga, Rafael (ASTR), *RT*, 255–2534

RYE

*Bello, Edward T. (ASTR), *TR*
Fogh, J.E. (AACR)
Tarnowski, G.S. (AACR)
Teller, M.N. (AACR)
*Wald, Arnold M. (ASTR), *TR*

ST. ALBANS

*Carr, John E., III (AACE)

SARANAC LAKE

*Gould, Richard G. (SSO), *S*

SCARSDALE (914)

*Abadir, Rushdy (ASTR), *RT*
*Escher, George C. (AACE, AACR, ASCO, SSO), *M*, 723-5039
Glidewell, O.J. (AACR)
*Hoffman, Wm. J. (SSO), *S*

SCHENECTADY (518)

*Archambault, Maureen K. (ASTR), *TR*
*Coolidge, Wm. D. (ASCO)
*Reilly, Charles J. (ASCO), *MO*, 372-1511

SNYDER

Kim, U. (AACR)

SPRINGVILLE

Takada, Y. (AACR)

STATEN ISLAND (212)

*Bartok, Stephen P. (ASTR), *RO*, 447-3010, ext. 507
*Meleka, Fikry M. (ASTR), *TR*

SUNNYSIDE (212)

Jacobson, Lillian E. (ARS, ASTR), 784-0045

SYOSSET

*Kolson, Harry (ASHNS, SHNS, SSO), *HNS*

SYRACUSE (315)

*Burdick, Daniel (ASCO, SSO), *S*, 476-9951
*Cooray, Neville C. (ASTR), *TR*
*Gale, Kenneth E. (ASCO, SSO), *S*, 476-5388
Gold, J. (AACR)
*Johnson, Worwood E. (ASHNS), *OT*, 476-7936
King, Gerald A. (ASTR), *TR*, 473-5276

*Rabuzzi, Daniel D. (ASHNS), *OT*, 473-4636
*Reed, George F. (ASHNS), *OT*, 473-4636
Ringrose, Thomas L. (ASTR)
*Rogers, Lloyd S. (AACE), *S*, 473-4550
*Sagerman, Robert H. (ARS, ASTR)
*Simon, Thomas R. (SSO), *PATH*, 478-6611

TONAWANDA

*Luhr, Alfred F., Jr. (SSO), *S*

UTICA

*Cramer, Irving (SSO), *S*
*Toksu, Esat A. (SHNS)

VALHALLA (914)

Weisburger, J.H. (AACR)
Williams, G.M. (AACR)
*Wolanske, Ann C.C. (ASTR), *R/TR*, 592-8500

WANTAGH (516)

*Craver, Lloyd F. (ARS, SSO), *M/MO*, 781-2294

WHITE PLAINS (914)

*Montroy, Robert E. (SHNS), *PLS*, 538-8779
*Rosen, David L. (ASCO), *M*, 949-4212

WHITESTONE

*Cole, Donald R. (ASCO), 767-5000

WILLIAMSVILLE (716)

*Kaufman, Jerome H. (ASCO), *MO*, 688-6883

WOODHAVEN (212)

*Martin, Daniel S. (AACE, AACR, ASCO), *S/ONC*, 849-0653

YONKERS (914)

*Petti, George H., Jr. (ASHNS), *OT/HNS*, 703-8588

NORTH CAROLINA

ASHEVILLE (704)

*Bagley, Carter S. (ASHNS), *OT*, 254-3517
*Cole, Warren H. (AACR, ASCO, SSO), *S*, 254-4475
*Costenbader, Wm. B., Jr. (ASHNS), *OT/HNS*, 254-3517
*Haslam, John B. (ASTR), *TR*, 255-4496

CHAPEL HILL (919)

*Bonanno, Joseph J. (ASTR), *RT*, 966-1101
*Brinkhous, Kenneth (AACE)
Kaufman, D.G. (AACR)
*Montana, Gustavo S. (ASTR), *RT*, 966-1101
*Newsome, James F. (AACE, AACR, ASCO), *S*, 966-4246
Pagano, J.S. (AACR)
Thomas, C.G., Jr. (AACR)

CHARLOTTE (704)

*Berkeley, Wm. T. (SHNS), *S*
*Edwards, E.F. (ASHNS), *OT*
*Pressley, C.L. (SSO)
*Scott, Walter P. (ARS, ASCO, ASTR), *RT/NM*, 373-2272
*Sternbergh, W.C. (SSO)

DURHAM (919)

*Abramson, Norman (ASTR), *RT*, 684-3742
Amos, D.B. (AACR), 684-4338

*Byhardt, Roger W. (ASTR)
*Cavanaugh, Patrick J. (ASTR)
*Creasman, Wm. (ARS, SGO), *ONC*
Day, E.D. (AACR)
*Evans, John C. (ARS, ASTR), *R*
*Georgiade, Nicholas G. (SHNS), *PLS/MXF*, 684-2894
*Hobart, Seth G., Jr. (ASHNS), *OT*
Kinney, T.D. (AACR)
Laszlo, J. (AACR)
*Noell, Karl Thomas (ASCO, ASTR), *RO*, 684-3742
*Ornitz, Robert D. (ASTR), *TR*
*Parker, Roy T. (SGO), *OG*, 684-2626
*Pickrell, Kenneth L. (SHNS, SSO), *PLS/ONC (head & neck)*
*Porter, F. Stanley (AACE), *PD*, 684-8111, ext. 3401
*Scruggs, Robert P., III (ASTR)
Seigler, H.F. (AACR)
*Shingleton, Wm. W. (AACE, AACR, SSO), *S*, 684-2282
*Wells, S.A., Jr. (AACR, SSO)
*Wharam, Moody D., Jr. (ASTR)
*Worde, Boyd T. (ASTR)

GREENSBORO (919)

*Cone, Donald (ARS), *R*, 379-4144
*Doyle, Owen W. (ASCO)

RESEARCH TRIANGLE PARK

Dixon, R.L. (AACR)
Woods, J.S. (AACR)

WINSTON-SALEM (919)

*Blake, Damon (ASTR), *RT*, 727-4981
*Cooper, Miles Robert (ASCO), *HEM*, 727-4300
*Feree, Carolyn R. (ASTR)
Gudson, J.P., Jr. (AACR)
*Hayes, Donald M. (AACE, AACR, ASCO), *M/HEM/ONC*, 727-4286
*Patterson, Richard B. (ASCO), *PD/HEM/ONC*, 727-4085

*Raben, Milton (ASTR), *RT*,
727–4981
Richards, Frederick, II (ASCO),
M/HEM, 727–4337
*Santos, Juan J. (ASTR)
*Spurr, Charles L. (AACE, AACR,
ASCO), *M/HEM/ONC*, 727–4354

NORTH DAKOTA

GRAND FORKS (701)

*Krech, W.G. (SHNS), *PLS*, 775–8121

OHIO

AKRON (216)

*Burnett, Harry W., Jr. (ARS, ASTR)
*Fairweather, Wm. H. (SHNS, SSO),
S, 666–3781
*Swenson, Franklin H. (ASTR), *TR*

CANTON

*Writz, Robert E. (ASTR), *TR*

CHAGRIN FALLS (216)

*Alexander, Fred W. (ASHNS), *OT*,
247–8348

CINCINNATI (513)

*Aron, Bernard S. (AACE, ARS,
ASTR), *RO*, 872–4775
*Ball, Thomas J., Jr. (ASCO), *M*,
921–5844
*Barrett, Charles (AACE)
*Coith, Robert I. (AACE)
*Compaan, Pearl J. (ASTR), *TR*
*Cotton, Robin I. (ASHNS),
OT/MXF, 872–7736
*Crocker, Dan (AACE)
*Dettmer, Cornelia M. (ASTR), *RT*,
369–2323
*Freckman, Herman A. (AACR, ASCO,
SSO), *M*, 381–0909
*Gall, Edward A. (AACE), *PATH*,
872–5633

*Griffin, George D.J. (ASCO), *S*,
281–2032
*Horwitz, Harry (AACE, ARS, ASTR),
TR, 872–4775
*Lampkin, Beatrice C. (AACE)
*LeClaire, Henri (ARS), *R*, 241–5560
*Longacre, Jacob J. (SHNS), *PLS*,
721–7556
*Marting, Esther C. (ASTR), *R*,
369–2323
*Meyer, Richard L. (ASCO, SSO),
M, 381–8440
*Milburn, Carol Swarts (ASTR), *RT*,
872–2636
*Pescovitz, Harold (AACE, SSO), *S*,
281–1252
*Saenger, Eugene L. (AACE, ARS),
R/NM, 872–4282
*Shehata, Wagih M. (ASTR), *TR*,
872–2636
*Shumrick, Donald A. (ASHNS,
SHNS), *OT*, 872–4155
*Will, John H. (AACE)
*Wozencraft, Jean P. (SSO)

CLEVELAND (216)

*Anderson, Robin (SHNS), *PLS*,
229–2200
*DeCosse, Jerome (AACE, SHNS,
SSO), *S*
*Desprez, John D. (SHNS), *PLS*,
421–8915
*Dyment, Paul G. (AACR, ASCO),
PD-HEM/ONC, 229–2200
*Friedell, Hymer L. (ARS, SSO), *R*,
791–7300
Goldblatt, H. (AACR)
Goldthwait, D.A. (AACR)
*Groppe, Carl W., Jr. (ASCO), *M*,
229–2200
*Hartwell, Shattuck W., Jr. (SHNS),
PLS, 229–2200
*Hewlett, James S. (ASCO), *M/
HEM-ONC*, 229–2200
*Kellermeyer, Robert W. (AACE)
*Kiehn, Clifford L. (SHNS), *PLS*,
421–8915

*Krieger, James (ARS, SGO), *G*,
229-2200
*Lavik, Paul S. (ASTR), *TR*,
791-7300
Lipsett, M.B. (AACR)
*Lulenski, Chester R. (SSO), *S*,
271-3232
Mandel, M.A. (AACR)
*Mansour, Edward G. (AACE, ASCO),
S/SO, 398-6000
*Pearson, Olof H. (AACR, ASCO, SSO),
M, 371-0133
*Pories, Walter J. (AACE, AACR,
ASCO), *S/TS*, 398-6000
*Reagan, James Williams (SGO),
PATH, 791-7300, ext. 313
*Rodriguez-Antunez, Antonio
(ARS, ASCO, ASTR), *RT,*
229-2200, ext. 526
*Rollins, Marvin (ARS, ASTR),
R, 696-4300, ext. 258
**Rossi, Edward P. (AACE), *OP*,
368-4260
*Sevilla, John L. (ASTR), *TR*,
791-7300, ext. 2176
**Stein, Murray (AACE), *OS*,
368-2538
*Storaasli, John P. (AACE, ARS,
ASTR), *R*, 791-7300, ext. 2177
*Topolnicki, Wladyslaw (ARS, ASTR),
RT/ONC, 398-6000, ext. 4434
*Tucker, Harvey M. (ASHNS),
OT-HNS, 229-2200
*Van Duzen, Dale (ASCO), 961-7344
*Weick, James J. (ASCO), *HEM*,
229-2200
*Wentz, W. Budd (SGO), *OG/GO*,
791-7300, ext. 364
*Zippert, Albert M. (SSO), *S*,
932-9506

COLUMBUS (614)

*Balcerzak, Stanley P., Jr. (AACR,
ASCO), *M*, 422-7581
*Bately, Frank (ARS, ASTR), *TR*
*Bonta, Joseph (SHNS, SSO), *S*,
263-1865
**Cavalaris, C.J. (AACE), *OP*,
422-6577

*Cerilli, James G. (AACE)
*Creedon, Patrick J. (SHNS), *RT*,
422-7548
*Ehlers, Gunther (ASTR), *R*
*Ertel, Inta J. (AACR, ASCO),
PD/HEM-ONC, 353-8841
*Hodgson, Sheila E. (ASTR), *TR*
*James, Arthur G. (ARS, SHNS, SSO),
S, 263-5469
*King, Gerald Wesley (AACR, ASCO),
M, 422-7581
Liss, L. (AACR)
*Lobuglio, Albert F. (AACR, ASCO),
M/HEM, 422-1540
*Miglets, Andrew W. (ASHNS), *OT*
*Minton, John P. (AACE, AACR,
ASCO, SSO), *S*, 422-5322
*Myers, Wm. G. (ARS)
*Neidhart, James Allen (AACR, ASCO),
M/HEM, 422-7581
*Newton, Wm. A., Jr. (AACR, ASCO),
M, 258-4875
*Sagone, Arthur L., Jr. (AACR, ASCO),
M, 422-7581
*Saunders, Wm. H. (ASHNS), *OT*,
422-4791
*Schloss, Charles (ARS)
Stevenson, Thomas D. (ASCO)
*Von Haam, Emmerick (AACE)
*Wilson, Henry E. (AACR, ASCO),
M/HEM, 457-9010
Yohn, D.S. (AACR)

DAYTON (513)

*Bretz, Giselle T. (ASTR), *TR*
*Keys, John (ASCO), *M*, 293-1117
*Marger, Donald (ASTR), *TR*,
222-5841
*Thompson, Nicholas J. (SGO), *OG*,
223-9942
*Ungerleider, James S. (ASCO),
M/HEM, 293-1117

ELYRIA (216)

*Berkebile, Robert (ARS, ASTR),
RT, 323-3221

*Sigalove, Wm. H. (ASCO), *M*,
323-3221

MASSILLON (216)

*Loeffler, R. Kenneth (ARS, ASTR),
TR, 832-9836

MIDDLETOWN (513)

*Gerber, David M. (SSO), *S*
422-2811

NEWARK

*Piatt, Arnold (ARS)

PARMA

*Jakubowycz, Alexander (ASTR), *TR*
*Salwan, Fayiz A. (SSO), *S*

SHAKER HEIGHTS

*Boukalik, W.F. (SSO), *S*

SOUTH EUCLID (216)

*Katz, Robert L. (ASHNS), *OT*,
291-0311

STEUBENVILLE

*Yobbagy, Jonathan J. (ASTR), *TR*

TOLEDO (419)

*Baibak, George J. (SHNS), *PLS*
*Blakemore, W.S. (AACR), 385-7461
*Cobau, Charles (ASCO), *M/ONC*,
479-8222
*Eggleston, Wm. D. (ASTR), *TR*,
473-1251
*Leighton, George A., Jr. (ASCO), *M*
*Robinson, E.K. (ASCO), *PD/HEM-
ONC*, 385-4661
*Robinson, Margaret G. (ASCO),
PD/HEM, 865-6522

TWINSBURG (216)

*Sevilla, John L. (ASTR), *TR*,
791-7300, ext. 2176

WORTHINGTON

*Fahey, Laurence J. (ASTR), *TR*

YOUNGSTOWN (216)

*Flynn, Wm. J. (ARS, SHNS, SSO),
HNS, 744-7944
*McDonough, John J. (ARS), *R*
Sheridan, Michael F. (ASTR), *RT*,
747-0751, ext. 224
*Soleimani, Parviz K. (ASTR), *TR*

OKLAHOMA

EDMOND

*Sartin, Michael A. (ASTR), *TR*
*Sukman, Robert (ASTR), *TR*

OKLAHOMA CITY (405)

*Acker, Stephen E. (ASTR), *TR*,
271-5642
Adams, G.D. (ASTR)
*Binkley, James S. (SHNS, SSO), *TR*
*Bogardus, Carl R., Jr. (ARS, ASTR), *R*
*Bottomley, Richard H. (AACR,
ASCO), *M*, 235-8331
*Dewar, James P., Jr. (SSO), *PATH*,
946-6414
Everett, M.A. (AACR)
*Gatchell, Frank G. (SHNS, SSO), *S*,
236-0641
*Graham, Wm. John (ASTR), *TR*,
751-3031
*Grozea, Petre N. (ASCO),
235-8331, ext. 381
*Hampton, James W. (ASCO), *M*,
235-8331
*Hoge, Arthur F., Jr. (ASCO), *G/M*,
271-4000
*Humphrey, G. Bennett (AACE, AACR,
ASCO), *PD/HEM*, 271-4412

*Lane, Daniel M. (AACE, ASCO), *PD*, 236–0641
*Maxwell, James D. (ASTR), *TR*
*Merrill, James A. (SGO), *OG*, 271–5000
*Moran, Willard B. (ASHNS), *OT*, 271–5504
*Nitschke, Ruprecht (AACE, ASCO), *PD*, 271–4412
*Resler, Donald R. (ASHNS), *OT*, 235–7561
*Richardson, David L. (ASTR), *TR*
Schilling, J.A. (AACR)
*Taylor, Thomas J. (ASTR), *TR*
*Walker, Ethan A., Jr. (ASHNS), *OT*, 236–0641
*Wine, Charles J. (ASHNS), *OT*, 236–0641
*Wizenberg, Morris J. (ARS, ASTR), *RO*

TULSA (918)

*Brickner, Theodore, Jr. (ARS, ASTR), *RT*, 627–2200
*Brownson, Richmond J. (ASHNS), *OT*, 663–5577
*Ellis, Robert George (ASTR), *TR*, 742–6541
*Garretson, Forrest D. (ASCO), *M/HEM*, 627–7200
Gooden, David S. (ASTR)
Horton, J. (AACR)
*Lhevine, Dave B. (ASTR), *RT*, 584–1351
Linscott, Joan S. (ASTR)
*Rosenthal, Avram E. (ASTR)
*Schnetzer, George W., III (ASCO), *HEM*, 584–7224
*Spann, Joe L. (SHNS), *S*, 584–6111
*Watt, Richard H., Jr. (ASCO), *M/ONC*, 749–7931

OREGON

BEAVERTON

Hsu, F.H. (AACR)

CORAVALLIS

Trout, Dale E. (ASTR)

EUGENE (503)

*Racely, Clay A. (ASTR), *R*, 686–6918

MEDFORD (503)

*Markee, Alan S. (ASTR)
*Ptacek, John J. (ASTR), *TR*, 773–6281, ext. 391

PORTLAND (503)

*Baker, Harvey W. (SHNS, SSO), *S*, 226–6071
Dawson, P.J. (AACR)
*Dennis, Daniel L. (SSO), *S*
*Everts, Edwin C. (ASHNS), *OT*, 225–8627
*Fletcher, Wm. S. (AACE, ASCO, SSO), *S*, 225–8478
*Galen, Wm. P. (ASCO), *M*, 228–6509
*Gallucci, John J. (ASTR)
*Goldman, Robert D. (ASCO), *M/HEM*, 292–0709
*Groshong, Leroy E. (ARS, ASCO, SHNS, SSO), *S*
*Hill, Dennis R. (ASTR)
*Horowitz, Irving J. (ASTR), *RT*, 223–6154
Hossman, Kenneth L. (ASTR)
*Hyman, Milton D. (ASTR), *R*
*Hyman, Selma B. (ASTR), *R*
*Krippaehne, Wm. W. (SSO), *S*
*Lee, J. Robert (ASTR), *RT*, 280–4161
*Lienert, Richard E. (ASTR)
*Lowy, Richard O. (ASTR), *RT*, 297–4411
*Molendyk, John M. (ASTR)
*Moss, William Thom (ARS, ASTR), *RT*, 225–8757
**Rickles, Norman H. (AACE), *OP*, 225–8903

*Simonton, Oscar C., Jr. (ASTR)
*Stevens, Kenneth R., Jr. (ASTR),
  TR, 225-8758
*Summers, Gordon W. (ASHNS),
  OT/HNS, 288-5861
Weber, G.H. (AACR)
*Wellings, Selton H. (AACE)
*Wilson, Nathaniel (SSO)

SALEM

*Allen, Kirby Lawrence (ASTR), TR
*Thompson, Margaret J. (ASTR), TR

PENNSYLVANIA

ABINGTON (215)

*Medinger, Fred (ARS, SSO)
*Tulsky, Emanuel G. (ASTR),
  R/RT, 885-3110

ALLENTOWN (215)

*Friedberg, Milton J. (SHNS),
  S/HNS, 433-4852
*Kim, Chung Han (ASTR), TR
*Prager, David (ASCO), HEM,
  433-6691
*Prorok, Joseph (ASCO), S, 439-8818
*Silon, Nathaniel (ASTR), RO,
  821-2283

ALLISON PARK (412)

*Connolly, David P. (SSO), S-ONC,
  566-1513

BALA CYNWYD

*Stanton, Leonard (ASTR)

BRYN MAWR (215)

*Pettit, Mary D. (AACE), OG,
  849-0400, ext. 4422
*Royster, Henry P. (SHNS)

CHELTENHAM

Kim, J.S. (AACR)

DANVILLE (717)

*Bates, James S. (SGO), OG
*Beecham, Clayton T. (SGO), OG,
  275-6296
*Beiler, David (ARS, ASTR), RT,
  275-6304
*Eyerly, Robert C. (SHNS, SSO), S
*Fazekas, John T. (ASTR), TR
*Vrabec, Donald P. (ASHNS), OT,
  275-6431

DARBY (215)

*Djerassi, Isaac (AACR), 586-5020

EASTON (215)

*Waltman, C.A. (AACR, SSO), S,
  252-6123

EDWARDSVILLE (717)

*Hora, James F. (ASHNS), OT,
  287-1148

ERIE (215)

*Demuth, Robert J. (SHNS), PLS/S,
  455-4496
Krohmer, Jack S. (ASTR)
*Scibetta, Mario P. (ASTR), R

GREENSBURG

*Ozarda, Ahsen T. (ARS, ASTR), R

HARRISBURG (717)

*Griff, Leonard C. (ASTR), R
*Herceg, Stephen J. (SHNS), PLS,
  233-4691

HERSHEY (717)

*Bartlett, G.L. (AACR), 534-8350
Kreider, J.W. (AACR)

*Lipton, Allan (AACR, ASCO), *M/ HEM*, 534-8390
*Miller, Stephen H. (SHNS), *PLS*, 534-8866
*Stryker, John A. (ARS, ASTR), *TR*

JOHNSTOWN

*McAneny, John B. (ASCO)

KENNETT SQUARE (215)

*Berkowitz, Irving M. (ASCO), *M*, 444-0180
*Ferrer, J.P. (ASCO)

LANCASTER (717)

Ebersole, John H. (ASTR), *RT/R*, 393-5801

MALVERN

Clark, W.H., Jr. (AACR)

MEADVILLE (814)

*Manning, Harry J. (ARS), *R*, 337-1261

MELROSE PARK

*Wolman, Irving (AACE)

PAOLI

*Lo Ponte, Marie A. (ASTR), *R*

PHILADELPHIA (215)

*Ainninger, George F. (ASTR), *RT*, 829-6254
*Aleo, Joseph J. (AACE)
*Aponte, Gonzalo (AACE)
*Asbell, O. Sucha (ASTR), *RT*, 448-8414
Atkins, Joseph P., Jr. (SHNS), *OT*, 829-5180

*Barry, Wm. (AACE), *M/HEM*, 221-4613
Baserga, R. (AACR), 221-3257
*Bellet, Robert E. (AACR, ASCO), *MO*, 722-1900
*Bennett, Hugh D. (AACE)
*Berwick, L. (AACR)
*Berkowitz, Irving M. (ASCO), *M*, 662-2407
*Bishop, Paul R. (ARS), *R*, 545-6476
*Bornstein, Richard S. (AACR, ASCO), *MO*, 927-3900
*Brady, Luther W., Jr. (AACR, ARS, ASCO, ASTR), *RT*, 448-8409
*Bransfield, John W. (ARS, ASCO)
*Breedis, C. (AACR), 259-0510
*Brennan, James T. (ASTR), *R*
*Brodovsky, Harvey S. (ASCO), *M/ ONC*, 829-7680
*Brodsky, Isadore (AACE, AACR, ASCO), *M/HEM*, 448-8026
*Burningham, Richard A. (ASCO), *M/HEM*
*Cameron, Charles S. (SSO), *S*, 448-7689
*Carabasi, Ralph A. (ASCO), *M*, 923-1096
*Cassileth, Peter A. (ASCO), *M*, 662-2433
Castro, Victoria G. (ARS), 722-1900, ext. 382
*Celebre, Joan A. (SGO), *OG*, 662-3312
*Chamberlain, Richard H. (ARS), *R*, 662-3030
*Clement, John A. (ASTR), *TR*
*Cohler, Alan (ASTR)
*Conroy, James F. (ASCO), *M*, 448-8026
*Cramer, Lester M. (SHNS), *PLS*, 221-3933
*Creech, Richard H. (ASCO), *M*, 722-1900, ext. 301
*Croll, Millard N. (ARS, ASTR), *R*
*Damsker, Jeffrey (ASTR)
D'Angio, G.J. (AACR)
*Davis, Lawrence W. (ARS, ASCO, ASTR), *RT*, 829-8814

*Day, John L. (ASTR)
*Demare, Paul M. (ASTR), *RT*,
 829-6527
*Dimitrov, N.V. (ASCO), *M*, (517)
 355-1855
*Donaldson, Milton H. (AACE, AACR,
 ASCO), *PD*, 546-2700
*Eisman, Sylvan (ASCO), *M*, 386-1414
*Engstrom, Paul F. (AACE, ASCO),
 M, 722-1900, ext. 301
Eskin, B.A. (AACR)
*Evans, Audrey E. (AACE, AACR,
 ASCO), *PD*, 387-6000
*Fineberg, Charles (AACE)
*Fishburn, Robert I. (ASTR)
Furth, J.J. (AACR)
Gasic, G. (AACR)
*Goepp, Carla E. (ASCO), *M*,
 829-6834
*Goldman, Leonard Irving (ASCO,
 SSO), *S*, 221-3624
*Goldsmith, Harry S. (SSO), *S*
Gorson, Robert O. (ARS), 829-7811
*Hann, Hie-Won L. (ASCO), *PD*,
 ASCO), *OG*, 545-4356
Hale, John (ARS), *R*, 662-3081
*Hamilton, Ralph (SHNS), *PLS*,
 662-2046
*Hann, Hie-Won L. (ASCO), *PD*,
 342-1000, ext. 456
*Harwick, Robert D. (SHNS, SSO),
 S, 221-3383
**Henefer, Edward (AACE)
Henle, W. (AACR)
Herbut, P.A. (AACR)
*Holroyde, Christopher Peter (ASCO),
 M, 649-1400
*Jackson, Laird G. (AACR, ASCO),
 M, 829-6955
*Jepson, Joanne H. (ASCO), *M/HEM*,
 849-0400, ext. 4791
*Kahn, Sigmund B. (AACE, AACR,
 ASCO), *M/HEM*, 448-8026
Koprowska, I. (AACR)
Koprowski, H. (AACR)
*Kramer, Simon (ARS, ASTR), *RT*,
 829-6702
*Lehr, Herndon B. (SHNS)

Leighton, J. (AACR)
*Lepanto, Philip B. (ASTR), *TR*,
 662-3071
*Lerner, Harvey J. (AACR, ASCO),
 S, 829-3583
*Levick, Stanley N. (ASCO), *ONC*,
 927-3900, 924-6030
*Lewis, George C. (ARS, SGO), *OG*
Linna, T.J. (AACR)
*Littman, Philip (ASTR), *TR*,
 662-3074
*Lloyd, Paul T. (AACE), *R*,
 748-1000, ext. 207
London, W.T. (AACR)
*McCracken, Stewart (ASCO), *M*,
 242-5077
Maguire, H.C., Jr. (AACR)
*Mansfield, Carl M. (ASTR)
*Mastrangelo, Michael J. (AACR,
 ASCO), *M/MO*, 722-1900
*Meadows, Anna T. (ASCO), *PD*,
 387-6000
*Mikuta, John J. (ARS, SGO), *OG*,
 662-3313, 662-3318
*Miller, Arthur S. (AACE), *OP*,
 229-8500, ext. 374
*Moss, N. Henry (SSO), *S*, 927-3131
*Nichini, Franco M. (ARS, ASTR),
 TR, 221-4234
*Norris, Charles M. (ASHNS), *OT*,
 223-4843
Nowell, P.C. (AACR)
*Parker-Popky, Janet A. (ASTR), *RT*,
 849-0400, ext. 4728
*Payne, Franklin L. (ARS)
*Pendergrass, Eugene P. (ARS), *R*,
 662-3035
*Popky, George L. (AACE)
*Pratt, Lindsay L. (ARS, ASHNS),
 OT, 829-6784
Prehn, R.T. (AACR)
*Putnam, Richard C. (AACR, ASCO,
 SSO), *M*, 642-6545
*Randall, Peter (SHNS)
Reichle, F.A. (AACR)
*Rhoads, Jonathan E. (AACR,
 SSO), *S*
*Robbins, Robert (ARS, ASTR), *R*

*Rominger, C. Jules (ARS, ASTR), *TR/NM*, 748-7595
*Rosemond, George P. (SSO), *S/TS*, 221-3621
*Schwartz, Emanuel (AACR, ARS), *R*, 655-8510
*Schwegman, Cletus (AACE)
*Serber, Wm. (ARS, ASTR), *RT*, 823-7447
*Seydel H. Gunter (ARS, ASTR), *RT*, 722-1900, ext. 381
*Sklaroff, David M. (ARS, ASTR), *RT*, 455-9577
*Smalley, Richard V. (ASCO), *M*, 221-4615
*Snow, James B., Jr. (ASHNS), *OT*, 662-2654
*Southam, Chester M. (AACR, ASCO, SSO), *MO*, 829-8874
*Southard, Martha E. (ASTR)
Sutnick, Alton I. (AACR, ASCO), *M*, 563-1365
*Talbot, Timothy R. (ASCO), *M/HEM*, 342-1000
*Teahan, Roscoe W. (SHNS), *S/ONC*, 844-6200
*Torpie, Richard J. (ASTR)
*Treat, Carmen L. (ASCO), *PD/HEM*, 563-8251
Tsou, K.C. (AACR)
Upton, G.V. (AACR)
Urback, F. (AACR)
Van Dyke, J.H. (AACR)
Van Scott, E.J. (AACR)
*Wampler, Stanley N. (ASTR)
Warren, G.H. (AACR)
Weinhouse, S. (AACR)
*Weiss, Arthur J. (AACR, ASCO), *M/MO*, 829-6952
Wheelock, E.F. (AACR)
*Whitaker, Linton A. (SHNS), *PLS*, 662-2048
*Woodward, Kent Thomas (ASTR), *RT*, 662-3033
Yamamoto, N. (AACR)
Yushok, W.D. (AACR)
Zeidman, I. (AACR)
*Zinninger, George F. (ASTR), *RT*, 829-9506

PITTSBURGH (412)

*Arena, Sebastian (ASHNS), *OT*, 566-1515
*Bress, Alan N. (ASCO), *MO*, 621-9117
*Bress, James C. (ASCO), *M*, 621-9117
*Clare, David W. (AACE), *S*
*Concannon, Joseph P. (ARS, ASTR), *RT*, 237-3456
*Deutsch, Melvin (ASTR)
*Dickinson, John T. (ASHNS), *OT*, 281-1565
*Diprimio, Joseph V. (ARS, ASTR), *R*
*Duerksen, Roger L. (ASHNS), *OT*, 621-2656
Fetterman, G.H. (AACR)
*Fisher, B. (AACR, SSO)
Fisher, E.R. (AACR)
*Frich, John C., Jr. (ASTR)
*Gaisford, John C. (SHNS), *PLS*, 681-5995
*Garrett, Wm. S. (SHNS), *PLS*, 621-1333
*Hanna, Dwight C. (SHNS), *PLS*, 681-5995
*Kaplan, Carl M. (ASTR), *R/RT*, 391-8800
*Leen, Raymond L. (ASTR)
*May, Mark (ASHNS), *OT*, 681-2300
*McAllister, John D. (ASCO, ASTR, SSO)
*Murphy, Arthur I. (SHNS, SSO), *S*
*Parsons, John D. (ARS, ASTR), *TR*
*Perryman, Charles R. (ARS)
*Pugh, Reginald P. (AACR, ASCO), *M*, 237-3630
*Richardson, George S. (SHNS), *PLS*, 681-5995
*Ripepi, Anthony C. (ASCO), *M*, 469-1000
*Rogow, Edward (ASTR), *TR*, 281-0317
*Ruefer, Raimund George (SHNS)
Schiffer, L.M. (AACR)
*Steichen, Felicien M. (SHNS), *S*, 683-1100, ext. 745
*Verbin, R.S. (AACE, AACR), *OP*, 624-3181

*Williams, Norman S. (ASTR), *RT*,
683-1100, ext. 581

PLYMOUTH MEETING

Trilol, V.A. (AACR)

POTTSTOWN

*Gowen, George F. (SHNS)

ROCHESTER (412)

*Wilkie, Louis J. (ARS), *R*, 728-2802

SAYRE (717)

*Boselli, Bruce (ASCO), *M/HEM*,
888-6666
*Carpender, J.W. (ARS, ASTR,
SSO), *R*
*Meyer, Kenneth K. (SSO), *S*

STRATFORD (215)

*Close, P. Henry (AACR, ASCO),
M, 688-3731

VILLANOVA (215)

*Blady, John V. (ARS, SHNS, SSO),
HNS, 564-4741

WEST READING (215)

*Lusch, Charles J. (ASCO), *M/HEM*,
374-4404
*Rowan, Noel M. (ASCO), *M/HEM*,
376-8004

WERNERSVILLE

*Faust, Donald S. (ASTR)

WEST CHESTER (215)

*Tyson, Russell R. (SSO), *S*,
436-9735

WILKES BARRE (717)

*Schulman, Norman (ASTR), *RO*,
823-1121, ext. 301

WILLIAMSPORT (717)

*Share, Frederick S. (ASTR), *RO*,
326-4191

YORK (717)

*Strockbine, Melvin F. (ARS, ASTR),
RT, 771-2211

RHODE ISLAND

PROVIDENCE (401)

*Alabala, Maurice (ASCO), *M/HEM*,
277-5395
*Allegra, S.R. (AACR), 331-3325
*Brenckman, Wayne Dewitt, Jr.
(ASCO), *M*, 521-5055
*Calabresi, Paul (AACR, ASCO),
M, 521-5055
*Coleman, George V. (AACE, SSO),
S, 421-4255
*Cummings, Francis J. (AACR, ASCO),
M, 521-5055
*Forman, Edwin N. (ASCO), *PD*,
277-5171
*Glicksman, Arvin S. (AACR, ARS,
ASCO, ASTR), *RT*, 277-5007
*Kadish, Sidney P. (ASTR), *TR*,
277-8311
*Kaplan, Stephen R. (ASCO), *M*,
521-5055
*Leone, Louis A. (AACE, AACR,
ASCO), *M*, 277-5991
*McDonald, Charles (ASCO), *DT*,
521-5055, ext. 400
*McDuff, Henry C., Jr. (SGO), *G*,
421-8420
*Randall, H.T. (AACR, SSO), *S*
*Rege, Vishram B. (ASCO), *M*,
277-5393
*Tefft, Melvin (AACR, ARS, ASCO,
ASTR), *R/RT*, 277-4000

*Triedman, Leonard J. (SHNS, SSO),
S, 421-2992
*Vohr, Fred (ASCO), M, 433-1150
*Waterman, George W. (ARS)
*Webber, Banice M. (ASCO, ASTR),
RT, 277-8311

RUMFORD

*Batchelder, Philip (ASCO)

WARWICK (401)

*Kaan, Sze Kin (ASCO), HEM,
737-1121

SOUTH CAROLINA

AIKEN (803)

*Rasmussen, Loton H. (ARS, SSO),
M, 649-6211, ext. 3435

CHARLESTON (803)

*Fenn, Jimmy O. (ASTR)
*Hagerty, Robert F. (SHNS, SSO),
PLS, 722-1985
*Harvin, James S. (SHNS), PLS,
792-4273
*Hawk, John C., Jr. (AACE, ARS,
SHNS, SSO), S, 577-7550
McIver, F.A. (AACR)
*Maguire, Carter P. (SHNS)
*Moore, Terence N. (ASTR), TR,
792-4255
*Morgan, Samuel K. (AACE)
*O'Brien, Paul H. (AACE, SSO),
S/ONC, 792-3276
*Othersen, Henry B., Jr. (AACE), S
*Putney, F. Johnson (ASHNS), OT,
792-3531
Roof, B.S. (AACR)
Travis, Elizabeth L. (ASTR),
792-4255
*Underwood, Paul B., Jr. (SGO),
OG, 792-2864
*Wallace, Keene M. (ARS, ASCO,
ASTR), M

COLUMBIA (803)

*Dennis, Edward J., III (SGO), OG,
765-7165
*Fishburne, Skattowe B., Jr. (ASCO),
M/HEM, 779-7104

GREENVILLE (803)

*MacComb, Wm. (ARS, SHNS, SSO),
S/HNS
*Martin, Mitz M. (ASTR), TR,
232-9703
*Terry, Lewis N. (ARS, ASTR),
RT/ONC, 232-9703

SPARTANBURG

*Hull, David C. (SSO), S

SOUTH DAKOTA

SIOUX FALLS

*Britt, Donald H. (ARS), R

VERMILLION (605)

*Jaqua, Richard A. (AACE), PATH,
677-5626
*Wegner, Karl H. (AACE)

TENNESSEE

CHATTANOOGA (615)

*Boxell, John F. (ASHNS), OT,
267-6738
*Dugan, Phillip (ASTR), TR/MO,
267-3341
*Hathaway, Harvey K. (ASHNS),
OT/HNS, 267-6738

FRANKLIN

Oldham, R.K. (AACR)

JOHNSON CITY (615)

*Brindley, Clyde O. (ASCO), M,
928-0281

*Avery, Robert Bruce (ASCO),
  HEM/ONC, 546-8521
*Comas, Frank (ARS, ASTR), *RT*,
  971-3701
*Johnson, Joe B. (ASTR)
Krauss, S. (AACR)
Lozzio, B.B. (AACR)
*Perry, Ronald H. (ASTR), *RT*,
  546-9484
Solomon, A. (AACR)
Wigler, P.W. (AACR)

MADISON (615)

*McSwain, Barton (AACE),
  S/S-PATH, 865-8876

MEMPHIS (901)

*Aur, R.J.A. (AACR), 525-8381
*Black, Wm. T., Jr. (SSO), *G*,
  726-1234
*Carroll, David S. (ARS), *R*,
  726-6026
*Cocke, Edwin W., Jr. (ASHNS, SHNS),
  OT, 525-4631
*Demere, McCarthy (SHNS)
*Fleming, Irvin D. (SHNS, SSO),
  S/ONC, 726-1287
*Grant, James A. (ASHNS), *OT/MXF*,
  522-3051
*Green, A.A. (AACR), 525-8381
*Gross, Charles W. (ASHNS), *OT*,
  528-5885
*Harris, Donald R. (ASTR), *RO*
*Hughes, Robert R. (SGO), *OG/GO*,
  527-6641, ext. 484 or 488
*Hustu, H.O. (AACR, ARS, ASTR),
  R/RT, 525-8381
*Jabbour, Charles E. (SHNS), *S*
*Johnson, H. Durell (ASCO), *PD*,
  388-2613
Johnson, W.W. (AACR)
Mauer, A.M. (AACR)
*Mauer, Alvin M. (AACE, AACR),
  PD
*Mills, Dan C. (ARS), *G*, (615)
  725-7891

*Neely, Charles L. (AACR, ASCO),
  HEM-ONC, 528-5817
*Nickson, James J. (AACR, ARS,
  ASCO, ASTR, SSO), *RT*, 523-
  2471, ext. 2400
*Page, Alfred (SSO), *S*
*Page, Gene R. (SHNS), *ONC*,
  525-5678
*Page, Roy C. (SSO), *S/ONC*,
  525-5678
*Pigott, John D. (SHNS, SSO),
  S/ONC, 725-0987
*Pratt, Charles Benton, III (AACR,
  ASCO), *PD*, 525-8381
*Rogers, S. (AACR), 528-6160
*Ruch, Robert M. (ARS), *OG*,
  527-6427
*Sabesin, Seymour M. (AACE)
*Simone, J.V. (AACR), *PATH*,
  525-8381
Soloway, M.S. (AACR)
*Votava, Charles, Jr. (ASTR)
Wood, J.L. (AACR)

NASHVILLE (615)

*Adkins, Robert B., Jr. (AACE)
*Banner, Robert L. (SSO), *SO*,
  322-2391
*Bernard, Louis J. (AACE, SSO)
*Bolden, Theodore E. (AACE), *OP*,
  327-6337
*Browne, Edward (AACE), *S/ONC*,
  327-6402
*Byrd, Benjamin F., Jr. (SSO), *S*,
  327-3418
*Cocke, Wm. (SHNS), *PLS*, 329-1056
**Harris, Perry F. (SHNS)
*Hartmann, Wm. H. (SSO), *PATH*,
  322-2294
*Orth, David N. (AACE)
*Perry, Frank A. (SHNS, SSO),
  S/SO, 327-6235
*Reynolds, Vernon H. (AACE)
*Rosenfeld, Louis (SHNS), *S*
*Sawyers, John L. (AACE), *S*,
  255-6311, ext. 274
*Stroup, Steven L. (ASTR)
*Walker, Matthew (AACE), *S*

*Wright, John K. (SHNS), *S*,
329-1291

FT. SAM HOUSTON (512)

*McCracken, Joseph D. (ASCO), *M*, 221-4287
*Saxena, V. Amod (ARS, ASTR)

FORT WORTH (817)

*Dirks, Donald C. (ASTR)
*Fredric, Shett Keyser (ASCO), *M*, 338-9291
*Hendrick, James W. (SHNS)
Tseng, Chun H. (ASTR)

GALVESTON (713)

*Bailey, Byron J. (ASHNS), *OT*, 765-2701
*Blocker, Truman G., Jr. (SHNS)
*Costanzi, John J. (AACR, ASCO), *M/HEM*, 765-1862
*Jennings, Frank L. (AACE), *PATH*, 765-2889
*Larson, Duane L. (SHNS), *PLS*, 765-2454
*Levin, Wm. C. (AACR, ASCO), *M/HEM*, 765-1164
*Lewis, Stephen R. (SHNS), *PLS*, 765-1255
*Lynch, John B. (ASCO, SHNS), *PLS*, 322-3451
*Olson, Marvin H. (ARS, ASTR), *RT*, 765-2531
*Panettiere, Frank Joseph (AACR, ASCO), *M*, 765-1862
*Pranab, Ray (ASTR), *TR*

HOUSTON (713)

*Alford, Bobby R. (ASHNS), *OT*, 790-4671
*Badillo, Jorge (SHNS), *S*, 224-7811
*Ballantyne, Alando J. (SHNS, SSO)
*Banker, Franklin (ASTR)
*Bardwil, John M. (SHNS, SSO), *S*, 526-6449
*Barkley, Howard Thomas, Jr. (ASTR)
*Benjamin, Robert S. (AACR, ASCO), *M*, 792-2926
*Benyesh-Melnick, M. (AACR)

*Blumenschein, George R. (AACR), *M/ONC*, 792-2696
*Bodey, Gerald P. (ASCO), *M*, 792-2920
*Burdette, Walter J. (AACE, AACR, ASCO), *S*, 523-2228
*Burgess, Michael A. (ASCO), 792-2688
*Busch, H. (ASCO)
*Butler, James (SHNS), *PATH*, 526-5411
*Byers, Robert M. (SHNS)
*Caderao, J.B. (ASTR)
*Cangir, Ayten (AACR, ASCO), *PD*, 792-2266
*Chamberlin, James A. (ARS, SSO), *HNS*, 522-0724
*Clark, R. Lee (AACE, ASCO, SHNS, SSO), *S*, 526-6411, ext. 231
*Collins, Vincent P. (ARS, ASTR, SSO), *RT*, 782-9515, ext. 251
*Colpitts, R. Vernon (ARS)
*Copeland, Murray M. (AACE, ARS, SHNS, SSO), *S*, 526-5411, ext. 525
*Dale, Sebron C. (ASCO), *M*, 792-2370
*DeBakey, M.E. (AACR), 526-2669
*Delclos, Luis (ARS, ASTR, SSO), *TR*, 526-5411, ext. 266
*Derrick, Wm. S. (SSO), *ANES*, 526-5411, ext. 300
*Dmochowski, Leon L. (AACR, ASCO), *V*, 792-3270
*Douglass, Charles C. (ASCO), *M*, 781-7120
**Drane, Joe B. (SHNS), 526-5411, ext. 507
*Durrance, Fred Y. (ASTR)
*Earl, David M. (ARS)
*Easley, James David (ASTR)
*Eckles, Nylene E. (AACR, ASCO), 526-5411, ext. 563
*Fechner, Robert E. (SSO)
*Feldman, Arnold (ARS, ASTR)
*Fernbach, Donald J. (AACR, ASCO), *PD/HEM/ONC*, 521-4122
*Fletcher, Gilbert H. (ARS, ASTR, SSO)

*Freeman, Bromley S. (SHNS),
  PLS, 795-5584
*Freireich, Emil J. (AACR, ASCO),
  M/HEM, 792-2660
*Fries, John G. (SHNS), *HNS*,
  522-0724
*Fuller, Lillian M. (ARS, ASTR,
  SSO), *RT*, 526-5411, ext. 553
*Goepfert, Helmuth (SHNS), *OT*,
  792-3255
*Guillamondegui, Oscar M. (ARS,
  ASCO, SHNS), *HNS*, 792-3255
*Gutierrez, Augusto E. (ARS, ASTR),
  RT
*Gutterman, Jordan U. (ASCO),
  M/HEM, 792-2676
*Harris, Herbert H. (ASHNS), *OT/
  HNS*, 526-4045
*Hart, Jacqueline S. (ASCO), *M*,
  526-5411, ext. 548
*Haynie, Thomas P., III (ASCO),
  M/NM, 792-2855
*Hersh, Evan (AACR, ASCO), *M*,
  792-2666
*Hickey, Robert C. (AACR, ARS,
  ASCO, SSO)
*Hill, C. Stratton, Jr. (ASCO), *M*,
  792-2844
*Hoaglin, Lester L., Jr. (ASCO), *M*,
  526-2051
*Hollander, N. (AACR)
*Howe, Clifton D. (AACR, ASCO),
  M, 792-3460
*Hrgovcic, Martin (ASCO), *M/HEM*,
  526-2051
*Hudgins, Philip T. (ASTR)
*Hussey, David H. (ARS, ASCO, ASTR)
*Jesse, Richard H. (ARS, ASTR,
  SHNS, SSO), *HNS*, 526-5411,
  ext. 395
*Johnson, Douglas E. (AACR, ARS),
  U, 792-3260
Jordon, G.L., Jr. (AACR), 790-4578
*Kaplan, Alan L. (SGO), *OG*,
  524-3049
*Kaufman, Raymond D. (SGO),
  OG, 529-4951
*Komorn, Robert M. (ASHNS), *OT*,
  797-0022

Landren, Robert C. (ASTR)
Lane, Montague (AACE, AACR,
  ASCO), *PD*, 790-4451
Levy, B.M. (AACR)
*Lindberg, Robert D. (ARS, ASTR),
  TR, 526-5411, ext. 266
Livingston, R.B. (AACR)
*McBride, Charles M. (SSO), *S*,
  526-5411, ext. 397
McCredie, Kenneth B. (AACR, ASCO),
  M/HEM, 792-2680
*MacDonald, Eleanor J. (ARS)
McKelvey, Eugene M. (AACR, ASCO),
  M, 792-2933
*Martin, John E. (SSO), *R*, 228-8561
*Martin, Richard (SSO)
**Matalon, Victor (SHNS)
*Mavligit, Giora M. (AACR, ASCO),
  M, 792-2121
Merino, Orlando R. (ASTR)
*Middleman, Edward L. (ASCO),
  M, 526-2051
*Miller, Lowell S. (ASTR), *RT*
*Moench, Howard C. (ASTR), *TR*,
  527-5000
*Montague, Eleanor (ARS, ASTR),
  RT, 526-5411, ext. 266
*Mountain, Clifton F. (ARS, ASCO,
  SSO), *S*, 792-3264
Nelson, Alvah J. (ASTR)
*Nelson, Robert S. (AACR, ASCO),
  M, 792-2828
*Newton, Berne L. (AACE, SSO),
  PATH, 526-3311, ext. 421
Orengo, A. (AACR)
*Price, Harry R. (ASCO), *M*,
  526-2051
Randerath, K. (ASCR)
*Rawson, Rulon W. (AACR, ASCO,
  SSO), *M*, 792-3020
*Rodriguez, Hector (SHNS, SSO), *SO*
*Rodriquez, Victorio (AACR, ASCO),
  M, 792-2924
*Romsdahl, Marvin M. (SSO), *S*,
  526-5411
*Root, Elihu N. (ASCO), *M*,
  526-2671
*Rutledge, Felix N. (ARS, SGO,
  SSO), *OG*, 526-5411, ext. 393

*Samuels, Melvin L. (AACR, ASCO),
M, 792-2830
Seman, G. (AACR)
*Sessions, Roy B. (ASHNS), OT,
790-4671
*Shalek, Robert J. (ASTR)
Shaw, C.R. (AACR)
*Shullenberger, C.C. (ASCO),
M/HEM, 792-2860
*Sinkovics, Joseph G. (AACR,
ASCO), M/ONC, 792-2820
*Smith, Frank E. (ASCO), M,
790-4461
*Smith, Julian P. (ARS, SGO)
*Spjut, Harlan J. (SSO)
*Starling, Kenneth A. (AACE, ASCO),
PD/HEM, 521-4122
*Stehlin, John S., Jr. (AACR)
*Sullivan, John Peter (AACR, ASCO),
M, 522-1711
*Sullivan, Margaret P. (AACE, ASCO),
PD, 526-5411, ext. 505
*Sutow, Wataru W. (ASCO), PD,
526-5411
*Taboada, Carlos F. (ASCO), M,
526-2671
*Tapley, Norah D. (ARS, ASTR)
*Tashima, Charles K. (ASCO), M,
792-2817
Taylor, H.G. (AACR)
*Tidwell, Thomas J. (ASTR)
*Topek, Nathan H. (ARS)
Trentin, J.J. (AACR)
Trujillo, J.M. (AACR)
Walborg, E.F., Jr. (AACR)
*Wall, John A. (ARS)
Ward, D.N. (AACR)
*Wharton, J. Taylor (ARS, SGO)
*White, Edgar C. (SSO)
*Withers, Hubert R. (ASTR)
Yeoman, L.C. (AACR)

LAKELAND AFB (512)

*Coltman, C.A., Jr. (AACR, ASCO),
M, 671-7311
*Rossoff, Arthur Harold (ASCO), M,
671-7511

*Skinner, Odis Duane (ASTR), R/RT,
671-7705

LUBBOCK (806)

*West, John T. (SSO), S/ONC,
762-3401

PASADENA (713)

*Brown, Gerald A. (SHNS), OT,
477-7000

PLAINVIEW (806)

*Long, John C., Jr. (SHNS, SSO), S,
293-4571

SAN ANTONIO (512)

*Aust, J. Bradley (AACE, ASCO,
SHNS), S, 696-6131
*Cruz, Anatolio B., Jr. (AACE, ASCO,
SHNS), S, 696-6151
*Decoursey, E. (SSO)
*Frazell, Edgar L. (SHNS, SSO), HNS,
227-6325
*Galbreath, Robert J. (AACE)
*Gregory, Ernest J. (ASCO), S,
696-3320
*Hills, Wm. J. (SHNS), S, 227-6325
*McGuire, Wm. L. (AACR, ASCO),
M, 696-6343
*Sears, David A. (AACE), M,
696-6526
*Smith, James R. (SHNS), S
*Thor, Daniel E. (AACR, ASCO),
PATH, 696-6501
*Weinberg, Paul (AACE)
*Whitecar, John P., Jr. (AACR, ASCO),
M, 227-6156
*Williams, Thomas Eugene (AACE,
ASCO), PD/PATH, 696-6251

TEMPLE (817)

*Bonnet, John (ASCO), M/HEM/ONC,
778-4451

*Palmer, Robert L. (ASCO), *HEM/
ONC/M*, 778-4451
*Riegler, Henry C. (SHNS), *S/HNS*,
778-4811

WACO (817)

*Canning, Lawrence (ASCO), *M/ONC*,
752-3444

UTAH

GRANGER (801)

*Christensen, Wm. R. (ARS), *R*,
298-9061

SALT LAKE CITY (801)

*Bragg, David G. (SSO), *R*, 581-7552
*Brown, Richard Clifton (ASTR), *RO*
*Cowan, Leland B. (SHNS, SSO), *SO*,
355-3991
*Dingman, David L. (SHNS)
*Dougherty, J.H. (AACR), 581-6308
*Eltringham, James R. (ASTR), *RT*,
581-8793
*Gunderson, Leonard L. (ASTR)
*Jackson, Henry M. (SSO), *S*, 364-5673
*Lahey, M. Eugene (AACE, AACR,
ASCO), *PD*, 581-7776
*McDivitt, Robert W. (SSO)
*Miles, C.P. (AACR)
*Plenk, Henry P. (ARS, ASTR), *RO*,
322-5105
*Quagliana, Joseph M. (AACE)
*Shaw, John A. (ASTR), *RO*,
322-1755
*Smart, Charles Rich (ASCO, SHNS,
SSO), *S*, 322-5666
*Snyder, Clifford C. (SHNS), *PLS*,
581-7719
*Stewart, J. Robert (ARS, ASTR),
581-8793
*Taylor, George W. (ASTR), *TR*
*Townsend, L.B. (AACR)
*Woolf, Robert M. (SHNS), *PS*,
322-1096
*Zbar, B. (AACR), 484-6757

VERMONT

BENNINGTON (802)

*Toolan, H.W. (AACR), 442-6361

BURLINGTON (802)

*Brown, G. Stephen (ARS, ASTR),
RT, 656-3506
*Coon, Robert W. (AACE), *PATH*
*Dickerman, Joseph David (ASCO),
PD, 656-2296
*Haines, Carleton R. (AACE, ASCO),
S/ONC, 656-3550
*Kun, Larry E. (ASTR), *R*
*Stevens, D.F. (AACR), 878-8345
*Yates, Jerome W. (ASCO), *M/ONC*,
656-3724

PITTSFORD (802)

*Lathrop, Frank D. (ASHNS), *OT*,
483-6430

VIRGINIA

ALEXANDRIA (703)

*Bateman, Jeanne C. (AACR, ASCO),
M/MO, 549-1130

ARLINGTON

*Richardson, H.L. (AACR)

CHARLOTTESVILLE (804)

Agarwall, Suresh K. (ASTR)
*Constable, Wm. C. (AACE, ASTR),
RO, (703) 924-5191
*Edgerton, Milton T. (SHNS), *PLS*,
924-5068
*El Mahdi, Anas M. (ASTR), *RT*,
(703) 924-5191
*Fitzhugh, G.S. (ASHNS), *OT/MXF*,
295-1181
*Goldstein, Gerald (AACE, AACR,
ASCO), *M*, 924-2627

*Horsley, J. Shelton, III (AACE, SSO), *S*, 924-2028
*Komp, Diane M. (AACR, ASCO), *PD*, 924-5105
*McLean, Walter C. (ASHNS), *OT*, 295-1181
*Rosenoff, Stephen (AACR, ASCO), *M*, 977-6212
*Ruffner, Winfred B., Jr. (AACE, ASCO), *M/MO*, 924-5067
*Shaeffer, James (ASTR), *R*
*Smith-Meyer, Ragnar (ASTR), *TR*
*Thornton, W. Norman, Jr. (SGO), *OG*, 924-2221

CULPEPER (703)

*Weaver, Delmar F. (ASHNS), *OT, MXF*, 825-0081

FALLS CHURCH (703)

Gargus, J.L. (AACR), 560-2519

MECHANICSVILLE

*Burke, Arthur W., Jr. (ASTR)

NEW PORT NEWS (304)

*Myles, John T. (ASTR), *TR*, 596-3081, ext. 386

NORFOLK (804)

*Adamson, Jerome (SHNS), *PLS*, (703) 623-1090
*Cross, James P., Jr. (ASHNS), *OT*, 623-0526
*Horton, Charles E. (SHNS)
*Mladick, Richard A. (SHNS), *PLS/MXF/HNS*, (703) 481-2612
*Rosato, Francis E. (AACE, ASCO), *S*, 441-3869
*Schechter, Gary L. (ASHNS), *OT*, 623-0526

PORTSMOUTH (804)

*Upton, Richard T. (SGO), *OG*, 397-6581

RESTON (703)

*Wright, B.S. (AACR), 860-1467

RICHMOND (804)

Aydar, Cetin K. (ASTR)
*Bilek, Frantisek S. (ASTR)
*Boyan, Charles P. (SSO), *ANES*, (703) 770-5263
*Coleman, Claude C. (SHNS), *PLS*, 285-0554
*Crawford, John N. (ASTR)
*Dabney, Wm. T., III (ASCO), *M/HEM*, 770-5184
*Dunn, Leo J. (ARS, SGO), *OG*, (703) 770-4111
*Elzay, Richard P. (AACE)
*Gill, John A. (ASHNS), *OT*, 320-1369
*Glover, John D. (ASTR), *RT*
*Goldman, I.D. (AACR), 770-4175
*King, E. Richard (ARS, ASTR), *RT*, 770-5138
*Kuperminc, Mario (ASCO), *M*, 825-9575
*Lawrence, Walter, Jr. (AACE, AACR, SHNS, SSO), *S*
*Markowitz, Martin (AACE)
*Mellette, Susan J. (AACE)
*Regelson, Wm. (AACR, ASCO), *M*, 770-5556
*Royster, R.L. (ASTR), *RT*
*Stickley, E. Eugene (ARS), 770-4341
*Terz, Jose Juan (SHNS, SSO), *S*, 770-4182
*Wampler, Galen Lee (ASCO), *M*, 770-4531
*Wassum, James A. (ASTR)

ROANOKE (703)

*Cole, John, Jr. (ASHNS), *OT,* 342-3461

*Haley, Harold B. (AACE, AACR, ASCO), *S*, 345-5363
*Lougheed, Marvin N. (ARS, ASTR), *R*
*Monaghan, Thomas W. (ASTR)
*Peterson, Charles H. (ARS)
*Trout, Hugh H., Jr. (SSO)

SALEM (703)

*Chakrovorty, Ranes C. (AACE, SHNS, SSO), *S*, 344-2021, ext. 221

VIRGINIA BEACH

*Degiorgi, Lucio S. (ASTR)

WINCHESTER (703)

*Boyd, Robert (SSO), *S*, 667-4830

WASHINGTON

BELLEVUE (206)

*Warner, Glenn A. (ARS, ASTR), *RO*, 292-2323

EDMONDS

Kent, Charles H. (ASTR)

MERCER ISLAND (206)

*Einstein, A.B., Jr. (AACR), 232-2678

RICHLAND

*Parker, Herbert M. (ARS)

SEATTLE (206)

*Bagley, C.M., Jr. (AACR), 329-3485
*Bean, M.A. (AACR), 624-1144
*Benditt, E.P. (AACE), *PATH*
*Bernstein, I.D. (AACR), 634-5427
*Berry, Herbert C. (ASTR)
*Chapman, W.H. (AACR), 543-4671
*Chard, Ronald L., Jr. (ASCO), *PD/ONC/HEM*, 624-5427

*Fefer, A. (AACR), 543-8556
Finley, John W. (AACE)
*Gerdes, Arthur J. (ASTR), *R*
*Goodell, Brian W. (ASCO), *M*, 329-6360
*Hafermann, Mark D. (ASTR), *TR*, 623-3700, ext. 348
*Hart, James E. (ASCO), *PD*
*Hartmann, John R. (AACE, AACR, ASCO), *PD/HEM/ONC*, 634-5427
*Hellstrom, I. (AACR)
*Hellstrom, K.E. (AACR)
*Hibbs, George G. (ARS, ASTR), *RT*, 292-2323
*Holcenberg, J.S. (AACR), 543-3268
Jones, Douglas (ASTR)
*Jones, Robert F. (AACE, SSO), *S/ONC*
*Novack, Alvin J. (SHNS), *HNS*, 682-4214
*Parker, Robert G. (AACE, ARS, ASTR), *RO*, 543-4895
*Rivkin, Saul E. (ASCO), *M/HEM*, 673-6600
*Taylor, Willis J. (ARS, ASTR), *R*
*Thomas, E.D. (AACR), 322-3140
*Weber, Edward L. (ASCO), *M/HEM/ONC*, 292-2323
*Wildermuth, Orliss (ARS, ASTR), *RT*, 292-2121
*Wotton, Peter (ASTR), *R*, 543-8897

SPOKANE

*Meekin, Francis A. (ASTR)
*Parson, E.F. (ASTR)
*Schmutz, Donald A. (ASTR)

TACOMA (206)

*Eliel, L.P. (AACR)
*Hays, Leonard L. (ASHNS), *OT/HNS*, 967-6622
*Origenes, M.L., Jr. (AACR), 572-6572
*Wallner, Paul E. (ASTR), *TR*
*Wong, Howard H. (ASTR), *RO*, 627-1181, ext. 313

WENATCHEE (216)

*Alexander, Donald W. (ASHNS), *OT*, 247-8348

YAKIMA

*Abbenhaus, James I. (SHNS), *OT*

WEST VIRGINIA

CHARLESTON (304)

*Gray, David B. (SHNS, SSO), *S/ONC*
*Lim, Romeo Y. (ASHNS), *OT*, 343-4371
*Litton, Clyde (SHNS)

HUNTINGTON

*Carey, James P. (SHNS, SSO), *S*

MARTINSBURG

*Hock-Ligeti, C. (AACR)

MORGANTOWN (304)

*Albrink, W.S. (AACR), 293-4469
*Jones, Barbara (AACR, ASCO), *PD/HEM/ONC*, 293-4451
**King, Ordie H., Jr. (AACE), *OP*, 293-2149
*Sprinkle, Philip M. (ASHNS), *OT*, 293-3233
*Tryfiates, G.P. (AACR), 293-4669
*Watne, A.L. (AACE, AACR, ASCO, SHNS), *S*, 293-3311
*Weiss, Raymond B. (ASCO), *M/ONC*, 292-4229
*Zimmermann, Bernard (SHNS), *S*, 293-3361

WHEELING (204)

*Castro, Leonides (ARS, ASTR), *TR*, 234-8561

WISCONSIN

BROOKFIELD (414)

*Turkington, R.W. (AACR), 786-4412

FOND DU LAC

*Parrish, John G. (ASTR)

GREEN BAY

*Mokrohisky, John F. (ASTR)

LA CROSSE (608)

Boge, R. Jerome (ASTR)
*Edland, Robert W. (ARS, ASCO, ASTR), *RT*, 785-2400, ext. 372
*Severeid, Larry R. (ASHNS), *OT*, 785-2400
*Weeth, John B. (AACR, ASCO), *M*, 785-2400

MADISON (608)

*Ansfield, Fred J. (AACE, AACR, ASCO, SSO), *M*, 262-1622
*Bosch, Antonio (ARS), *TR*, 262-2474
*Brandenburg, James H. (ASHNS), *OT*, 262-6846
*Bryan, George T. (AACR, ASCO, SSO), *MO*, 262-2110
*Buchler, Dolores A. (AACE, ASCO, ASTR), *OG/R*, 262-1961
*Caldwell, Wm. (ARS, ASTR), *RT*, 262-2477
*Carr, Richard M. (ASCO), *M/HEM*, 255-9414
*Davis, Hugh L., Jr. (ASCO), *M*, 262-1622
*Dibbell, David G. (SHNS)
*Dudiak, Stephen (ASTR)
*Goldfarb, S. (AACR), 262-2929
*Greenberg, Alvin J. (ASTR)
*Johnson, Robert O. (AACR, ASCO), *S*, 262-1626
*Kajiwara, K. (AACR), 262-1902

*Kline-Puletti, Joyce C. (ASTR), *R*
*Korbitz, Bernard C. (ASCO), *M/HEM/ ONC*, 252-8000
*Korst, Donald (AACR, ASCO), *M*. 263-4771
*Kubinski, H.A. (AACR), 262-6950
*Mackman, Sanford (ASCO), *S/ONC*, 255-6731, ext. 343
*Mohs, F.E. (AACR), 262-2803
*Mueller, G.C. (AACR), 262-1226
*Puletti, Joyce C. Kline (ASCO), *RT*, 262-2477
*Ramirez, Guillermo (AACR, ASCO), *ONC*, 262-1622
*Richards, Marcia J.S. (ASTR), *RO*, 262-2477
Rusch, H.P. (AACR)
*Samp, Robert J. (AACE)
*Schroeder, John M. (ASCO), *ONC*, 257-0561
*Wirtanen, George W. (ASCO, ASTR), *R*, 262-2477
*Wiley, Albert Lee, Jr. (ASCO, ASTR), *RT/NM*, 262-2477

MARSHFIELD (715)

*Banerjee, Tarit Kumar (ASCO), *M*, 387-5416
*Greenlaw, Robert H. (ASTR), *TR*, 387-1711

MIDDLETON (608)

*Gollin, Frank F. (ASCO, ASTR), *RT*, 233-5040

MILWAUKEE (414)

*Berridge, Frank (SSO), *S*, 463-1220
*Borella, L.D. (AACR), 344-7100
*Cox, James D. (ARS, ASTR)
*DeCosse, J.J. (AACR)
*Donegan, William Laurence (SHNS), *S*, 257-5226
*Fetherston, William (SGO), *OG*, 271-5152
*Fidler, Alan B. (ASTR)

*Filmanowicz, Edward (ASCO), *M/HEM/ONC*, 771-9870
*Gingrass, Ruedi P. (SHNS), *S*, 771-7730
*Greenberg, Maurice (ASTR), *R*
*Grueninger, Anthony (ASTR), *TR*, 271-2325
*Hurley, John D. (AACE, ASCO), *S*, 933-5066
*Kallas, Gerald J. (ASCO), *M*, 278-8290
*Kinzie, Jeanie J. (ASTR)
*Marks, Stanton A. (ASTR)
*Mattingly, Richard F. (SGO), *OG*
*Pattillo, R.A. (AACR), *OG*, 257-5567
*Pinkel, D. (AACR), 344-7100
*Stafl, Adolf (SGO), *OG*, 257-5560
*Wilson, Jesse F. (ARS, ASTR), *R*

SHEBOYGAN (414)

*Hoon, James R. (ASCO), *S*, 457-4461

WAUWATOSA (414)

*Gramling, Joseph J. (AACE), *S*, 771-1361

International

ARGENTINA

BUENOS AIRES

*Caubarrere, Alfredo N. (ASTR), *R*
*Cerisola, Jose A. (SHNS)
*Gruart, Federico (SHNS), *S/HNS*
*Maissa, Pedro A. (ARS)
*Marino, Hector (SHNS), *PLS*, 83-0365
*Pradier, Roberto N. (SHNS)
*Samengo, Luis A. (SHNS)
Schavelzon, Jose (ARS, SSO)
*Viacava, Enrique (SHNS)
*Yoel, Jose (SHNS)

CORDOBA

*Suarez, Osvaldo G. (SHNS)

MENDOZA

*Rufino, Carlos D. (SHNS)

SANTE FE

*Bertotti, Jorge A. (SHNS)

AUSTRALIA

FITZROY

*Millar, Hugh S. (ASHNS), *OT*

SIDNEY

*Indyk, John Sol (SHNS), *S*, 274–309
*Newton, Noel C. (SHNS)
*Poole, Allan G. (SHNS), *S/HNS*
*Sheridan, Brian F. (SHNS)

VICTORIA

*Ewing, Maurice Rossie (SHNS), *S*

BELGIUM

BRUSSELS

*Dor, Pierre (SHNS), *HNS/ONC*,
    (02) 343-39-88
*Tagnon, H.J. (ASCO, SSO), *MO*,
    (322) 382-766

GENT

*Matton, Guido E. (SHNS), *PLS*,
    22/2300

BRAZIL

BAHIA

*De Almeida, Joao Soares (ASTR), *TR*
*Telxelra, Luis C. (ASTR)

RIO DE JANEIRO

*Coutinho, Filho Alberto (ASTR),
    TR, (021) 260-0791
*De Marsillac, Jorge (SHNS)
*Dornelles, J. Jacques (SSO), *S*
*Lima, Victor A. (SHNS), *HNS*,
    255-0253
*Machado, Osolando J. (ARS, ASTR)
*Pinto, Vieira A. (ASCO)
*Santos-Silva, Moacyr Alves Dos A.
    (ARS, ASCO, SSO)
*Vierrira, Antonio P. (ASTR)

SAO PAULO

*Barbosa, Jorge F. (SHNS), *HNS*
*Barreto, Lins Jose R. (ASTR)
*Franca, Juiz C. (SSO)
*Gentil, Fernando C. (ARS, SHNS,
    SSO), *SO*, (0100), 278-8811
*Lederman, Marcos V. (ASTR), *R*
*Libonati, Sergio B. (ASTR), *TR*
*Pinto, Paulo E. (ASHNS, ASTR), *R*
*Roxo Nobre, Mathias O. (ARS,
    ASTR), *RT*, 278–88–11

CANADA

ALBERTA

Calgary (403)

*Barnes, Priscilla (ASTR), 263–0770

Edmonton (403)

*Band, Pierre R. (ASCO), *M/ONC*,
    452-6454
*Khaliq, Abdul (ASCO), *M*, 433-9461
*McCarten, Alan B. (SHNS), *S*,
    433-0904
*MacDonald, R. Neil (ASCO), *M/HEM*,
    433-3498
*McGowan, David (ASTR), *R/ONC*,
    433-9461
*MacLean, Wm. A. (SHNS, SSO),
    S/ONC, 429-6911
*Mallen, Richard W. (ASHNS), *OT*,
    433-6111

Pearson, James G. (ASTR)
*Tamaoki, T. (AACR), 432-3835
*Urtasun, R.C. (AACR, ASCO), *TR/R*, 433-9461

Manning (403)

*Nundy, Dhirenda M. (SHNS), *S*, 624-2551

BRITISH COLUMBIA

Vancouver (604)

*Cosbie, W.G. (ASCO)
*Flores, Albino (ASTR)
*Gibson, John M.W. (ARS, ASTR), *TR*, 874-9321
*Noble, R.L. (AACR), 228-3867
*Plenderleith, Ian H. (ASCO), *M*, 874-9321
*Robins, R. Edward (SHNS)
*Trapp, Ethylyn (ASTR)

MANITOBA

Winnipeg (204)

*Cooke, Robert L. (SSO), *S*, 774-6541
*Giles, James M. (ASTR), *RO*, 786-4731
Henderson, J.S. (AACR), (204) 783-3537
Hryniuk, W.M. (AACR)
Johnson, Richard J. (ARS, ASTR)
Karasewich, Eugene G. (SSO)
Levitt, Martin (AACR, ASCO)
McLellan, Wm. (ASTR)
*Penner, Donald (SSO), *PATH*
*Riese, Karl Theodore (SHNS, SSO), *S*, 233-1421
*Wallbank, A.M. (AACR)
*Walton, Richard J. (ARS, ASTR), *RT*, 774-6511, ext. 7604

NEW BRUNSWICK

St. John

*Smith, George D. (ASTR)

NOVA SCOTIA

Halifax (902)

*Aquino, Jose (ASTR), *TR/NM*, 429-7473
*Cunningham, Robert (ASTR), *RT*, 429-7473

ONTARIO

Hamilton (807)

*Dent, P.B. (AACR)
*Green, Lloyd S. (ARS)
*Lane, G. Alan (SHNS)
*Stratmanis, Ingrid Z. (ARS, ASTR), *TR*, 389-1371

Kingston (705)

*Burr, R.C. (ARS)
*Enns, Arthur G. (ASTR)
Kaufman, N. (AACR)
*Lott, J. Stewart (ARS, ASTR), *TR*, (613) 542-2877
*Sterns, Ernest E. (SHNS), *S*, 542-6920

London (519)

*Banerjee, Prabhat (ASTR), *TR*, 432-5241
*Fetterly, John C. (ASTR)
*Heeneman, Hans (ASHNS), *OT*, 432-9973
*Mackenzie, Donald A. (SHNS), *S*, 672-2120
*Thomson, Dugald H. (ASTR), *TR*
*Walker, I.G. (AACR), 679-2363
*Wallace, A.C. (AACR), 679-3022
*Watson, Thomas A. (ARS, ASTR), *TR*, 432-5241
*White, David F. (ASCO), *M*, 432-5241, ext. 385

Ottawa (613)

*Catton, Gordon (ARS, ASTR), *TR*, 728-3745
*Harris, Jules (AACR, ASCO), *M*, 231-2085
*Henderson, Ian W.D. (ASCO), *S*, 996-7332

*Hirte, Wolfgang E.O. (ASCO), *M*,
725-4361
*Klaassen, David J. (ASCO), *M*,
728-3745
*Rapp, Edna F. (ASCO), *M*, 738-3745
*Stewart, T.U.M. (AACR), 231-3168
*Stoddart, T. Glen (ARS, ASTR), *TR*,
728-3745

Thunder Bay

*Harger, William A. (ASTR)
*Riches, John (ASCO)

Toronto (416)

*Ash, Clifford L. (ARS, ASTR), *TR*,
924-0671, ext. 266
*Bartlett, Glenn S. (SHNS)
*Beale, Francis A. (ASTR)
*Bergsagel, Daniel E. (AACR, ASCO),
M/HEM, 924-0671, ext. 424
*Bush, Raymond (ASTR), *TR*,
924-0671
*Cannell, Douglas E. (ARS), *OG*,
423-4240
*Clark, Roy M. (ASTR), *RT*, 924-0671
*Conen, P.E. (AACR), 239-6338
*Curtis, John E. (AACE, AACR,
ASCO), *M/HEM*, 924-0671
*Fitzpatrick, Peter J. (ASTR), *TR*,
924-0671, loc. 445
*Jenkin, Richard D. (ASTR), *PD/TR*,
924-0671, ext. 442
*Johns, Harold E. (ARS), 924-0671,
ext. 336
*McCulloch, E.A. (AACR), 924-0671
*Mustard, Robert A. (ARS, SHNS)
*Palmer, John A. (SHNS), *S*, 921-6765
*Peters, M. Vera (ARS, ASCO, ASTR),
R, 924-0671
*Rider, Walter D. (ARS, ASTR), *RT*
*Rosen, Irving B. (SHNS), *S*, 596-4656
*Simpson, Wm. J. (ASTR)
*Taylor, R.M. (AACR), 961-7223
*Till, J.E. (AACR), 924-0671
*Wookey, Harold W. (SHNS)

Windsor (519)

*Maus, John H. (ARS, ASTR), *TR*,
253-7455
*Mok, George (ASTR)

QUEBEC

Chicoutimi (418)

*Genest, Leopold E. (ARS, ASTR),
TR/NM, 549-2195, ext. 581

Cote du Palais (418)

*Dionne, Louis (SSO), *S*, 694-5352

Montreal (514)

*Audet-Lapointe, Pierre (AACE, SSO)
*Ayoub, Joseph I.G. (ASCO), *HEM*,
937-8511, ext. 656
*Blais, Madeline (ASCO), *M/HEM*,
876-7964
*Boileau, Guy (ASCO), *M/HEM*,
876-7078
*Bouchard, Jean (ARS, ASTR)
*Bricout, Phillippe (ASTR), *TR*,
845-5178
*Cantero, A. (AACR), 866-7285
*Chevalier, Louise (ASCO), *PD*,
937-8511, ext. 392
*DelVecchio, Pierre (ASTR)
*Dufresne, Origene M. (ARS)
*Franchebois, Pierre (SHNS), *S*
*Hadzic, Ejub (ASTR), *R*
*Hazel, Joseph J. (ARS, ASTR), *R*
Lewis, M. (AACR)
*Mansell, Peter Wm. (ASCO), *S*,
842-1251, ext. 1803
*Margolese, Richard G. (ASCO), *S*,
697-3813
*Methot, Yuan (ARS, ASTR), *NM*,
876-6580
*Palmer, John D. (SHNS, SSO), *S*,
933-4432
*Pierce, Carleton B. (ARS)
*Perras, Colette (SHNS, SSO), *PLS*,
737-3015
*Poisson, Roger (ASTR)
*Roman, Ted (ARS)

*Sedlezky, Isadore (ARS), *R*,
 342–3111
*Shibata, Henry R. (SSO), *S*, 842–1231
*Skoryna, S.C. (AACR), 392–4860
*Tabah, Edward J. (ARS, SHNS, SSO),
 S, 932–4224
*Tremblay, G. (AACR), 842–1251
*Webster, John H. (ASTR), *TR*,
 (716) 845–3172

Quebec (418)

*LaPointe, Henri (ARS)
*Raymond, Paul E. (ASTR), *R*
*Thibault, Maurice (ARS, ASTR)
*Turcot, Jacques (SHNS), *S*, 522–7670

Sherbrooke

*Brailovsky, C. (AACR)

SASKATCHEWAN

Regina (306)

*Barclay, Thomas H.C. (SHNS), *SO*,
 537–9851

Saskatoon

*Brown, Esther (ASTR)
*Burkell, Charles (ASTR)

CHILE

SANTIAGO

*Rahausen, Albert (ARS, ASCO, SHNS)

CHINA, REPUBLIC OF

TAIPEI

*Chiang, Tze Chun (ASTR)
*Hung, Wen-Chih (SHNS)

COLUMBIA

BARRANQUILLA

*Lujan, Hernando E. (ASTR), *RT*

BOGOTA

*Ariza, Alvaro (ASTR)
*Constantin-Jimenez, Enrique (ASTR)
*Gaitan-Yanguas, Mario (ARS, ASTR,
 SSO)
*Hakim, Alejandro (SHNS)

CALI

*Aljure, Fortunato (SHNS, SSO)
*Palma, Jaime (ASCO), *M*, 661996

MANIZALES

*Arango, Cesar (ASTR)

COSTA RICA

SAN JOSE

*Camacho, Alvsro Manuel (ASTR)
Guevara-Barahona, Claudio (ASTR), *R*
*Gutierrez, Carlos M. (SHNS)
Hutt, G. Herbert (SSO)
*Nunez, Raphael (SSO)
*Perez, Vinicio (ASTR)

DENMARK

COPENHAGEN

*Clemmesen, Johannes (AACE)

HILLEROD

*Hansen, Heine H. (ASCO), *M*

EGYPT

CAIRO

*Sebai, Ismaile (SHNS)

EL SALVADOR

SAN SALVADOR

*Diaz-Bazan, Narciso (ARS, SSO)
*Mayen, Jose (ASTR)
*Toruno, Helmo R. (ASTR)

FRANCE

BORDEAUX

*Portmann, Georges (SHNS)

MONTPELLIER

*La Marque, J. Paul (ASCO)
*Romieu, Claude (SHNS, SSO)

NANCY

*Chardot, Claude (SHNS)

PARIS

*Ennuyer, Auguste (ARS)
*Israel, Lucien (ASCO), *M*, 260–77–00
*Leroux, Robert J. (SHNS)
*Moyse, P. (SHNS)

GERMANY

ESSEN

*Roettinger, Erwin M. (ASTR), *TR*

HAMBURG

*Zehm, Siegfried Johannes (SHNS), *OT*

MAINZ

*Scheunemann, H. (SHNS), *MXF*

GREECE

ATHENS

*Papaioannou, Anaxagoras (SHNS,
   SSO), *S*
*Razis, Dennis V. (SSO), *M*

GUATEMALA

GUATEMALA CITY

*Del Valle, Bernardo S. (ARS, ASCO,
   SHNS, SSO)
*Escobar, Carlos A. (ARS, ASTR), *RT*
*Galvez, Armando (SSO)

HAITI

PORT AU PRINCE

*Chevallier, Charles (SSO)

HONG KONG

KOWLOON

*Wang, Raymond S. (SHNS), *PS*

INDIA

AGRA

Srivastava, Sarda P. (SHNS)

BOMBAY

*Hiranandani, Lokhumal H. (ASHNS,
   SHNS), *OT*
*Jussawalla, Durab J. (SSO)
*Kothary, Pramod M. (SHNS), *S*
*Meher-Homi, Dady R. (SHNS, SSO)
*Mehta, Asok R. (SHNS), *S*
*Paymaster, Jal (SHNS, SSO)

MAHARASHTRA

*Gosavi, Dattatraya K. (SHNS), *S*

MADRAS

*Doraiswami, K.R. (ARS, *R*, 86641

MIRAJ

*Gosavi, Dattatraya K. (SHNS),
   699-Miraj

IRAN

SHIRAZ

*Haghighi, Parvix (SSO)

TEHRAN

*Akbar, Ghaffarian (ASTR), *RT*

IRAQ

BAGHDAD

*Talib, Hussein (ASCO), *S*, 89001

IRELAND

DUBLIN

*Mullins, Gordon M. (ASCO), *MO*

ISRAEL

JERUSALEM

*Hochman, Avraham (ASCO), *M/R*,
  02-6-2643

NABLUS

*Masri, Fayeg (SSO)

SAVYON

*Merenfeld, Ruben (ARS)

TEL AVIV

*Schindel, Jehuda (ASHNS), *HNS/OT*,
  (03) 222561

ITALY

FLORENCE

*Alajmo, Ettore (ASHNS), *OT*

MILAN

*Bonadonna, Gianni (ASCO), *M*, 2390
*DeLena, Mario (ASCO), *M*
*Veronesi, Umberto (AACE)

ROME

*Nervi, Carlo (ARS, ASCO, ASTR,
  SSO), *TR/M*, 495-6741, ext. 282
*Turano, Luigi (ARS)

JAPAN

CHIBA

*Majima, Hisashi (ASCO), *M*

KENYA

NAIROBI

*Levin, Arthur G. (ASCO), *M*, 2-4026

KOREA

CHOLA PUK DO

*Seel, David J. (SHNS, SSO), *S*

TAEGU CITY

Suh, Chul Sung (ARS)

LEBANON

BEIRUT

*Salem, Philip A. (ASCO), *M*, 340460

MEXICO

CUAHTEMOC Y PASTEUR

*Albores-Saavedra Jorge (SHNS),
  PATH, 578-45-08

GUADALAJARA

*Ramirez-Jaime, Casimiro (ARS,
  ASTR), *ONC*, 13-19-72
Riebeling, Manuel (ASCO, SSO)
*Sernia, Graciela M. (ASTR)

MEXICO CITY (905)

De La Garza, Jaime (ASCO), *M*,
  593-1890
*Garcia, German (ARS)
*Garza, Roberto C. (SHNS), *ONC*
*Krause, Luis G. (SHNS), *S/HNS*,
  534-7514
*Navarro, Lopez Efrain (ASTR)

*Noriega, Jose (ASTR), *RT*, 5-78-60-51
*Perches, Rudolfo D. (ASTR)
*Zalce, Horacio (SHNS, SSO)

MONTERREY

*Alaniz-Camino, Francisco (SHNS), *RT*

PISO

*Hasfura, Guilermo (ASTR)

NETHERLANDS

AMSTERDAM

*Snow, Gordon B. (ASHNS, SHNS),
  OT

LEIDEN

*Zwaveling, Albert (ASCO), *S*

NIJMEGEN

*Van Den Broek, Paul (ASHNS),
  OT/HNS

NORWAY

OSLO

*Berdal, Peter (SHNS)

PANAMA

PANAMA

*Aviles, Enero (AACE, SHNS, SSO), *S*

PARAGUAY

ASUNCION

*Riveros, Manuel (SHNS)

PERU

LIMA

*Caceres, Eduardo (SHNS, SSO), *SO*
*Pinillos-Ganoza, Luis (ASTR)

*Plaza, Felipe L. (SHNS)
*Reusche, Juan (ASTR)
*Rodriquez, Walter A. (SHNS)
*Salem, Louis E. (SHNS, SSO)
*Soto, Oscar (ARS)
*Travezan, Rodrigo (SHNS)

PHILIPPINES

MANILA

*Sarmiento, Augusto P. (SHNS, SSO)

PORTUGAL

LISBON

Tavares, Maria Aida (ARS)
*Vilhena, Mario (ARS)

PUERTO RICO

MEDELIN

Llamas, Augusto J. (ASTR)

PONCE

*Correa, Jose N. (ASTR)
*Vicens, Enrique A. (ASHNS), *OT*

RIO PIEDRAS (809)

*Pantoja, Enrique (ASTR), *R*, 765-7070

SAN JUAN (809)

*Frias-Monserrate, Antonio E. (ASCO),
  PD/HEM-ONC, 766-0205
**Harris, Norman O. (AACE)
*Llamas, Augusto J. (ASTR), *R*
*Marcial, Victor A. (ARS, ASTR), *PD*,
  767-0350, ext. 214
*Nadal, Hector M. (SHNS), *S*, 722-2016
*Rojas, Raul A. (ASCO)
Sorrentino, Rafael (AACE)
Sqepsenwol, J. (AACR)
*Tome, Jose M. (ASTR)
*Ubinas, Jeanne (ASTR)
*Velez-Garcia, Enrique (ASCO),
  MO/HEM, 764-1800

SANTURCE (809)

*Vallecillo, Luis A. (ARS, SHNS, SSO),
S, 723-3975

SRI LANKA

MAHARAGAMA

*Cooke, Reginald R. (SHNS)

SOUTH AFRICA

PRETORIA

*Falkson, G. (ASCO), M, 47-2050
*Falkson, H.C. (ASCO), M, 47-2050
*Sloane, Alec M. (ASCO), M, 36709

SPAIN

BARCELONA

*Galofore, Manuel (SHNS), S
*Raspall, Guillermo (SHNS), HNS/MXF

MADRID

*Alonso-Artieda, Miguel (SHNS)
*Die Goyanes, Alfredo (SHNS, SSO),
S/ONC, 274-3992

SWEDEN

DANDERYD

*Jacobsson, Folke (ARS)

LUND

*Landberg, Torsten G. (ASTR), TR

STOCKHOLM

*Hamberger, Carl Axel (SHNS)
*Kottmeier, Hans L. (ARS)

SWITZERLAND

BERN

*Zuppinger, Adolph (ARS)

NUSSBAUMEN

Wideroe, Rolf (ARS)

ZUG

*Friedman, Milton (ASTR)

ZURICH

*Haab, Otto (ASCO), M/HEM,
01-44-11-85

TANZANIA

MOSHI

*Holmes, Frederick F. (AACE)

THAILAND

BANGKOK

*Punyahotra, Vichit (SHNS)
*Thongphiew, Prakob (SHNS), S

DHONBURI

Smerasuta, Amnuey (SSO)

TURKEY

ANKARA

*Firat, Dincer (ASCO), M, 242240,
ext. 1815

IZMIR

*Deger, Nebil (ASTR), R

UNITED KINGDOM

ENGLAND

AYLESBURY, BUCKS

*Hadfield, Geoffrey J. (SHNS), S

HASLEMERE, SURREY

*Negus, Sir Victor (SHNS)

HEDON, YORKSHIRE

*Williams, Richard G. (ASHNS), *OT*

LIVERPOOL

*Littlewood, Martin (SHNS), *PLS*
*Stell, Philip M. (SHNS)

LONDON

*Chauser, Barry M. (ASTR)
*Eisert, Donald R. (ASTR)
*George, Phyllis (SSO), *S*
*Lederman, Manuel (ARS)
*Matthews, David N. (SHNS)
*Raven, Ronald W. (SHNS)
*Shaw, Henry J. (SHNS, SSO)
*Singleton, John M. (SHNS)
*Snelling, Margaret D. (ARS)
*Wallace, David (ARS, ASCO)
*Westbury, Gerald (SHNS)
Wood, C.A. (ARS)

NEW CASTLE

*Way, Stanley A. (SGO), *OG*

SCOTLAND

DUMFRIESSHIRE

*Paterson, Ralston (ARS)

EDINBURGH

*McWhirter, Robert (ASCO)

GLASGOW

*Porter, E. Humphrey (ARS), *RT*

ST. ANDREWS, FIFE

*Maran, Arnold G. (ASHNS, SHNS), *OT*

VENEZUELA

CARACAS

*De Lima, A. Rodriguez (SHNS)
*Garcia, Ramon (ASTR)
*Gyorfi, Margarita (ARS), *TR*
*Marquez, Armando (SSO), *S*
*Millan, Ramon J. (ASTR)
*Paz, Otto (ARS)
*Ravelo, Jose A. (SHNS)
*Rivero, Modesto (ARS)
*Rodriguez-Griman, Oscar A. (SSO)

MARACAIBO

*Padilla, Jose L. (ASTR)

MERIDA

*D'Lacoste, P. Guillermo H. (ASTR), *R*

YUGOSLAVIA

ZAGREB

*Padovan, Ivo (SHNS)

GEOGRAPHICAL LISTING OF CANCER RESEARCH SPECIALISTS

United States of America

ALABAMA

Bennett, L.L., Jr.
Brockman, R.W.
Casey, A.E.
Crispens, C.G., Jr.

Griswold, D.P., Jr.
Hill, D.L.
Haramoto, R.
Lampkin-Asam, J.M.
Laster, W.R., Jr.

Lloyd, H.H.
Mellett, L.B.
Montgomery, J.A.
Murad, T.M.
Myers, G.H., Jr.
Nelson, J.A.
Sani, B.P.
Schabel, F.M., Jr.
Schmidt, L.H.
Simpson-Herren, L.
Skipper, H.E.
Struck, R.F.
Wheeler, G.P.
Wilkoff, L.J.

ARIZONA

Woods, M.W.

ARKANSAS

Bower, R.K.
Jackson, C.D.
King, C.M.
Oleson, J.J.

CALIFORNIA

Abraham, S.
Alfred, L.J.
Apple, M.A.
Aronow, L.
Baker, D.G.
Bartlett, G.R.
Bern, H.A.
Bischoff, F.
Blair, P.B.
Bloom, E.T.
Bonavida, B.
Bryson, G.
Byfield, P.E.
Cardiff, R.D.
Chee, D.O.
Cohn, M.
Conzelman, G.M., Jr.
DeCarvalho, S.M.
DeOme, K.B.
Dodge, A.H.
Dorfman, R.I.

Egan, M.L.
Faulkin, L.J., Jr.
Feldman, M.K.
Fieldsteel, A.H.
French, F.A.
Friedkin, M.E.
Furst, A.
Golub, S.H.
Gupta, R.K.
Hackett, A.J.
Harris, J.W.
Hayflick, L.
Hochstein, P.
Kallman, R.F.
Kaplan, N.O.
Kelly, L.S.
Khwaja, T.A.
Kirkman, H.
Lennette, E.H.
McCoy, T.A.
Manning, J.S.
Marshall, G.J.
Masouredis, S.P.
Mendelsohn, M.L.
Momparler, R.L.
Mustacchi, P.
Nandi, S.
Nicolson, G.L.
Nicolson, M.A.O.
Nyhan, W.L.
Ohno, S.
Orlando, R.A.
Oshiro, L.S.
Pace, D.M.
Patt, H.M.
Peters, J.H.
Pilgrim, H.I.
Riggs, J.L.
Robins, R.K.
Rouser, G.L., Jr.
Salinas, F.A.
Sassenrath, E.N.
Sauberlich, H.E.
Scholler, J.
Sheikh, K.M.A.
Sherman, M.R.
Shimizu, C.S.N.
Silver, H.K.B.
Siperstein, M.D.

Smith, H.S.
Sobel, H.
Stoner, G.D.
Strong, L.C.
Sykes, J.A.
Wellings, S.R.
Winters, W.

COLORADO

Block, M.H.
Cohen, S.S.
Jacobs, B.B.
Jordan, R.T.
Lehman, J.M.
Moore, G.E.
Prasad, K.N.
Puck, T.T.
Sneider, T.W.
Snyder, S.P.

CONNECTICUT

Agrawal, K.C.
Ambellan, E.H.
Clarke, D.A.
Cobb, J.P.
Creasey, W.A.
Fischer, J.J.
Gardner, W.U.
Handschumacker, R.E.
Petrea, I.
Prusoff, W.H.
Reiskin, A.B.
Roth, J.S.
Sartorelli, A.C.

DELAWARE

Lunger, P.D.

DISTRICT OF COLUMBIA

Breyere, E.J.
Criss, W.L.
Feller, W.F.
Harshbarger, J.C.
Hollinshead, A.C.
Klubes, P.

Lavrin, D.H.
Mandel, H.G.
Melendez, L.V.
Morris, H.P.
Pradham, S.N.
Saslaw, L.D.

FLORIDA

Bergs, V.V.
Brada, Z.
Brill, E.
Cory, J.G.
Dunning, W.F.
Frankel, J.W.
Groupe, V.
Hofer, K.G.
Radomski, J.L.
Schyltz, J.
Sigel, M.M.
Stein, G.S.

GEORGIA

Akamatsu, Y.
Bain, J.A.
Bresnick, E.
Cutroneo, K.R.
Glazer, R.I.
Groth, D.P.
Kinkade, J.M., Jr.
Murphy, V.V.
Popovic, V.
Ragland, W.L., III
Scott, D.F.
Stevens, C.D.

HAWAII

Furusawa, E.
Matsumoto, H.

ILLINOIS

Brown, E.R.
Casto, B.C.
Chandra, S.
Daniels, E.W.
Das Gupta, T.K.

Davis, J.R.
DeSombre, E.R.
Dolowy, W.C.
Dray, S.
Duff, R.G.
Finkel, M.P.
Gershbein, L.L.
Hadler, H.I.
Harvey, R.G.
Honig, G.R.
Hurban, Z.
Hung, P.P.
Jensen, E.V.
Jungmann, R.A.
Kahan, B.D.
Kaltenbach, J.P.
Lloyd, E.
Lombard, L.S.
Moon, R.G.
Nora, P.F.
O'Connor, T.E.
Peraino, C.
Price, J.M.
Reilly, C.A., Jr.
Rotkin, I.D.
Sky-Peck, H.H.

INDIANA

Beck, L.V.
Chen, T.T.
Hodes, M.E.
Johnson, I.S.
Levine, A.G.
Mason, E.J.
Morton, J.L.
Sweeney, M.J.

IOWA

Gal, E.M.
Steele, W.J.

KANSAS

Humphrey, L.J.

KENTUCKY

Flesher, J.W.

Goldenberg, D.M.
Swim, H.E.

LOUISIANA

Arcos, J.C.
Argus, M.F.
Hornung, M.O.
Kasten, F.H.
Morgan, L.R., Jr.
Rothschild, H.

MAINE

Fraenkel-Conrat, J.
Hauschenka, T.S.
Kaliss, N.
Stevens, L.C., Jr.

MARYLAND

Abbott, B.J.
Ablashi, D.V.
Abrell, J.W.
Adamson, R.H.
Aurelian, L.
Bachur, N.R.
Bandyopadhyay, A.K.
Barrett, M.K.
Bassin, R.H.
Borsos, T.
Bourke, A.R.
Brown, A.M.
Bruan, W.R.
Chang, K.S.S.
Chirigos, M.A.
Cho-Chung, Y.S.
Chopra, H.C.
Dawe, C.J.
Dean, J.H.
DiPaolo, J.A.
Douros, J.D.
Dunkel, V.C.
Ebert, P.S.
Engle, R.R.
Evans, G.H.
Fidler, I.J.
Gantt, R.
Gelboin, H.V.

Geran, R.I.
Gerber, P.
Glick, J.L.
Goldin, A.
Gross, M.A.
Hatt, W.T.
Hanna, M.G., Jr.
Heine, U.I.
Hennings, H.
Hertz, B.
Hillman (Matthews), E.A.
Hisaoka, K.K.
Hsu, Y.C.
Ihle, J.N.
Jones, D.H.
Jerina, D.M.
Johns, D.G.
Kaiser, H.E.
Kakefuda, T.
Kende, M.
King, T.J.
Klein, M.
Kline, I.
Kohn, K.W.
Kouri, R.E.
Kramarsky, B.
Kramer, S.P.
Kripke, M.L.
Kuff, E.L.
LaBrosse, E.H.
Law, L.W.
Leiter, J.
Ludlum, D.B.
McCoy, J.L.
Manaker, R.A.
Mantel, N.
Mead, J.A.R.
Merwin, R.M.
Millar, F.K.
Mishra, L.C.
Moloney, J.B.
Nadkarni, M.V.
Neubauer, R.H.
Ohanian, S.H.
Oliverio, V.T.
Owellen, R.J.
Payne, W.W.
Pazmino, N.H.
Peacock, A.C.

Pearson, J.W.
Pederson, P.L.
Phillips, L.A.
Pienta, R.J.
Itha, P.M.
Pittillo, R.F.
Poiley, S.M.
Poirier, L.A.
Price, P.J.
Priori, E.S.
Rabinovitz, M.
Rapp, H.J.
Rice, J.M.
Richman, D.J.
Rosenberg, S.A.
Rubin, D.J.
Sanel, F.T.
Sanford, B.H.
Sanford, K.K.
Sarin, P.S.
Sarngardharan, M.G.
Schepartz, S.A.
Schidlovsky, G.
Schlom, J.
Schneider, W.C.
Schneiderman, M.A.
Schrecker, A.W.
Shelton, E.
Shibley, G.P.
Sibal, L.R.
Smith, G.H.
Smith, W.W.
Sobert, H.A.
Squire, R.A.
Stansly, P.G.
Straube, R.L.

MASSACHUSETTS

Adams, R.A.
Baril, E.F.
Bernfeld, P.
Bogden, A.E.
Booth, B.A.
Cohen, S.M.
Daniel, M.D.
Desai, L.
Eckner, R.J.
Essex, M.

Fishman, W.H.
Foley, G.E.
Friedman, O.M.
Geyer, R.P.
Handler, A.H.
Hilgar, A.G.
Hughes, W.L.
Israel, M.
Krishan, A.
Kupchik, H.
Lazarus, H.
Linder, M.C.
Mautner, H.G.
Meader, R.G.
Merker, P.C.
Modest, E.J.
Reif, A.E.
Rosenoer, V.M.
Rule, A.H.
Russfield, A.B.
Sivak, A.
Smith, E.E.
Soloway, A.H.
Steckerl, F.
Stephenson, M.L.
Suit, H.D.

MICHIGAN

Al Saadi
Baker, L.H.
Bhuyan, B.K.
Brooks, S.C.
Chen, Y.M.
Colburn, N.H.
Duboff, G.S.
Essner, E.S.
Gerstacker, C.A.
Goodman, J.I.
Hanka, L.J.
Horwitz, J.P.
Kessel, D.
Kim, J.C.S.
Kithier, K.
Li, L.H.
McCormick, J.J.
Maher, V.M.
Meites, J.
Neil, G.L.

Reynolds, M.M.D.
Rich, M.A.
Rivera, E.M.
Rowe, N.H., Jr.
Ruddon, R.W.
Simpson, W.L.
Soule, H.D.
Stulberg, C.S.
Swenberg, J.A.

MINNESOTA

Barry, E.J.
Gokcen, M.
Malejka-Giganti
McKinnell, R.G.
Mizuno, N.S.
Nagasaw, H.T.
Sheppard, J.R.
Sladek, N.E.
Song, C.W.

MISSISSIPPI

Gentry, G.A.

MISSOURI

Blumenthal, H.T.
Cutts, J.H.
Hill, H.Z.
Lin, H.S.

NEBRASKA

Banerjee, M.R.
Cavalieri, E.L.
Clayson, D.B.
Dubes, G.R.
Langenbach, R.J.
McCarthy, R.E.
Mirvish, S.S.
Raha, C.R.
Rogan, E.G.
Ryan, W.L.
Scholar, E.M.
Shubik, P.
Somogyi, A.
Stenback, F.

NEVADA

Cramer, J.W.

NEW HAMPSHIRE

Lubin, M.

NEW JERSEY

Ahmed, M.
Bieber, S.
Borman, A.
Briody, B.A., Jr.
Brown, H.D.
Came, P.E.
Conney, A.H.
Coriell, L.L.
Foley, E.J.
Fu, S.C.J.
Gitterman, C.O.
Hansen, H.J.
Hirschberg, E.
Lasfargues, E.Y.L.
Lea, M.A.
Leathem, J.H.
McBride, T.J.
Mayyasi, S.A.
Moore, D.H.
Munroe, J.S.
Nichols, W.W.
Raska, K.F.J., Jr.
Reilly, H.C.
Spencer, H.J.

NEW MEXICO

Loftfield, R.B.
Reyes, P.
Stroud, A.N.

NEW YORK

Ackerman, N.B.
Albrecht, A.M.
Atten, L.M.
Andrews, E.J.
Argyris, T.S.
Back, N.

Balis, M.E.
Barclay, M.
Barclay, R.K.
Bardos, T.J.
Bekesi, J.G.
Belman, S.
Bendich, A.
Bertram, J.S.
Biedler, J.L.
Bloch, A.
Blumenson, L.E.
Bock, F.G.
Borek, C.G.
Borenfreund, E.
Bradner, W.T.
Bross, I.D.J.
Brown, G.B.
Buffett, R.J.
Burger, C.L.
Burns, F.J.
Cappuccino, J.G.
Carruthers, C.
Chheda, G.B.
Chmielewicz, Z.F.
Chou, T.C.
Chu, T.M.
Cohen, A.I.
Coligan, J.E.
Creaven, P.J.
Danishefsky, I.
Dave, C.
Deschner, E.E.
Dounce, A.L.
Eidinoff, M.L.
Ely, C.A.
Fiegelson, P.
Fiala, E.S.
Fiel, R.J.
Fishman, M.M.
Fissekis, J.D.
Fjelde, A.
Fondy, T.P.
Fowler, E.H.
Fox, J.J.
Freedman, L.S.
Fried, J.
Friend, C.
Fugmann, R.
Gabelman, N.

Giner Sorolla, A.
Goldfeder, A.
Goldschmidt, B.M.
Graham, R.M.
Green, S.
Greenberg, S.S.
Grindey, G.B.
Grossman, S.H.
Grunberger, D.
Curtoo, H.L.
Hacker, B.
Hakala, M.T.
Hamilton, L.D.
Hebborn, P.
Hilf, R.
Hoffman, D.
Hollander, V.P.
Horwitz, S.B.
Huang, C.C.
Hutchison, D.J.
Hutner, S.H.
Kim, J.H.
Klein, E.
Kopelovich, L.
Korman, S.
Korytnyk, W.
Kreis, W.
Laskowski, M.
Lee, K.M.
Libby, P.R.
Lilly, F.
McGarry, M.P.
Makulu, D.R.
Mandl, I.
Mashburn, L.T.
Mike, V.
Miller, L.L.
Mirand, E.A.
Miroff, G.
Moroson, H.
Mukai, F.H.
Munson, B.R.
Muschel, L.H.
Novikoff, A.B.
Noyes, W.F., III
Paigen, K.
Parshley, M.S.
Parsons, D.F.
Pecora, P.F.
Philips, F.S.

Pine, M.J.
Pogo, B.G.T.
Popp, F.D.
Pressman, D.
Prutkin, L.
Rakieten, N.
Reddy, B.S.
Reid, A.F.
Roberts, J.
Rosen, F.
Rosenkranz, H.S.
Salser, J.S.
Sarcione, E.J.
Saroff, J.
Schmid, F.A.
Schwartz, H.S.
Schwartz, M.K.
Segal, A.
Shellabarger, C.J.
Shigeura, H.T.
Simpson, C.L.
Sinha, D.
Sirotnak, F.M.
Skipski, V.P.
Slack, N.H.
Smith, C.G.
Spar, I.L.
Spiegelman, S.
Srivastava, B.I.S.
Stock, C.C.
Stohrer, G.
Stolfi, R.L.
Suguira, K.

NORTH CAROLINA

Bigner, D.D.
Bo, W.J.
Bonar, R.A.
DeChatelet, L.R.
deSerres, F.J.
Elion, G.B.
Falk, H.L.
Haughton, G.
Hitchings, G.H.
Hooker, C.W.
Irvin, J.L.
Levy, N.L.
Lieberman, M.W.
McCarty, K.S.

Metzgar, R.S.
Mohanakumar, T.
Nichol, C.A.
Pearlman, W.H.
Rall, D.P.
Rundles, R.W.
Steffee, C.H.

NORTH DAKOTA

Cornatzer, W.E.

OHIO

Cook, E.S.
Denlinger, R.H.
Deodhar, S.D.
Epstein, S.S.
Koestner, A.
Lavik, P.S.
Ledinko, N.
Lessler, M.A.
Liebelt, A.G.
Liebelt, R.A.
Liss, L.
Mattheis, E.B.
Myers, W.G.
Petering, H.G.
Shamberger, R.J.

OKLAHOMA

Cantrell, J.L.
Griffin, M.J.
Kampschmidt, R.F.
Kizer, D.E.
Kollmorgen, G.M.
Leach, F.R.
Nordquist, R.E.
Olson, R.L.
Patterson, M.K., Jr.

OREGON

Beaudreau, G.S.
Brooks, R.E.
Siegel, B.V.
Siegel, J.I.M.

PENNSYLVANIA

Auerbach, V.H.

Blumberg, B.S.
Castor, L.N.
Ciaccio, E.I.
Creech, H.J.
Devlin, T.M.
Diamond, L.
Edmonds, M.P.
Eng, C.P.
Forbes, P.D.
Freed, J.J.
Glaser, R.
Green, E.U.
Gregory, F.J.
Griswold, D.E.
Hampton, A.
Havas, H.F.
Hilleman, M.R.
Jeejeebhoy, H.F.
Kalf, G.F.
Lausch, R.N.
Litwack, G.
Loeb, L.A.
Lotlikar, P.
Magee, P.N.
Marshak, R.R.
Merkow, L.P.
Mezger Freed, L.
Millman, I.
Moorehead, P.S.
Ove, P.
Peck, R.M.
Poel, W.E.
Rapp, F.
Roosa, R.A.
Rubin, B.A.
Rutman, R.J.
Sarma, D.S.R.
Schwartz, A.G.
Shatton, J.B.
Shinozuka, H.
Sorof, S.
Studzinski, G.P.
Swern, D.

RHODE ISLAND

Chu, M.Y.W.
Fischer, G.A.
Heppner, G.H.
Laux, D.C.

Leduc, E.H.
Parks, R.E., Jr.
Quevedo, W.C., Jr.

SOUTH CAROLINA

Anderson, N.G.
Baggett, B.

TENNESSEE

Bahner, C.T.
Bucovaz, E.T.
Chiu, J.F.
Clapp, N.K.
Coogin, J.H., Jr.
Cox, R.
Girardi, A.J.
Granoff, A.
Griesemer, R.A.
Hnilica, L.
Hsie, A.W.
Irving, C.C.
Kaplan, A.S.
Kenney, F.T.
Lijinsky, W.
Murphy, M.J., Jr.
Novelli, G.D.
Park, J.
Price, R.A.
Regan, J.D.
Roberts, D.
Selkirk, J.K.
Sharma, R.K.
Snyder, F.L.

TEXAS

Abell, C.W.
Barranco, S.C., III
Biesele, J.J.
Bowen, J.M.
Butel, J.S.
Cameron, K.L.
Chan, J.C.
Chang, J.P.
Choi, Y.C.
Drewinko, B.
Finney, J.W.
Furlong, N.B.

Gehan, E.A.
Giovanella, B.C.
Griffin, A.C.
Haas, F.L.
Ho, D.H.W.
Hurlbert, R.B.
Hwang, K.M.
Kimball, A.P.
Kit, S.
Liau, M.C.
Lin, A.J.
Loo, T.L.
McCormick, K.J.
Macdonald, E.J.
McDonald, H.G.
Medina, D.
Melnick, J.L.
Moore, E.C.
Nishioka, K.
Olson, M.O.J.
Prager, M.D.
Prestayko, A.R.
Randerath, E.
Rao, P.N.
Reeves, W.J., Jr.
Ro-Choi, T.S.
Romsdahl, M.M.
Shetlar, M.R.
Starbuck, W.C.
Stenback, W.A.

UTAH

Dethlefsen, L.A.
O'Neill, F.J.
Steinmuller, D.

VERMONT

Jaffe, J.J.

VIRGINIA

Banks, W.L., Jr.
Costa, G.
Elford, H.L.
Friedman, M.A.
Hopkins, H.A.
Kaplan, A.M.
Looney, W.B.

Lynch, C.J.
McCuen, R.W.
MacLeod, R.M.
Munson, A.E.
Somers, K.D.

WASHINGTON

Evans, C.A.
Fletcher, T.L.
Riley, V.T.
Santisteban, G.A.
Scribner, J.D.
Shearer, R.W.
Sikov, M.R.
Staga, T.J.
Smuckler, E.A.
Spackman, D.H.

WEST VIRGINIA

Fiala, S.

WISCONSIN

Baumann, C.A.
Boutwell, R.K.
Brown, R.R.
Clifton, K.H.
Heidelberger, C.
Johnson, B.M.
Kasper, C.B.
Lower, G.M., Jr.
Miller, E.C.
Miller, J.A.
Peterson, A.R.
Pitot, H.C.
Potter, V.R.
Rose, D.P.
Skibba, J.L.

Canada

Auersperg, N.
Axelrad, A.A.
Balir, D.G.R.
Beer, C.T.
Berozi, I.
Bertalanffy, F.D.
Brox, L.W.
Bruce, W.R.

Cass, C.E.
Colter, J.S.
Daoust, R.
Darcel, C.Q.
de Lamirande, G.
Farber, E.
Frei, J.
Gold, P.
Goldenberg, G.J.
Grad, B.
Hall, R.H.
Henderson, J.F.
Hillcoat, B.L.
Hoshino, K.
Howatson, A.F.
Inch, W.R.
Isler, H.
Jellinck, P.H.
Jerry, L.M.
Karasaki, S.
Leblond, C.P.
Lemonade, P.
LePage, G.A.
McCredie, J.A.
Morgan, J.F.
Nazar, R.N.
Nigam, V.N.
Perdue, J.F.
Peterson, A.R.P.
Ritchie, A.C.
Robins, M.J.
Scholefield, P.G.
Selye, H.
Siminovitch, L.
Stich, H.F.
Sutherland, R.M.

International

BRAZIL

Brentani, R.

ISRAEL

Bergmann, E.
Gross, J.

SWITZERLAND

Leuchtenberger, C.

D

Some Cancer Statistics

CANCER AROUND THE WORLD, 1972-1973

Age-Adjusted Death Rates Per 100,000 Population for Selected Cancer Sites for 44 Countries

Country	All Sites Male	All Sites Female	Oral Male	Oral Female	Colon & Rectum Male	Colon & Rectum Female	Lung Male	Lung Female	Breast Female	Uterus Female	Skin Male	Skin Female	Stomach Male	Stomach Female	Prostate Male	Leukemia Male	Leukemia Female
United States	157.2(21)	106.1(21)	4.6(10)	1.5(8)	18.9(17)	15.1(15)	48.9(9)	10.8(5)	22.4(12)	8.4(32)	2.4(10)	1.4(18)	7.5(40)	3.7(43)	14.4(11)	7.1(4)	4.3(15)
Australia	158.1(20)	100.0(26)	3.9(16)	1.3(13)	20.1(14)	17.4(8)	44.5(12)	6.7(14)	19.9(15)	7.3(35)	4.5(1)	2.6(1)	13.9(35)	7.0(38)	15.7(7)	6.7(10)	4.4(13)
Austria	191.1(5)	124.3(8)	4.0(15)	0.7(35)	23.9(2)	16.8(12)	52.3(7)	6.5(15)	19.2(17)	15.1(6)	2.2(12)	1.7(8)	33.2(8)	17.3(9)	14.3(12)	6.1(19)	4.3(18)
Bulgaria	128.3(28)	81.0(34)	1.6(38)	0.6(41)	8.6(30)	6.9(32)	36.2(22)	6.4(16)	11.2(29)	7.6(37)	1.7(21)	1.1(26)	31.0(11)	18.2(6)	6.3(35)	4.3(30)	3.5(26)
Canada	157.0(23)	109.4(19)	4.5(12)	1.4(10)	21.9(8)	18.2(7)	43.3(14)	8.0(10)	23.9(7)	8.0(34)	1.8(19)	1.3(21)	13.7(36)	6.3(40)	14.2(13)	7.0(6)	4.5(7)
Costa Rica	123.7(32)	111.2(17)	3.0(23)	0.8(29)	4.5(38)	5.1(37)	9.6(39)	4.3(29)	8.3(36)	18.2(4)	1.6(22)	0.7(35)	49.5(3)	30.1(3)	8.0(31)	3.9(35)	4.5(8)
Chile	157.8(21)	133.3(3)	2.5(31)	0.9(32)	7.8(32)	8.0(29)	18.5(31)	4.6(28)	12.2(26)	21.8(2)	1.1(32)	1.1(27)	57.4(2)	30.7(2)	11.5(23)	3.9(36)	3.3(28)
Czechoslovakia	204.1(2)	110.9(18)	3.3(18)	0.7(36)	21.4(11)	14.2(16)	62.9(6)	5.5(21)	8.6(35)	11.7(16)	2.4(8)	1.6(11)	33.5(7)	17.3(8)	10.1(26)	6.5(13)	4.4(11)
Denmark	170.2(15)	132.1(4)	2.1(35)	0.9(27)	23.1(5)	18.5(6)	46.4(10)	9.8(8)	26.3(4)	13.2(13)	2.6(6)	1.9(5)	16.4(30)	8.5(32)	13.4(17)	7.4(2)	4.9(1)
El Salvador	26.7(43)	42.7(42)	0.9(43)	0.3(43)	1.4(43)	1.6(42)	1.8(43)	0.6(44)	1.1(42)	6.5(39)	0.4(40)	0.2(42)	5.6(43)	10.1(25)	1.2(42)	2.9(40)	1.9(40)
England & Wales	184.3(8)	119.6(12)	2.8(29)	1.3(14)	21.7(10)	17.0(11)	73.5(2)	13.4(3)	27.1(3)	8.9(28)	1.6(23)	1.4(19)	17.5(27)	9.6(27)	11.8(22)	5.6(23)	3.7(25)
Finland	182.9(9)	99.1(27)	2.3(32)	0.9(28)	11.4(26)	10.4(24)	64.3(5)	4.1(32)	15.0(22)	7.3(38)	2.8(5)	1.6(12)	27.4(16)	14.1(16)	13.5(16)	7.0(5)	4.8(3)
France	187.0(7)	98.5(28)	13.4(2)	1.0(20)	20.3(12)	13.8(18)	33.6(24)	3.4(37)	17.9(19)	9.7(24)	1.5(27)	1.2(23)	16.6(29)	7.9(34)	14.8(9)	6.8(9)	4.4(10)
Germany, F. R.	178.0(12)	121.2(10)	2.2(33)	0.6(38)	22.4(7)	17.4(9)	46.0(11)	4.7(27)	19.7(16)	11.1(18)	1.8(18)	1.4(20)	28.7(15)	15.1(12)	15.0(8)	6.2(16)	4.4(12)
Greece	124.5(31)	75.3(38)	1.4(42)	0.5(42)	6.0(36)	5.5(35)	35.8(23)	6.0(17)	12.0(27)	6.0(40)	0.9(33)	1.0(30)	13.3(38)	7.8(35)	6.6(34)	6.9(7)	4.3(14)
Hong Kong	170.7(14)	96.8(29)	19.8(1)	7.0(1)	12.9(25)	9.3(25)	41.3(18)	20.0(1)	9.7(32)	9.8(23)	0.7(38)	0.6(37)	16.3(32)	9.1(28)	2.1(40)	3.2(38)	2.4(38)
Honduras	30.6(42)	45.9(41)	0.3(44)	0.1(44)	1.0(44)	0.2(44)	5.0(44)	0.8(43)	6.3(41)	8.4(30)	0.2(42)	0.1(43)	7.0(41)	6.6(39)	0.8(43)	1.6(43)	1.3(41)
Hungary	182.6(10)	125.6(7)	4.6(11)	0.9(24)	19.1(16)	15.5(14)	43.1(15)	8.2(9)	17.5(21)	16.8(7)	2.5(7)	2.0(4)	38.1(4)	18.6(5)	14.7(10)	6.2(15)	4.2(20)
Iceland	114.6(37)	93.8(30)	1.8(37)	0.7(34)	17.4(20)	9.3(25)	11.1(37)	7.4(11)	14.1(24)	5.9(41)	0.7(39)	0.1(43)	31.6(9)	14.9(13)	3.8(37)	4.9(28)	4.7(5)
Ireland	158.0(19)	122.1(9)	3.3(17)	2.0(5)	21.8(9)	18.4(6)	39.1(21)	11.9(4)	23.9(8)	7.7(36)	1.9(16)	1.7(10)	22.8(19)	13.8(17)	13.9(17)	6.2(18)	4.3(16)
Israel	121.5(33)	118.8(13)	1.5(40)	0.8(30)	13.1(24)	12.1(23)	23.1(28)	7.2(12)	25.2(5)	5.3(42)	1.2(31)	1.1(7)	15.7(33)	9.0(29)	7.5(32)	6.2(17)	4.3(16)
Italy	173.3(13)	103.0(23)	6.0(6)	1.0(21)	17.3(21)	12.8(21)	40.9(19)	5.1(25)	18.3(18)	11.2(17)	1.6(26)	1.0(31)	29.3(14)	14.2(15)	10.9(25)	6.9(8)	4.6(6)
Japan	141.2(25)	89.9(32)	1.5(39)	0.6(39)	10.1(28)	7.6(32)	17.7(32)	5.6(20)	4.6(41)	9.8(22)	0.6(36)	0.5(38)	59.6(1)	31.1(1)	2.1(39)	4.1(33)	3.3(31)
Luxembourg	200.7(3)	120.8(11)	6.2(5)	1.4(11)	23.1(6)	17.0(11)	64.5(4)	5.7(19)	21.1(13)	9.8(22)	2.3(11)	0.9(32)	21.6(21)	10.8(21)	13.6(15)	5.0(27)	3.3(29)
Mauritius	80.4(38)	57.4(40)	2.9(25)	0.8(31)	7.6(33)	4.4(39)	15.1(33)	2.2(41)	6.0(38)	16.4(8)	0.0(44)	0.3(40)	16.4(31)	7.1(37)	3.2(38)	3.2(42)	0.8(42)
Mexico	55.2(40)	71.0(39)	2.0(36)	0.6(37)	2.8(40)	3.8(40)	7.0(39)	4.2(30)	8.8(34)	12.4(14)	0.8(37)	0.7(34)	9.7(39)	8.6(31)	5.5(36)	2.5(41)	2.2(39)
Netherlands	186.9(7)	160.2(1)	2.0(36)	0.7(33)	18.4(18)	16.1(13)	67.5(3)	4.0(34)	29.9(1)	10.5(21)	1.7(20)	1.5(17)	22.0(20)	10.7(23)	22.9(1)	12.5(1)	4.3(17)
New Zealand	162.4(16)	114.4(15)	3.1(21)	1.2(16)	25.6(1)	20.8(1)	42.8(16)	10.1(6)	23.5(11)	8.6(29)	4.5(2)	2.2(2)	14.4(34)	6.2(41)	15.8(6)	6.6(12)	4.8(2)
Northern Ireland	159.8(17)	117.1(14)	3.3(17)	1.1(14)	21.8(9)	18.4(6)	50.7(8)	10.1(7)	23.7(10)	9.1(26)	1.3(29)	1.0(29)	20.1(24)	10.7(22)	11.0(24)	6.0(20)	4.0(23)
Norway	133.2(27)	101.4(25)	3.0(24)	0.9(26)	15.8(22)	13.0(19)	19.5(30)	4.1(33)	17.7(20)	8.2(33)	3.0(3)	1.6(13)	20.0(25)	10.0(26)	16.3(5)	6.4(14)	4.3(19)
Panama	75.4(39)	76.1(37)	3.1(20)	1.4(9)	4.3(39)	5.0(38)	11.0(38)	3.1(38)	6.6(37)	17.5(6)	0.3(41)	0.2(41)	13.5(37)	7.6(36)	8.7(28)	3.7(37)	2.4(37)
Philippines	49.8(41)	39.9(43)	4.4(13)	1.9(6)	2.8(41)	2.3(41)	5.2(41)	2.5(40)	4.7(40)	4.7(40)	0.8(35)	0.4(39)	6.0(42)	4.1(42)	1.4(41)	3.0(39)	2.6(36)
Poland	158.3(18)	102.9(24)	4.7(9)	1.0(22)	10.0(29)	8.1(28)	40.8(20)	5.1(24)	12.3(25)	14.2(11)	1.9(17)	1.6(15)	36.7(5)	15.6(11)	8.3(30)	5.5(24)	3.9(24)
Portugal	127.1(29)	91.1(31)	5.3(8)	1.0(19)	14.1(23)	12.9(20)	14.3(34)	3.1(39)	14.3(23)	12.3(15)	2.0(14)	1.6(16)	33.5(6)	19.0(4)	13.0(18)	5.8(21)	4.2(21)
Puerto Rico	119.5(35)	80.3(35)	10.2(3)	2.1(4)	7.2(34)	6.3(34)	14.3(35)	5.9(18)	8.8(34)	12.4(14)	0.8(37)	0.7(36)	19.0(26)	8.1(33)	12.6(19)	5.5(25)	3.3(27)
Romania	126.2(30)	146.5(2)	2.9(26)	1.0(23)	6.7(35)	6.3(34)	27.8(26)	5.4(22)	10.2(31)	17.9(5)	1.6(24)	1.2(24)	30.3(12)	13.6(18)	8.4(29)	4.6(29)	3.2(30)
Scotland	205.0(1)	128.4(6)	2.9(28)	1.3(12)	23.2(3)	19.4(2)	84.1(1)	16.0(2)	27.5(2)	8.4(31)	1.9(15)	1.7(6)	20.8(23)	11.7(19)	12.2(20)	5.3(26)	3.0(32)
Spain	137.4(26)	87.2(33)	3.2(19)	0.6(40)	13.2(23)	10.2(27)	27.5(27)	4.0(35)	11.4(28)	9.0(27)	1.3(30)	0.7(33)	26.2(17)	14.3(14)	11.9(21)	4.3(31)	3.4(20)
Sweden	114.7(24)	111.7(16)	2.7(30)	1.2(15)	18.4(19)	13.9(17)	22.6(29)	5.4(23)	20.2(14)	9.1(25)	2.4(9)	1.6(14)	17.2(28)	9.0(30)	21.1(2)	6.6(11)	4.7(4)
Switzerland	178.8(11)	108.7(20)	6.6(4)	0.9(25)	20.2(13)	18.2(2)	33.4(23)	4.2(31)	23.8(9)	10.7(19)	2.9(4)	1.7(9)	21.2(22)	10.6(24)	19.3(3)	7.1(3)	4.5(9)
Thailand	29.4(44)	19.6(44)	2.2(34)	1.1(18)	1.7(42)	1.2(43)	3.3(42)	1.3(42)	4.0(44)	3.0(44)	0.1(43)	0.0(44)	2.0(44)	0.9(44)	0.2(44)	4.1(34)	3.4(20)
Uruguay	200.6(4)	131.7(5)	5.8(7)	1.1(17)	19.5(15)	19.2(3)	42.6(17)	3.9(36)	24.0(6)	14.7(10)	2.1(13)	1.0(28)	31.4(10)	15.8(10)	17.6(4)	5.8(22)	4.2(22)
Venezuela	116.0(36)	104.0(22)	2.9(27)	2.5(3)	5.0(37)	5.4(36)	14.2(36)	6.8(13)	9.6(33)	25.5(1)	0.0(44)	1.1(25)	29.7(13)	17.7(7)	9.5(27)	4.0(34)	3.0(33)
Yugoslavia	120.4(34)	78.4(36)	3.1(22)	0.7(34)	8.4(31)	7.0(31)	30.1(25)	4.9(26)	10.3(30)	10.6(20)	1.6(25)	1.3(22)	23.0(18)	11.4(20)	7.4(33)	4.3(32)	3.0(35)

NOTE: Figures in parentheses are order of rank within site and sex group.

Source: World Health Statistics Annual 1972-1973.

Mortality for the Five Leading Cancer Sites in Major Age Groups by Sex, United States — 1975

UNDER 15		15–34		35–54		55–74		75+	
MALE	FEMALE	MALE	FEMALE	MALE	FEMALE	MALE	FEMALE	MALE	FEMALE
Leukemia	Leukemia	Leukemia	Breast	Lung	Breast	Lung	Breast	Lung	Colon & Rectum
648	505	746	540	10,070	8,344	40,924	15,867	12,226	11,174
Brain and Nervous System	Brain and Nervous System	Brain and Nervous System	Leukemia	Colon & Rectum	Lung	Colon & Rectum	Colon & Rectum	Prostate	Breast
420	333	426	522	2,496	4,102	12,700	11,830	10,835	7,404
Lympho- and Reticulosarcoma	Bone	Testis	Brain and Nervous System	Pancreas	Colon & Rectum	Prostate	Lung	Colon & Rectum	Lung
64	73	402	324	1,326	2,430	8,299	10,851	8,426	3,582
Bone	Kidney	Hodgkin's Disease	Uterus	Brain and Nervous System	Uterus	Pancreas	Uterus	Stomach	Pancreas
54	48	391	303	1,254	2,397	6,216	5,515	3,037	3,367
Kidney	Connective Tissue	Skin	Hodgkin's Disease	Stomach	Ovary	Stomach	Ovary	Pancreas	Uterus
44	35	252	230	1,057	2,371	4,799	5,690	3,031	2,935

Source: Vital Statistics of the United States, 1975

Mortality for Leading Causes of Death: United States, 1975

Rank	Cause of Death	Number of Deaths	Death Rate Per 100,000 Population	Percent of Total Deaths	Rank	Cause of Death	Number of Deaths	Death Rate Per 100,000 Population	Percent of Total Deaths
	All Causes	1,892,879	888.9	100.0					
1	Diseases of Heart	716,215	336.2	37.8	9	Suicide	27,063	12.7	1.4
2	Cancer	365,693	171.7	19.3	10	Diseases of Infancy	26,616	12.5	1.4
3	Stroke	194,038	91.1	10.3	11	Homicide	21,310	10.0	1.1
4	Accidents	103,030	48.4	5.4	12	Emphysema	18,795	8.8	1.0
5	Influenza & Pneumonia	55,664	26.1	2.9	13	Congenital Anomalies	13,245	6.2	0.7
6	Diabetes Mellitus	35,230	16.5	1.9	14	Nephritis & Nephrosis	8,072	3.8	0.4
7	Cirrhosis of Liver	31,623	14.8	1.7	15	Ulcers	6,743	3.2	0.4
8	Arteriosclerosis	28,887	13.6	1.5		Other & Ill-defined	240,655	113.3	12.8

Source: Vital Statistics of the United States, 1975.

How to Estimate Cancer Statistics Locally

Community Population	Estimated No. Who are Alive, Cured of Cancer	Estimated No. Cancer Cases Under Medical Care in 1978	Estimated No. Who Will Die of Cancer in 1978	Estimated No. of New Cases in 1978	Estimated No. Saved from Cancer in 1978	Estimated No. Who Will be Eventually Develop Cancer	Estimated No. Who Will Die of Cancer if Present Rates Continue
1,000	7	4	1	3	1	250	150
2,000	15	9	3	6	2	500	300
3,000	22	13	4	8	3	750	450
4,000	30	18	6	11	4	1,000	600
5,000	37	21	7	14	5	1,250	750
10,000	74	43	15	28	9	2,500	1,500
25,000	185	107	37	70	23	6,250	3,750
50,000	370	215	75	140	47	12,500	7,500
100,000	740	430	150	280	93	25,000	15,000
200,000	1,480	860	300	560	186	50,000	30,000
500,000	3,700	2,150	750	1,400	465	125,000	75,000

NOTE: The figures can only be the roughest approximation of actual data for your community. It is suggested that every effort be made to obtain actual data from a Registry source.

Reference Chart: Leading Cancer Sites, 1978*

SITE	ESTIMATED NEW CASES 1978	ESTIMATED DEATHS 1978	WARNING SIGNAL IF YOU HAVE ONE SEE YOUR DOCTOR	SAFEGUARDS	COMMENT
BREAST	91,000	34,000	LUMP OR THICKENING IN THE BREAST, OR UNUSUAL DISCHARGE FROM NIPPLE.	REGULAR CHECKUP. MONTHLY BREAST SELF-EXAM.	THE LEADING CAUSE OF CANCER DEATH IN WOMEN.
COLON AND RECTUM	102,000	52,000	CHANGE IN BOWEL HABITS; BLEEDING.	REGULAR CHECKUP INCLUDING PROCTOSCOPY, ESPECIALLY FOR THOSE OVER 40.	CONSIDERED A HIGHLY CURABLE DISEASE WHEN DIGITAL AND PROCTOSCOPIC EXAMINATIONS ARE INCLUDED IN ROUTINE CHECKUPS.
LUNG	102,000	92,000	PERSISTENT COUGH, OR LINGERING RESPIRATORY AILMENT	80% OF LUNG CANCER WOULD BE PREVENTED IF NO ONE SMOKED CIGAR-ETTES.	THE LEADING CAUSE OF CANCER DEATH AMONG MEN AND RISING MORTALITY AMONG WOMEN.
ORAL (INCLUDING PHARYNX)	24,000	8,000	SORE THAT DOES NOT HEAL. DIFFICULTY IN SWALLOWING.	REGULAR CHECKUP.	MANY MORE LIVES SHOULD BE SAVED BECAUSE THE MOUTH IS EASILY ACCESSIBLE TO VISUAL EXAMINATION BY PHYSICIANS AND DENTISTS.
SKIN	10,000**	6,000	SORE THAT DOES NOT HEAL, OR CHANGE IN WART OR MOLE.	REGULAR CHECKUP, AVOIDANCE OF OVEREXPOSURE TO SUN.	SKIN CANCER IS READILY DETECTED BY OBSER-VATION, AND DIAGNOSED BY SIMPLE BIOPSY.
UTERUS	48,000***	11,000	UNUSUAL BLEEDING OR DISCHARGE.	REGULAR CHECKUP, INCLUDING PELVIC EXAMINATION WITH PAP TEST.	UTERINE CANCER MORTALITY HAS DECLINED 65% DURING THE LAST 40 YEARS WITH WIDER APPLICA-TION OF THE PAP TEST. POSTMENOPAUSAL WOMEN WITH ABNORMAL BLEEDING SHOULD BE CHECKED.
KIDNEY AND BLADDER	45,000	17,000	URINARY DIFFICULTY. BLEEDING – IN WHICH CASE CONSULT DOCTOR AT ONCE.	REGULAR CHECKUP WITH URINALYSIS.	PROTECTIVE MEASURES FOR WORKERS IN HIGH-RISK INDUSTRIES ARE HELPING TO ELIMINATE ONE OF THE IMPORTANT CAUSES OF THESE CANCERS.
LARYNX	9,000	3,000	HOARSENESS – DIFFICULTY IN SWALLOWING.	REGULAR CHECKUP, INCLUDING LARYNGOSCOPY.	READILY CURABLE IF CAUGHT EARLY.
PROSTATE	57,000	21,000	URINARY DIFFICULTY	REGULAR CHECKUP, INCLUDING PALPATION.	OCCURS MAINLY IN MEN OVER 60, THE DISEASE CAN BE DETECTED BY PALPATION AT REGULAR CHECKUP.
STOMACH	23,000	15,000	INDIGESTION.	REGULAR CHECKUP.	A 40% DECLINE IN MORTALITY IN 25 YEARS, FOR REASONS YET UNKNOWN.
LEUKEMIA	22,000	15,000	LEUKEMIA IS A CANCER OF BLOOD-FORMING TISSUES AND IS CHARACTERIZED BY THE ABNORMAL PRODUCTION OF IMMATURE WHITE BLOOD CELLS. ACUTE LYMPHOCYTIC LEUKEMIA STRIKES MAINLY CHILDREN AND IS TREATED BY DRUGS WHICH HAVE EXTENDED LIFE FROM A FEW MONTHS TO AS MUCH AS TEN YEARS. CHRONIC LEUKEMIA STRIKES USUALLY AFTER AGE 25 AND PROGRESSES LESS RAPIDLY.		
LYMPHOMAS	33,000	21,000	THESE CANCERS ARISE IN THE LYMPH SYSTEM AND INCLUDE HODGKIN'S DISEASE AND LYMPHOSARCOMA. SOME PATIENTS WITH LYMPHATIC CANCERS CAN LEAD NORMAL LIVES FOR MANY YEARS. FIVE YEAR SURVIVAL RATE FOR HODGKIN'S DISEASE INCREASED FROM 25% TO 54% IN 20 YEARS.		

*All figures rounded to nearest 1,000.   **Estimate new cases of non-melanoma skin cancer about 300,000.
***If carcinoma in situ is included, cases total over 88,000.
INCIDENCE ESTIMATES ARE BASED ON RATES FROM N.C.I. THIRD NATIONAL CANCER SURVEY 1969-71.

Trends in Age-Adjusted Cancer Death Rates Per 100,000 Population 1953-55 to 1973-75

Sex	Sites	'1953-55	1973-75	Percent Changes	Comments
Male	All Sites	136.0	160.2	+ 18	Steady increase mainly due to lung cancer.
Female	All Sites	116.4	107.5	– 8	Slight decrease.
Male	Bladder	5.1	4.9	– 4	Slight fluctuations; overall no change.
Female	Bladder	2.1	1.4	*	Some fluctuations; noticeable decrease.
Male	Breast	0.3	0.3	*	Constant rate.
Female	Breast	22.3	23.0	+ 3	Slight fluctuations; overall no change.
Male	Colon & Rectum	19.3	18.6	– 4	Slight fluctuations; overall no change.
Female	Colon & Rectum	18.3	14.9	– 19	Slight fluctuations; noticeable decrease.
Male	Esophagus	3.7	4.1	*	Slight fluctuations; overall no change in both
Female	Esophagus	0.9	1.1	*	sexes.
Male	Kidney	2.9	3.7	+ 28	Steady slight increase.
Female	Kidney	1.6	1.7	*	Slight fluctuations; overall no change.
Male	Leukemia	6.8	6.9	+ 1	Early increase, later leveling off.
Female	Leukemia	4.7	4.2	– 11	Slight early increase, later leveling off and decrease.
Male	Lung	24.0	51.7	+115	Steady increase in both sexes due to cigarette
Female	Lung	4.1	12.3	+200	smoking.
Male	Oral	4.6	4.8	*	Slight fluctuations; overall no change in both
Female	Oral	1.2	1.6	*	sexes.
Female	Ovary	7.4	7.3	– 1	Slight fluctuations; overall no change.
Male	Pancreas	7.1	8.5	+ 20	Steady increase in both sexes, then leveling off.
Female	Pancreas	4.4	5.2	+ 18	Reasons unknown.
Male	Prostate	13.6	13.7	+ 1	Fluctuations all through period; overall no change.
Male	Skin	2.4	2.6	*	Slight fluctuations; overall no change in both
Female	Skin	1.5	1.5	*	sexes.
Male	Stomach	15.8	7.2	– 54	Steady decrease in both sexes; reasons unknown.
Female	Stomach	8.1	3.5	– 57	
Female	Uterus	16.6	8.1	– 51	Steady decrease.

*Percent changes not listed because they are not meaningful.